How We Heal

How We Heal

Nutritional, Emotional, and Psychospiritual Fundamentals

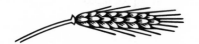

Douglas Morrison

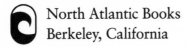
North Atlantic Books
Berkeley, California

Published by
North Atlantic Books
P.O. Box 12327
Berkeley, California 94712

Cover art by Divit Cardoza
Illustrations by Sergei Ponomarov
Cover and book design by Paula Morrison
Printed in the United States of America

How We Heal: Nutritional, Emotional, and Psychospiritual Fundamentals is sponsored by the Society for the Study of Native Arts and Sciences, a nonprofit educational corporation whose goals are to develop an educational and crosscultural perspective linking various scientific, social, and artistic fields; to nurture a holistic view of arts, sciences, humanities, and healing; and to publish and distribute literature on the relationship of mind, body, and nature.

North Atlantic Books' publications are available through most bookstores. For further information, call 800-337-2665 or visit our website at www.northatlanticbooks.com.

Substantial discounts on bulk quantities are available to corporations, professional associations, and other organizations. For details and discount information, contact our special sales department.

Library of Congress Cataloging-in-Publication Data
Morrison, Douglas, 1960–
    How we heal: nutritional, emotional, and spiritual fundamentals / by Douglas Morrison
        p. cm.
    ISBN 1-55643-362-X (trade paper . alk. paper)
    1. Healing. 2. Healing—Nutritional aspects. 3. Healing—Psychological aspects. 4. Healing—Religious aspects. 5. Health attitudes. 6. Health. I. Title.

RA776.5.W94 2001
615.5—dc21

00-049011

1 2 3 4 5 6 7 8 9 / 06 05 04 03 02 01

Dedicated to my wonderful parents,
Beverly and Archie Morrison;
to my beloved children, Meghan and Andrew;
and to the God Within All Life.

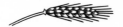

Acknowledgments

I WISH TO EXPRESS MY GRATITUDE TO JOHN WHITMAN RAY, FOUNDER OF the modality known as Body Electronics. Many years of close study with this pioneer have been a wonderful opportunity for me, and certainly my understanding of many of the principles expressed in this book has been greatly influenced by my studies with him. I admire and applaud his dedication and pursuit of truth over many years.

This book has certainly not come out of a vacuum, and I am also grateful to the many authors, living and otherwise, who have taken the time to write the wonderful books quoted or referenced here. In particular, I would like to offer many thanks to the late Weston A. Price, author of the monumental work *Nutrition and Physical Degeneration* and also the Price-Pottenger Nutrition Foundation for helping keep the research of Weston Price, Francis Pottenger, Melvin Page, and many related researchers available to all of us for these many years.

I would also like to thank Anthony Collier and the National Enzyme Company for their permission to reprint the "Condensed Summary and Conclusions" from *Food Enzymes For Health and Longevity* by Edward Howell. Thanks also to Bernard Jensen, David Pesek, and Harri Wolf for their kind permission to include their iridology charts, and to Jack Tips for permission to use his sclerology chart. These four men have all made wonderful contributions to the twin disciplines of iridology and sclerology, and it is an honor to feature their excellent eye charts.

And I would like to thank Tom Quackenbush, who liked my first book *Body Electronics Fundamentals* enough to put me in touch with his publisher, North Atlantic Books, and to recommend my book to them. Thanks also to Richard Grossinger at North Atlantic Books for helping me to get this book out to a larger audience. And a special thanks to Michele Chase for a wonderful job editing this book and for all her helpful feedback during the process. Thanks also to Sergei Ponomarov for his fine illustrations, and to Paula Morrison for her excellent design of the book.

I would also like to give thanks to each of the following for taking the time to read and make helpful comments upon certain writings which have made it into this present work as the chapter on Weston Price: Graham Bennett, Kyle Grimshaw-Jones, Peter Brotherton, and Andrew Duffy. And thanks to John Whitman Ray and Peter Brotherton for similar assistance with the eventual chapters on biological transmutations and on melanin and monopoles. And thanks to Wayne Slack for his assistance and suggestions on the section concerning the work of Johann Grander. Thanks also to Alan Meyer for his assistance with those portions of the book dealing with microbes and with the Grainfields products.

I would like to thank all who have organized Body Electronics seminars for me over the years, as well as all who have attended these seminars. It has been my pleasure and privilege to work with each of you.

Many thanks to Eleanor Butler and her staff at Enzymes International for their support and assistance over the last fifteen years. Thanks also to Alan and Kate Meyer and their staff at AGM Foods for their help over the last five years. And also thanks to Roy Kupsinel for his support and assistance over the years.

A special thanks goes to Louis Frick and Kris Limont for distributing my first book, *Body Electronics Fundamentals,* ever since I left the United States in 1996.

This book has also benefited greatly from the opportunity I have had over the past few years to discuss many of these ideas with some of my closest friends. I would like in particular to thank Peter Brotherton, Graham Bennett, Kyle Grimshaw-Jones and Danielle Ryan for this.

And a very special thanks to my parents, Beverly and Archie, who provided me with a good set of values by their actions as well as their words.

May *How We Heal* help to pass on to all who read it at least a few of the many blessings that I have received over my years of study and teaching. I hope that reading it will be as enjoyable as writing it has been. And more importantly, I hope that the material may be applied with great benefit by all who read these words.

Douglas Morrison
November 16, 2000

Author's Note

A new truth is a new sense, for with it comes the ability to see things we could not see before—and things which cannot be seen by those who do not have that new truth.
Weston Price

Principles don't change; our understanding of them does.
Stephen Covey

THIS BOOK IS BASED UPON MY RESEARCH AND EXTENSIVE EXPERIENCE. The views expressed are mine unless indicated otherwise. It is my intention to understand and express truth to the best of my ability, and both my understanding and expression may differ from that of others.

While I believe everything stated herein to be accurate to the best of my own current understanding, the reader is advised to carefully weigh all that is contained in this book (or any other book for that matter) and to seek proper medical assistance whenever necessary. Nothing in this book is intended to replace consultation with health care professionals.

I firmly believe that each of us must ultimately be responsible for our own health and wellness. Ready access to a variety of viewpoints and an open exchange of ideas and opinions will help us to achieve this end. Let us exchange ideas in a spirit of unity in diversity because none of us has full understanding or all the answers to life's questions.

This book is offered solely for educational purposes. Therefore, neither the author nor the publisher assumes any responsibility for the use that any reader makes of the information it contains. The reader is simply urged to consider the material presented and to use it at their own risk.

Contents

PART FOUR: OUTER MANIFESTATION AND INNER ESSENCE

List of Figures

Preface

EXPERIENCING A VARIETY OF HEALTH CHALLENGES IN EARLY ADULTHOOD and not satisfied with what conventional medicine had to offer me, I began to look for answers and assistance elsewhere. I became acquainted with a modality known as Body Electronics in 1985, and quickly became impressed by its benefits for me and for others. After spending several years intensively studying Body Electronics with its founder, Dr. John Whitman Ray, I began to teach seminars about it in early 1988. Since that time I have had the opportunity to teach Body Electronics seminars throughout the United States, Europe, Australia, Africa and New Zealand.

Some readers will be familiar with my previous book, *Body Electronics Fundamentals*. I wrote it between 1991 and 1993 because at that time there was little available in writing about Body Electronics, and many of my students had requested a basic book on the subject. *Body Electronics Fundamentals* was originally self-published in 1993, with a second printing following in 1994. A Flemish/Dutch version (expertly translated by Brigitte Quanten) followed in 1996. Other enthusiastic students of Body Electronics undertook translations into German, Finnish, French and Swahili, although none of these have yet made it into print. *Body Electronics Fundamentals* was intended as a comprehensive introduction to Body Electronics, and all in all, I think it has served that purpose fairly well over the years. But as time has gone by, I have felt some things needed alteration, expansion, or in some cases, deletion. This was particularly true with respect to the nutritional recommendations, which did not reflect the most up-to-date information. In particular, I felt it extremely important to include the work of Dr. Weston Price and his classic *Nutrition and Physical Degeneration*, a book with which I did not become familiar until after writing *Body Electronics Fundamentals*. To say that the work of Weston Price has changed my views on nutrition would be a great understatement.

In the seven years since *Body Electronics Fundamentals* first appeared,

I have had much time to reflect upon its shortcomings as well as its good points. I have also had the opportunity to take to heart many helpful comments from readers. Rather than simply updating the original book, I have decided to expand its scope and purpose considerably. *How We Heal* is intended to present many of the basic principles of health and healing more comprehensively than was attempted in *Body Electronics Fundamentals*. While many of these principles are essential to understanding as well as practicing Body Electronics, they are equally valid without any reference to that particular healing modality. As such, they have the potential to be of great assistance to any who desire to understand the nature of health and healing. They can be applied with great benefit by individuals for their own benefit as well as by practitioners/educators for the benefit of others.

No assumption will be made in *How We Heal* that the reader has any prior knowledge of Body Electronics. Those who wish to further investigate Body Electronics should seek out a Body Electronics practitioner or teacher. The basics can be learned in a seminar taught by a certified instructor or in a local cooperative pointholding group. For further written explanation, Dr. John Whitman Ray gives detailed information in the first three books in the *Logic In Sequence Series,* known as *The Laws of Perfection, The Healing Crisis,* and *The Electrification of Matter.* In addition, his booklet *The Patient's Guide to Body Electronics* presents many of the basics of his nutritional program. Dr. Ray has been researching and refining the field of Body Electronics since the early 1950s. May we each be blessed according to the desires of our heart, and may those who embark upon the pathway of individual responsibility outlined herein find it rewarding.

May this book help shed some light on the path of each of its readers, and may it help each of you who reads it to find those truths for which you are searching. And while I hope this book will help many of you to find answers, I hope that it also helps you to discover some new questions.

Prologue

We must not cease from exploration and the end of all explor-
ing will be to arrive where we began and to know the place for
the first time.

T. S. Eliot

I know of no more encouraging fact than the unquestionable
ability of man to elevate his life by a conscious endeavor.

Henry David Thoreau

The Possibility of Healing

AS AN ACTIVE CHILD, I EXPERIENCED ANY NUMBER OF MINOR INJURIES. While fortunately never badly hurt, I certainly had my fair share of cuts, bruises, sprains and assorted consequences of my boisterous nature and that of my friends. I grew up a few houses away from my elementary school in a neighborhood full of children, and there was rarely a shortage of playmates or activities. I remember from a young age being fascinated by the way the body repaired itself: no matter how severe the injury, without fail the body would naturally return to a "good as new" condition after days or weeks, with no special effort on my part. For example, if I fell on the pavement while playing basketball, a considerable portion of skin might be scraped off my arm or leg. The blood would soon dry and turn into a scab. The skin and tissue underneath would gradually fill in, and sooner or later the scab would fall off. At first, the new skin underneath would be of a distinctly different texture and color than the skin around it. Yet given more time, the corresponding part of the arm or leg would indeed end up good as new.

A fall off my bicycle after hitting a patch of sand might result in a big

---

bruise on my shin with a swollen bump the size of a large egg. The bruise would change in color, size and tenderness and the bump would gradually become smaller, and eventually, they would both pass away as if nothing had ever happened.

Once, sitting on my sled and steering with my feet as I came down a steep and icy hill, I managed to sprain my ankle so severely I could not stand on it without intense pain. I had to crawl most of the way home through the snow. Yet in a short time, the ankle also felt good as new.

Another time, I was struck on my skate by an ice hockey puck. This so damaged my big toenail that it turned a purple to black color underneath, and over the next week or two, it fell off. Yet even as this was happening, I remember watching intently as a nice new big toenail grew in place underneath. While this whole process was not without its discomforts, it was exciting to watch as it unfolded.

Another time, I was struck in the eye by a stick. Apparently this ruptured a blood vessel, for the white of my eye turned completely blood red. I kept close track of my eye in the mirror over the next week, and within a few days of the injury, the blood in the eye started to disappear and the white to reappear in patches. Once again, given enough time, my eye was good as new. A broken thumb while playing street hockey at age thirteen healed in a similar fashion within a week or two.

While this process of healing was fascinating to me, as a child I pretty much took it for granted that the body would simply fix itself when injured: it never occurred to me that any of these injuries would not heal. Perhaps I might have looked at things differently had I suffered anything more severe than these injuries. But the only childhood injuries that seem to have left any visible mark upon me were two instances where I had stitches as a result of deeper cuts. Other than the slight scars from the stitches, my body just seemed to naturally repair whatever damage I managed to inflict upon it, as far as I knew, with neither effort nor direction on my part.

Then at sixteen, I had my first knee injury. I tore the medial meniscus cartilage in my right knee while playing soccer. I injured both knees several times over the next few years, both in soccer and in wrestling. Both knees had similar tears in the medial meniscus cartilage, and there was ligament damage as well, especially in the right knee. These knee injuries were a turning point for me in many ways. For here were injuries which for whatever reason my body did not fully heal. Certainly they did heal to some extent, for I was able to continue with sports for a few more years. But unlike my childhood injuries, my knees never seemed to return to good as new. I resigned myself to the fact that I had "bad knees" and that this would probably be so for the remainder of my days. While there was doubtless a part of me that still remembered my earlier experiences of healing so readily, somehow this part was largely ignored. Gradually I became accustomed to frequent swelling, discomfort, and aches in my knees, often for little apparent reason.

Over the next few years the condition of my knees continued to deteriorate. Eventually I had to stop running, as my knees could no longer handle the stresses involved. Hiking with a backpack was next to go, as walking downhill also proved too much for my knees. Within another year, even hiking downhill without a backpack proved too painful. Finally, around the time I turned twenty-four, simply standing for any amount of time resulted in much discomfort and swelling in the knees. This was an intolerable situation to me, and I felt I had to do something about it. Being largely unaware of any other options, I had surgery on my right knee, which was in the worst shape of the two.

I remember meeting with my surgeon a few months after the operation and asking him some questions. I began to wonder why, if the cartilage had been torn seven or eight years previously, it was still torn, as test results confirmed. It seemed to me that broken bones did not stay broken, and many other things in the body fixed themselves without much fuss. I could not understand why cartilage should be any different. So I asked my surgeon why. His first answer was simply "because it can't." As this answer shed little light upon my question, I next asked why not and his answer was "because it does not have enough blood supply." Thinking I was starting to get somewhere, I asked why cartilage did not have enough blood supply, and the answer was "because it doesn't." After a few more unsuccessful attempts at finding a question whose answer would shed some light on my confusion, our appointment was over, and I went home feeling quite puzzled. I could not understand how some parts of the body like bones seemed to heal so easily, while others like cartilage just did not seem to heal, even after years. While I could accept that my surgeon had never seen or heard of it happening, I could not accept that it was impossible for my knees to heal. I knew that even if I could not find a single person who had ever seen or heard of torn cartilage healing, this did not mean that it was impossible. I chose to believe that it was possible, whether or not anyone else did.

A few months after this conversation, I consulted a Rolfer to see if he could help me with back problems that I had been having the previous five years. I had sprained my back in a motor vehicle accident at age nineteen, and since that time had gone through many periods of severe back pain that were quite incapacitating at times. As I was explaining my health history, I mentioned my knee problems. He said without hesitation, "Well, you should try pointholding for your knees." (Pointholding is another name for the technique of Body Electronics.) For some reason, I got extremely excited the moment he said "pointholding," so I asked him how it worked. His brief answer was something like, "Well, you eat these high prana foods, you drink this swamp water, these friends of mine press on certain points on your body, and then your knees grow back." He said this all very casually, as though it were unremarkable. While I had clung to the belief that my knees could indeed heal, this was the first modality I had yet heard of that not only agreed that such healing was possible but offered a method.

A short time later I contacted his friends, and I began my involvement with Body Electronics. My healing process over the next few months is described in excerpts from a brief testimonial I once wrote:

Let me cover some of the more obvious physical transformations in my body as a result of my involvement in Body Electronics. Physical healing is a blessing in itself, but it is never accomplished in the absence of an even greater blessing: change of consciousness. My physical healing, as welcome as it has been, has truly been minor compared to the much greater gift of continually expanding freedom from the subtle entanglements of my own patterns of resistance and judgment. These are, of course, the very things that led to the physical problems in the first place. My initial impetus to begin was chiefly the condition of my knees.

Prior to commencing Body Electronics, both my knees were in very poor shape with very little flexibility in either: I was able to bend them to roughly about ninety degrees before it became too painful to bend further. This ninety degree bending of the knees was without any weight on the leg. With my weight on the legs, I could not even bend that far without some pain. The right knee was more painful and less flexible than the left, and while each felt unstable, the right knee was worse. In brief, I had a "bad" knee (left) and a "worse" knee (right). I relied heavily upon my arms in getting in or out of a chair. Lateral motion caused great pain in the knees, and I was unable to run or go hiking. In addition to the knee problems, I had often suffered from severe back problems since being in an automobile accident at age nineteen. After most meals, I had also been experiencing abdominal discomfort, often quite severe, and constipation. At the time, however, I was blissfully unaware of the full extent of my digestive problems. Yet these problems had been growing rapidly worse in the previous six months. While I had various other physical problems, the knees, back and digestion were the most obvious, and apparently the most severe.

I began to follow the recommended dietary and supplement program in late June of 1985. Being intent on getting the best results possible, I followed the recommended nutritional program fanatically. As a result, I went into a pretty intense healing crisis or cleansing reaction almost immediately. I learned quite quickly one aspect of the healing crisis: you'll usually feel worse before you feel better. I felt truly awful for weeks at a time. Virtually every bowel movement that I had over the next four months (and these were frequent, often six or more times a day in contrast to my previous constipation) came out of me as black as could be. I also experienced headaches, fatigue, weakness and assorted aches and pains.

Within two or three weeks, I was shocked when during an especially explosive bout of diarrhea I passed quite a number of strange looking things into the toilet. They were each approximately one centimeter in diameter, and generally of a whitish or grey color, with black or brown tentacles or feelers attached to them. People in Body Electronics politely refer to them as "fuzzies." These are carcinoid tumors, and they are frequently found in people's intestines. (Years later, I had a student, a surgeon who was originally from India but had relocated to the United States. In discussing these fuzzies with me, she made an interesting observation. During her training and surgical practice in India, she had rarely come across the so-called fuzzies. Yet once she came to the United States, she began to find them in the intestines of many of her patients. This suggests that diet plays a factor in their formation.) I had heard about fuzzies prior to this. But it was quite sobering to see them floating in the toilet and realize that these had come from my own body. Only when I saw these first few fuzzies did it really become obvious to me that my knee troubles were the least of my problems.

My persistent abdominal distress and constipation were the outer symptoms of a far more serious problem. I was inspired by the appearance of fuzzies to redouble my efforts on the nutritional program I was following. As a result, the intensity of the healing crises increased, and I began to pass fuzzies frequently. While I initially counted them, this eventually became absurd, even to an applied mathematics major! My best estimate would be that I passed in excess of three thousand fuzzies over the next four months. (After the first few months, I continued to pass fuzzies on occasion over the next few years, but eventually stopped. My intestines continued to improve, and eventually they returned to a fine state of function.)

I had my first pointholding session about the time I began passing fuzzies. A month later I traveled to Wisconsin to take four weeks of Body Electronics seminars with Dr. Ray. There I had my points held frequently. As a result, nerve supply, circulation, endocrine function, and eventually spinal and cranial symmetry, were all greatly improved. By the end of this series of seminars, less than four months after beginning, I experienced some wonderful changes in my knees as well. I now had full flexibility in both knees. I could easily and comfortably bring my heels all the way to my buttocks when standing. I could sit back on my heels with ease and without any pain. The pain upon lateral motion was greatly reduced. As for the strength of the knees, I could now do a deep knee bend on one leg (either leg) with no pain or discomfort. This was quite a change from having to use my arms to get in and out of a chair. It was as if the knees had never been injured.

I have not since this time had any invasive testing procedures done on my knees to verify what has happened inside them. I am simply happy to have good knees, and see little reason to cut them open or inject radioactive dye into them to satisfy somebody else's curiosity. But about fifteen months later, at another Body Electronics seminar, I did have my knees examined and manipulated by an orthopedic surgeon who was there. In his opinion, the torn cartilage in the left knee had healed completely. (The left knee had never undergone any surgery.) He also stated that the cartilage was whole and untorn in the right knee. Thus, the cartilage had apparently regenerated or grown back where it had been surgically removed. (It is conventionally believed that cartilage, having little or no blood supply, is incapable of repairing itself, which, given my experience, appears to be a matter of opinion rather than fact.) He did report a small degree of instability in some of the ligaments in the right knee laterally, which I do believe.

It quickly became obvious to me that knees healing was only one small demonstration of what was possible. My faith in the ability of the body to heal itself was renewed. While in childhood it had seemed as if all I needed to do was sit back and let it happen, I now realized that to some extent I had to make it happen as well. Since that time, I have attempted to better understand what is necessary to regain and maintain health. I have studied and taught Body Electronics extensively for many years and have studied and considered much related material as well. On a regular and consistent basis I have seen other people regain their own health. In the process, my own understanding of health and healing has continued to expand and grow.

Health is indeed a precious gift. Perhaps we do not all receive this gift in equal measure, yet we each receive our own portion. Many of us take our health for granted, at least until we lose it. As will be discussed more extensively later in this book, often it is our very lack of appreciation for our health that plays a significant role in its loss. Also, it would appear that maintaining our health is actually far easier than regaining it once it has been squandered. This might be likened to the fact that it takes far more effort to climb up a hill once we have descended than it would be to simply maintain our position at its summit. This is not meant to imply that maintaining health is automatic or effortless; rather, that it takes much less effort to maintain a given level of health than to rise to that level from a lesser level.

Some will wonder, in light of the above, whether there are limits to healing. I have received hundreds of inquiries from people wanting to know if I have ever seen a particular condition heal. I do not have a simple answer for that question. I can say that I have seen things that I would once have considered impossible. Perhaps in one or more cases I have seen a particular condition heal. Yet to me, this does not mean that whomever is asking will get the same result. As I once read, "It is not the disease with the patient that is important; rather it is the patient with the disease." Not everyone will get the same result, and with some conditions I have seen nothing of major consequence happen. However, this in no way indicates to me that healing is impossible. Difficult, perhaps, but not impossible. I choose to remain open to the possibility of healing, while acknowledging that it may not happen easily or even at all. And even if it has never happened before, somebody has to be the first to do it.

I do not have a full understanding of health and healing, and I do not believe I have yet met anybody who does. Yet nonetheless, it is possible to present some of the principles of healing, with practical suggestions as to how they may be effectively applied.

It is not my intention in this book to prove the truth of these principles. Indeed, a great many of them would be extremely difficult to prove or disprove completely. Rather, it is my intention to help people to remain open to possibilities. The principles and suggestions in this book are intended to help people come to a good understanding of health and healing, and to offer practical guidance as to how health can be maintained or regained in keeping with these principles.

Many of these principles of health are explored in detail in the first section of *How We Heal*. A basic model is presented, considering the physical, emotional, and mental bodies and many of the principles pertaining to them individually and in conjunction with one another. Various other influences from the Hereditary Level, the Soul Level and the Entity Level are introduced and discussed. The presence and role of *crystals* within the body are examined. The central role of *resistance* is covered in detail. Many of the basic requirements of health and healing are enumerated: love, forgiveness, gratitude, faith, nutrition, elimination, exercise, sleep, water, light and darkness, air and breathing, and prayer. And the healing crisis is considered in great detail.

In the second section of *How We Heal* the subject of nutrition is extensively covered. While it must be stressed that nutrition alone is seldom the answer to our health challenges, nutrition almost invariably comprises part of the answer to many such challenges. This section will begin with a broad overview of many principles of nutrition prior to delving into many of the specifics. Patience and a proper attitude are among the principles considered in this overview. Other topics highlighted include cleansing and building, assimilation and elimination, and many of the psychological factors involved in improving one's diet. The work of Dr. Weston Price and his classic *Nutrition and Physical Degeneration* is presented in a separate chapter. Food quality is covered as well as food quantity, timing and frequency of meals, and food combinations. The assimilation of nutrients is highlighted, with emphasis upon the roles of enzymes and friendly microbes. Essential nutrients and their sources are covered. There are separate chapters on what sorts of foods to eat as well as what sorts of foods not to eat. The use of natural supplements is also addressed. And finally, degenerative disease is explored in the context of its relationship to faulty nutrition and various related factors.

In the third section, the modality of Body Electronics is introduced and presented in detail. Briefly, Body Electronics is a healing modality that includes the use of a method of sustained acupressure commonly referred to as *pointholding* in conjunction with a program of nutrient saturation to help bring about the regeneration of the body. While the principles of health and healing presented in this book have broad application and can be applied with great benefit quite independently of Body Electronics, I have chosen to present Body Electronics in considerable detail for two main reasons: it offers a practical example of a particular healing modality wherein these principles can be applied, and it happens to be the modality in which I am personally most experienced and hence in the best position to offer as a model of these principles. This section includes much of the basic theory and practice of Body Electronics.

In the final section of the book, we return to a broader model of health and healing. Many of the nuts and bolts of health and healing related to a simple model have been presented in earlier sections. It then becomes possible to reexamine and explore the original simple model at a far deeper level. A chapter on Iridology and Sclerology is included in this section, as well as an introduction to the process of biological transmutation. The broader model presented here effectively ties together much of the previous material in the book, examining in detail the interplay between the physical, emotional, and mental levels and exploring the very essence of creation and uncreation.

PART ONE

Health and Healing

Chapter One

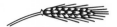

Coming Out of the Shadows to a Different Way of Looking at Reality

The mind once expanded to the dimensions of a larger idea never returns to its original size.
Oliver Wendell Holmes

The significant problems we face cannot be solved at the same level of thinking we were at when we created them.
Albert Einstein

Chasing Shadows

A FEW YEARS AGO, I WAS IN A LARGE PARKING LOT SHORTLY AFTER dark playing with a group of young children, including my own. It was brightly lit, and we each cast distinct shadows upon the ground. As these children were all familiar with the game of tag, I taught them a variation I call "shadow tag." In regular tag, the idea is to touch the other person's body with your hand. For shadow tag, I asked the children to try to get their shadow to tag or touch my shadow. As can be imagined, after awhile the children focused far more intently upon their own shadows and mine than upon their bodies or anyone else's. Shadows soon became more real than the bodies that cast them. Eventually, as the children became more focused upon the shadows and less aware of their own bodies, there began to be a number of near collisions. At this point, rather than wait for an actual collision, I decided it might be a good idea to find something else to do.

They were all still pretty intrigued by the shadows. So we stood with our backs to the light and cast long shadows on the ground. I began to move my body around so as to make my shadow do amusing things. To my surprise, these fairly young children did not at first understand how I could get my shadow to move about as it was. They all understood that there was some connection between their body and their shadow, especially after the game of shadow tag. But the exact nature of this connection was still not obvious to them. So I told them all to look at their shadows, and find the shadow's hands and the shadow's head. Then I asked them to make the shadow's hands touch the shadow's head. Try as they might, none of them could quite figure it out at first. I told them it was so simple that I could do it with my eyes shut. And then, as these young children watched with amazement, I shut my eyes and simply touched my own hands to my head, and naturally, my shadow did the same. As soon as they saw me do it, it was obvious to all how easy it really was. Our shadows, of course, will simply do whatever our bodies do.

We may find it amusing that these children did not at first realize that the shadow simply follows the body. We may find it funny that they placed so much attention upon their shadows that their own bodies virtually ceased to be apparent to them, such that they came very close to colliding with each other while playing shadow tag. Yet I would suggest that in the field of health most of us have little more understanding than these children. For the physical body (and indeed the entire physical universe) is in many ways simply a shadow of something else. The physical body cannot exist without this something else any more than our shadow can exist without our body. Trying to make the shadow's hands touch the shadow's head without taking the body that casts the shadow into account is quite absurd. In the same way, trying to heal the physical body without taking this something else into account is absurd. This analogy suggests that the vast majority of health modalities (orthodox, alternative, natural, holistic, or otherwise) are by and large chasing shadows and ignoring what casts the shadows.

Trying to Explain Shadows Solely in Terms of Shadows

SHADOWS CAN BE EXPLAINED IN TERMS OF CERTAIN BASIC ELEMENTS: light, an object to cast the shadow, and somewhere for the shadow to fall. But suppose we were asked to explain shadows without reference to either light or objects to cast shadows: suppose we were asked to explain shadows solely in terms of shadows. I do not think this would be easy, possible, or meaningful.

Suppose for the time being that we accept this idea that the physical body, as well as the entire physical universe, is indeed the shadow of something else. If this is so, there can be no more possibility of explaining what goes on in the physical universe solely in terms of the physical universe than there is of explaining shadows solely in terms of shadows. If we are ever going to understand the physical body, we are going to need to understand the nature of the something else referred to above. For otherwise we continue to chase shadows endlessly.

In Search of This "Something Else"

THE HUMAN BODY IS CONTINUALLY REPAIRING AND REPLACING ITSELF at the cellular level and beyond. While different tissues are completely replaced at different rates, over time the entire body is replaced. In other words, on a physical level, nothing remains permanently. So if a person has a scar that persists over time, it is a scar that is being continually remade, right along with the rest of the body. It is not the same scar from one year to the next, at least not in a physical sense. This is because as the body replaces itself, it follows a certain consistent pattern. This pattern can in some manner change over time, at least within certain parameters. We grow and age, for example, while remaining fundamentally recognizable to ourselves and others.

We might then consider just where this pattern may be found, as well as how it can be altered. Some might suggest it is within our DNA. Yet it is hard to imagine how that could account for a scar. It seems absurd to think that the pattern for a scar was lying hidden in the DNA for years, and would only be expressed physically after some sort of injury. It seems more logical to think that while the body follows some sort of pattern, in some manner this pattern can be changed to account for injuries, a phenomenon which would be extremely difficult to account for in terms of DNA.

I would suggest that looking within the physical universe for the pattern that the body follows is chasing shadows. It is like trying to explain shadows only in terms of shadows. This pattern must be found elsewhere, not in the physical universe at all. It is simply *reflected into* the physical universe. We might say that the pattern the body follows is the something else mentioned earlier. This something else might be likened to a blueprint, and the physical body might be said to repair and replace itself in accordance with this blueprint. While it might include the information in our DNA, this blueprint would not be limited to that information only. It would be capable of change. And it would not be found within the physical universe at all.

On Scars Disappearing

SUPPOSE A PERSON HAD AN OPERATION AT AGE TWENTY-FIVE. SUPPOSE their abdomen was opened up for the surgery and then sewed or stapled shut at its conclusion. Suppose that as this healed, an obvious scar formed, and twenty years later, at forty-five, this scar is still obvious. Most people would explain the scar as a result of the surgery. And if asked how long the scar is likely to remain there, most would assume that if it is still present after twenty years, it is permanent.

Yet, after twenty years, the cells of the body have been replaced many times over. In other words, on a physical level, nothing remains from the time of the surgery. The cells now forming the scar were never touched by the surgeon's knife. Nor were these cells present as the incision healed. So if a scar still exists, it is a scar that is being continually remade, right along with the rest of the body. Clearly up until age twenty-five, the pattern of this individual did not involve an abdominal incision scar. In fact, for the first twenty-five years of their life, this person had no difficulty continually making an abdomen without any scar. Yet ever since the surgery, a scar has been made over and over in the area where the incision was made. It is as if, since the time of the surgery, this individual has lost the ability to make a scarless abdomen. Or we could say that somehow or another their blueprint has changed such that it now includes a scar on the abdomen. Most people would probably consider it quite impossible for this scar to disappear, or at least not in a short time. That's a sensible position if we try to understand the scar only in terms of the physical universe. But suppose we look at things from the perspective of this blueprint. If a scar can be added to the blueprint, we might consider the opposite possibility: a scar can also be deleted from the blueprint. If the addition of the scar to the blueprint is responsible for the body continuing to generate the scar from one year to the next, then perhaps the removal of the scar from the blueprint would lead to the disappearance of the scar from the physical body. Let us clarify this with an analogy.

The Analogy of the Overhead Projector

CONSIDER AN OVERHEAD PROJECTOR. WHEN A TRANSPARENCY WITH A certain image is placed upon it and it is switched on, this image is projected upon a screen. Suppose we place an initial transparency of a body without any scars upon the projector and project the image upon the screen. Now suppose a transparency containing a scar is superimposed upon the initial transparency. Naturally, the image upon the screen will now have a corresponding scar, and if this second transparency is then removed, the scar will immediately disappear from the image on the screen. If we understand the operation of the projector, neither seeing the scar appear nor subsequently seeing it disappear from the screen would be in any way mysterious to us. Yet if a scar abruptly disappeared from our own body or someone else's, most of us would be quite astounded. I would suggest, however, that how the process works might be no more mysterious than using an overhead projector and removing a single transparency from a stack of transparencies.

In this analogy, we can equate our physical body with the image projected upon the screen, with the screen being the physical universe. The blueprint that our body is following would then be the combination of the transparencies placed upon the projector. (The projector itself, the source of light, might be equated with God, whom some might term the ultimate source of all light. And just as the images on transparencies can only be projected onto a screen in the presence of light, perhaps it is only God and the light of God manifesting through our individual blueprints that creates our physical bodies in the first place.)

To expand this analogy, there might be one or more transparencies holding information equivalent to our genetic information. For those who believe in reincarnation, other transparencies might represent those aspects of our previous existences which are being expressed in this one. And any event of life that alters the overall blueprint (such as the scar related to the surgery) would be represented by a separate transparency. Thus, we would each have a stack of transparencies superimposed upon one another. As a result of this, we would each project a particular image onto the screen. Put another way, we would each have a unique and changeable blueprint, and our physical body would be the outer result or reflection of this blueprint.

In this analogy, the projector, the light, the transparencies, the image on the screen and the screen itself are all equally apparent and real to any observer. But in our own situation, for the most part it is only the physical body and the universe that seem real to us most of the time. For many of us, neither the blueprint nor the light nor even God seems real in comparison to our own bodies or the outer physical universe around us. Just as in my story of children and shadows children became oblivious to their own bodies when they focused upon their shadows, so do we become oblivious to the blueprint when our attention is continually directed towards the physical body and the physical universe. One might say that we get so lost in the shadows that we become oblivious to how shadows are formed in the first place. We cease to be aware of anything other than the outer, oblivious not just to the existence of the inner but to the fundamental fact that the outer is a reflection of the inner.

ALTERING THE IMAGE ON THE SCREEN

Our unawareness of how our bodies are created leads us astray when we seek to improve their function or health. Suppose we were asked to change the image upon the screen by removing the scar from it. To go back to our

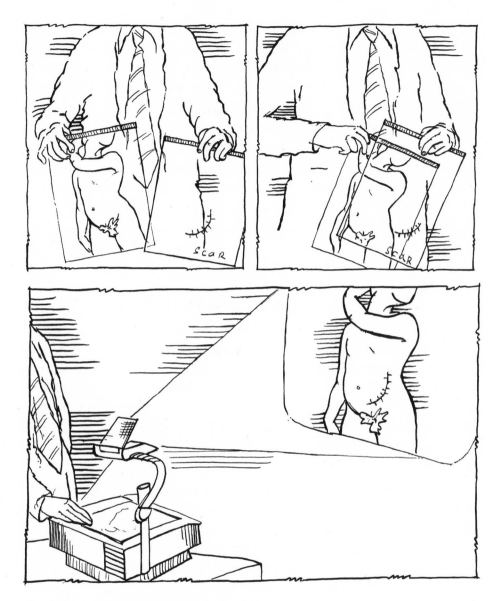

Figure 1: The Overhead Projector

analogy, the simplest way would be to locate and remove the corresponding transparency. And this would not be mysterious to most people watching, as long as they could see projector, light, image, and screen, and understood which was causing which.

Yet imagine if someone else with the same assignment were completely unaware of the projector, the light, or the transparencies and only aware of the image on the screen and the screen itself. They might approach the screen and try to erase the scar from the image on the screen. They might try and cover it up by writing on the screen with a magic marker, white-out, or white paint. They might even cut or burn away that part of the screen where the scar was present. Anyone watching these efforts who was aware of the projector, light and transparencies (and understood their workings) would probably be struck by how much easier it would be to just remove the correct transparency and tempted to help the person to do so. Yet if this person were unaware of the light, projector, or transparency, it might be difficult to assist them.

HELPING ANOTHER SEE HOW

Some might appreciate the assistance offered, and might at least consider the possibility of something other than screen and image. Some might be readily able to see the projector, light and transparencies as soon as these were pointed out to them; indeed for some it would simply be a matter of looking in the direction indicated. However, others might not be able to see the light, projector, and transparencies upon first look. And yet with time and assistance, these might eventually become quite obvious. Still others, perhaps despite the best efforts of all involved, might remain unable to see the light, projector or transparencies for a much longer time.

Some people might be so convinced that there was nothing other than the screen and the image, that any talk of light, projector or transparency might be met with ridicule, disbelief or even complete contempt. The light, projector and transparencies would remain undiscovered mainly because they never looked for them, or perhaps if they did search for them, they might not be able to see them anyway. For often the very fact that we consider something impossible renders it invisible, at least to us, because our belief systems are powerful indeed. They do not merely shape how we see things; often they determine what we can see in the first place.

A New Truth

To those who are unwilling to consider the possibility that anything else exists besides the physical universe, many of the ideas in this book will be of no more use than talk of light, projectors and transparencies would be to someone who believes that only the screen and the images upon it are real. Yet others, when alerted to the possibility that there is more than just the screen and image, might be willing to consider this possibility. It is the intention of this book to help any who are interested to do so. For as Weston Price has expressed it, a new truth is a new sense, for with it comes the ability to see things we could not see before—and things which cannot be seen by those who do not have that new truth.

One can follow the light from the screen back towards the projector, and in so doing find the projector as well as the transparencies. In a similar fashion, the physical body and the physical universe will often serve as a good starting point from which to lead back to both blueprint and God. Indeed for many, the physical is the only possible starting point for this journey, for it is initially the only thing of which we are aware. In our analogy, it is a simple matter to alter the image on the screen however we desire, so long as we have located the relevant transparencies. If we are able to eventually access our own blueprint, the next step is to understand how to alter it. Perhaps the best way to delete something from the blueprint is to understand how it was added in the first place. This will require a broader model which shall be presented next.

Chapter Two

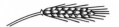

A Basic Model to Consider

The ancestor to every action is a thought.
Ralph Waldo Emerson

Physical healing is a pleasant side effect of consciousness change.
Douglas Morrison

Contempt prior to complete investigation will enslave the soul to ignorance.
Anonymous

HEALTH IS A PRECIOUS GIFT AND FAR SIMPLER TO MAINTAIN THAN it is to regain once lost or squandered. A multitude of factors determine or influence our health, including physical ones such as nutrition, genetic inheritance and lifestyle. However, important as these physical factors may be, our emotional and mental states also play an immense role in determining our state of health. Through an understanding of how these mental, emotional, and physical factors are related, we may see how disease is developed in the body in the first place. Once we understand how disease is created, it becomes clearer how health can be regained and maintained. Just as importantly, we can understand how disease can be prevented.

The Physical, Emotional, and Mental Bodies

LET US BEGIN BY CONSIDERING A SERIES OF THREE MUTUALLY CONNECTED levels which we shall refer to as the mental, emotional and physical bodies. These three bodies may be thought of as interdependent and continually interactive with each other, yet they are distinguishable from each other. One might also say that these bodies interpenetrate each other. While each body influences the others to a varying degree, there is a hierarchy wherein the physical body is encompassed by the emotional body which in turn is encompassed by the mental body. Thus, the mental body may be thought of as the highest of these three levels followed by the emotional and then the physical, respectively. Conditions which exist on a higher level will eventually be made manifest on a lower level, and any condition which exists on a lower level will have originated on the higher levels. The fundamental dictum which must be borne in mind when we deal with these three levels is quite simple: *Thought is senior to substance.* Thus, all outer or physical conditions originate on the mental level. The manner in which this occurs will be discussed below. For now let us just realize that the condition of the physical body is dependent upon that of the emotional and mental bodies. True permanent healing of the physical body cannot occur without addressing the underlying causes on the emotional and mental levels.

THE PHYSICAL BODY

It is useful to consider the physical, emotional and mental bodies and how they interact with one another. The physical body is the tangible vehicle of flesh and blood with which we are all familiar and with which most of us identify almost completely. The physical body exists primarily in the realm of matter. Next is the emotional body, which in most cases is quite firmly fused with the physical body as a result of tremendous resistance and considerable levels of suppressed emotion. The emotional body is a more subtle or finer vehicle, of which most people are ordinarily less aware than they are of the more tangible physical vehicle. Yet each of us is somewhat aware of its existence, although we may not think of it much. This more

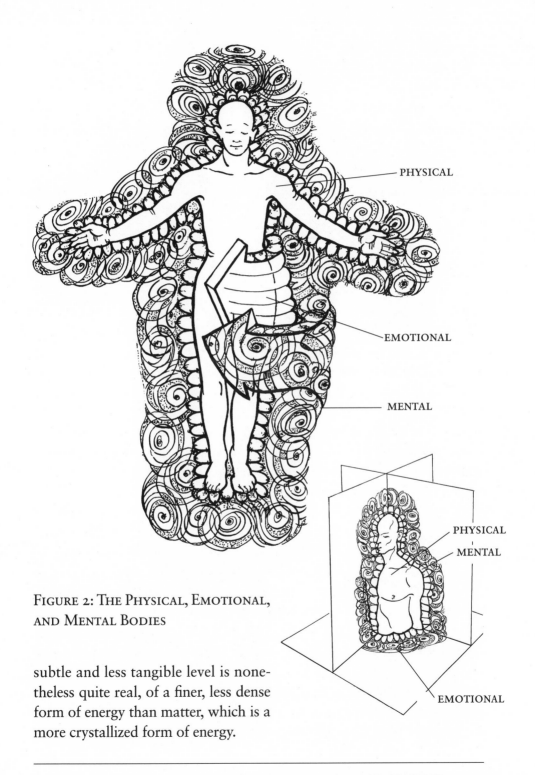

PHYSICAL

EMOTIONAL

MENTAL

PHYSICAL
MENTAL

EMOTIONAL

FIGURE 2: THE PHYSICAL, EMOTIONAL,
AND MENTAL BODIES

subtle and less tangible level is nonetheless quite real, of a finer, less dense
form of energy than matter, which is a
more crystallized form of energy.

```
┌─────────────────────────────────────────────────────────────┐
│  FIGURE 3: THE SCALE OF EMOTIONS                              │
├─────────────────────────────────────────────────────────────┤
│  LEVEL OF EMOTION              ENDOCRINE GLAND                │
│      1. Enthusiasm             Pineal                         │
│      2. Pain                   Pituitary                      │
│      3. Anger                  Thyroid/Parathyroid            │
│      4. Fear                   Thymus/Heart                   │
│      5. Grief                  Pancreas/Adrenals              │
│      6. Apathy                 Spleen                         │
│      7. Unconsciousness        Gonads                         │
│                                                               │
└─────────────────────────────────────────────────────────────┘
```

THE EMOTIONAL BODY

The function of the emotional body can be well understood by a careful study of the *scale of emotions*.[1]

The Scale of Emotions

A Scale of Emotions runs from top to bottom as follows: Enthusiasm, Pain, Anger, Fear, Grief, Apathy, and Unconsciousness. Let us briefly define and examine each of these seven levels, noting that we may find ourselves on different points on the scale depending upon the area of life.

1. Enthusiasm: At the top of the Scale of Emotions, we are free from all judgment and resistance and capable of seeing things as they are and making choices. Neither true choice nor free agency is really possible in the absence of enthusiasm, for wherever there is less than enthusiasm, there is resistance. This resistance automatically removes the possibility of full awareness in the given situation, for whenever there is any degree of resistance we are no longer capable of undistorted perception. We cannot be free, or really make free choices, if we are not fully aware of what our choices actually are. Many times we think we have free agency, and yet really we are simply playing out old tapes of preconditioned reactive behavior. Enthusiasm is the level at which we can receive the experiences of life and accept them as they are without resistance. The emotion of enthusiasm is said to

be associated with the pineal gland, which helps regulate the entire endocrine system.

2. Pain: At the pain level, we are no longer enthusiastic with respect to some area of life; we are in a state of resistance. Although our level of awareness is still fairly high, we are unwilling to lovingly receive the full experience. However, our experiences are but a reflection of our own inner creative essence as expressed in patterns of thought, feeling and spoken word. Our resistance to these experiences is the source of our pain, whether the pain is physical, emotional or otherwise. We wish things to be other than they really are, and we react with contraction, and this causes pain. The pituitary gland resonates to the emotion of pain.

3. Anger: At this level, we have become completely identified with a single point of view. We therefore consider all other points of view wrong, if we can even see them at all. Thus, there is no reason in anger but simply justification that allows us to remain angry and to defend our point of view in the face of all perceived opposition. While our awareness is considerably diminished at this point, there is greater awareness here than at the lower levels of the scale. Anger corresponds to the thyroid and the parathyroid glands.

4. Fear: At this level, we are unwilling to tolerate what we find uncomfortable. We remove ourselves from what appears to be the source of our problem, often by running away from it. We do this because we are afraid, and we also fail to realize that this outer manifestation is not truly the source of our discomfort. Rather, the situation is simply the reflection of our own suppressed patterns of thought, word, and emotion. Though we are capable of being somewhat causative in our environment at the level of anger or above, from the level of fear on down, through our own resistance to life's experiences we relegate ourselves to being the effect of our own resisted creations. Fear is the midpoint of the Scale of Emotions. Above the fear level, we have some ability to see ourselves as capable of changing our environment, or being causative. Below the fear level, we mainly see ourselves as being the effect of our environment. At the fear level, while we do not see ourselves as capable of changing anything, we do see ourselves as capable of running away. However, we can run but we can never truly hide, for the source of our apparent problem is not without but within. And as such, the outer manifestation of this resisted inner essence will be drawn to us in

some form with great exactness even though we try to escape. Hence, in the words of Job, "That which I have feared has come upon me." The emotion of fear is associated with the thymus gland as well as the heart.

5. Grief: At this level, we are the classic victim, a state we maintain through justification and denial. We feel perfectly justified in believing that our problems are caused by something outside of ourselves beyond our control. We are not at all pleased with whatever it is that we are resisting; in fact at the grief level we are often in considerable distress about it. We may sob and moan, we may feel quite sorry for ourselves. We may make many of those around us miserable as well, for indeed misery loves company. Yet we will fail to see that we are at all responsible for our situation. And since we place the problem outside of ourselves, we simultaneously place its solution outside ourselves. In so doing, we remain a victim and avoid assuming responsibility for our own creative efforts. The only way we can get clear of the problem is perhaps to get somebody else to solve it for us. At grief, the pancreas and adrenals are involved.

6. Apathy: At this level, there is nearly total denial of our own ability to do anything. This is where the "I can't" word patterns typically flourish. We are almost entirely incapacitated through denial of our own ability to do anything. We feel that we cannot do anything about our situation, so why try. Thus, the tendency is to simply shut out that which is resisted. This eventually brings us down into the level of unconsciousness. The spleen is associated with apathy.

7. Unconsciousness: Here we are totally identified with matter and almost totally lack awareness. We simply react continually to a given situation on the basis of a broad array of reactive patterns. However, there is a certain level of balance and/or stability achieved thereby. The appropriate expression might be that ignorance is bliss. For here we are largely unaware of problems; thus, they appear to be resolved. This, then, is the counterfeit for enthusiasm. At the level of enthusiasm, we have resolved all resistance through total awareness and unconditional love, thus transmuting the resistance of the emotional body in the area of consideration. Whereas at the level of unconsciousness, the resistance is not truly resolved but simply submerged, apparently no longer an issue for us. At the level of unconsciousness, the gonads are involved.

Seven Levels within the Seven Levels

Within each of these seven levels of emotion we find all seven levels as well. For example, at the level of unconsciousness we have levels of enthusiasm, pain, anger, fear, grief, apathy, and unconsciousness, and at the level of apathy we also have each of these seven levels. This continues for each of the other levels up to and including enthusiasm. This seven within seven model underscores the great key to transmuting all resistance on the emotional body: enthusiasm. For at each of the seven levels, the top of that level is always the level of enthusiasm. Hence, we overcome each of the various emotions by experiencing it with total enthusiasm. Enthusiasm is basically synonymous with unconditional love. (Enthusiasm comes from Greek, with the literal meaning "God in you." As "God is love," it might be fair to define enthusiasm as also "love in you.") Enthusiasm transmutes the various emotions, each in turn.

There is a vast difference between fully experiencing an emotion by encompassing it with enthusiasm versus covering up the painful emotion and blotting it out from our awareness by concentrating on enthusiasm to the exclusion of the emotion. In other words, the goal is to feel what we actually feel with enthusiasm. The goal is not to feel enthusiasm instead of feeling what we actually feel. If we feel each emotion with love or enthusiasm, this will lead to freedom from the bondage of continued resistance, whereas focusing upon love or enthusiasm instead of what we really feel will perpetuate the already considerable levels of resistance. For it is difficult to transmute that which we refuse to acknowledge in the first place. It is essential to our progress that this concept be understood fully. That which we exclude through continued resistance, or that which we refuse to encompass with unconditional love, will halt our progression.

THE MENTAL BODY

That which we embrace with enthusiasm is transcended, bringing us eventually up through the entire scale of emotions and on to the mental body.

The Outer Is the Reflection of the Inner

The mental body cannot be comprehended fully without the crucial under-

FIGURE 4: SEVEN LEVELS WITHIN EACH OF THE SEVEN LEVELS

ENTHUSIASM
- Enthusiasm
- Pain
- Anger
- Fear
- Grief
- Apathy
- Unconsciousness

PAIN
- Enthusiasm
- Pain
- Anger
- Fear
- Grief
- Apathy
- Unconsciousness

ANGER
- Enthusiasm
- Pain
- Anger
- Fear
- Grief
- Apathy
- Unconsciousness

FEAR
- Enthusiasm
- Pain
- Anger
- Fear
- Grief
- Apathy
- Unconsciousness

GRIEF
- Enthusiasm
- Pain
- Anger
- Fear
- Grief
- Apathy
- Unconsciousness

APATHY
- Enthusiasm
- Pain
- Anger
- Fear
- Grief
- Apathy
- Unconsciousness

UNCONSCIOUSNESS
- Enthusiasm
- Pain
- Anger
- Fear
- Grief
- Apathy
- Unconsciousness

standing that the physical body and indeed the entire physical universe is but the outer manifestation of consciousness, a reflection of the inner essence. In a very real sense each of us is a cocreator of the universe, for the various conditions which arise on the outer level are simply reflections of what already exists on the inner level in patterns of thought, word, and emotion. Another way of expressing this is "as a man thinketh in his heart, so is he."

Thought patterns are the sensory aspect of each experience: the when, where, who, what and how. Emotional patterns are the emotion or emotions associated with a given experience. Word patterns are the verbal or mental utterances associated with the patterns of thought and emotion. When thought patterns, word patterns, and emotional patterns are held in a continual state of creation, whether consciously by choice or unconsciously through our subtle or not so subtle resistances, they will eventually come into manifestation in the outer world. The principle is that *what we resist will persist,* and for this reason no true permanent physical healing can occur without a change of consciousness. If the underlying patterns are not encountered and transmuted, then any other changes we effect will be at best temporary. The outer symptoms will eventually reappear if the inner causes remain intact.

Resistance and Duality

Healing at the mental body level necessitates overcoming the resistances in the physical and emotional bodies, in the area of consideration at least, so that we are now capable of considering and encompassing the various dualities involved. A duality is a pair of apparent opposites: night/day, hot/cold, good/bad, and so on. In the physical world there is opposition in all things, hence duality is a constant consideration. At the mental level we are capable of simultaneously viewing both sides of a given duality. When this is done from a position of unconditional love and forgiveness we can then encompass that particular duality.

Resistance originates at the mental body level when we make a judgment, identifying with one side of the duality to the exclusion of the other, thus setting in motion the long chain of resistance. Once we resist an area of life, from that point on we will draw to ourselves via the Law of Attraction similar experiences which we will tend to resist on the basis of our previous resistances. That resistance already exists in some area renders us unable to view this area impartially. Another way of saying this is that we believe things to be a certain way, so we see things that way. This is what judgment is all about. Any judgment takes us out of the now to where we cannot see what truly *is* but simply what we expect to see. Another way to phrase this fundamental truth would be to say that believing is seeing. Making judgments that form our beliefs and restrict our seeing has many consequences for our health and well being.

The Formation of Crystals

THE EVENTUAL END RESULT OF RESISTANCE, WHETHER AT THE MENTAL or emotional level, is the formation of what we term *crystals* located throughout the tissues of the physical body. These may be thought of as organic computer chips, which function as storehouses of suppressed thought, word and emotion. Modern science tells us that it is possible to store vast amounts of information in a manmade computer chip, and in the same way, the capacity for information storage in these organic computer chips may be virtually limitless. The implications of holding these crystals within the physical body are numerous on many levels. On the physical level they hinder the free flow of cerebrospinal fluid or CSF and consequently impede nerve supply and circulation. Other repercussions include lymphatic congestion, poor supply of nutrition to various tissues, poor elimination of wastes from these tissues, and diminished electrical potential in the tissues, thus increasing their susceptibility to invasion by bacteria, parasites, and viruses. This sad progression continues ever downward if the cause is not removed. It is important to understand that the crystals themselves are *not* the cause, but a result. The true cause lies not on the physical level but in our consciousness. Eventually the process may culminate in chronic disease, the proliferation of abnormal tissue, cancer, or other physical problems if the cause is left intact for a sufficient length of time.

Beyond the physical ramifications, other areas are worth considering. Each of us exists in a sea of light or information, these being states of frequency and vibration. The vast majority of that which is all around us is imperceptible, for the crystals block the light, thus rendering us incapable of perceiving. Therefore, the crystals operate as a sort of stimulus-response mechanism whereby we are rarely in the now, because most of what is happening all around us never makes it to our awareness. The bulk of this information is simply intercepted by the crystals, which then trigger various patterns of predetermined behavior with computerlike precision. Hence, most of the time when we think we are exercising our free agency, we are simply acting on the basis of ingrained reactive patterns which are locked into the crystals.

Moving Back Towards Freedom and Health

THIS STATE OF AFFAIRS MAY APPEAR BLEAK. YET IT IS POSSIBLE TO TURN this whole sequence around and undo that which we ourselves have set in motion. We have enslaved ourselves through our own judgments. Hence, it is within our power to uncreate this enslavement. Whatever we have brought into a state of creation, we also have the power to uncreate.

UNPROGRAMMING AND REPROGRAMMING

It is important to clearly distinguish between unprogramming and reprogramming. In unprogramming we get to the root of the judgment and transmute it, thus restoring free agency and choice. In reprogramming only the outer behavior is changed by covering it up or overpowering it with yet more programming, thus driving the cause further into unconsciousness. If we consider the analogy of the overhead projector used previously, unprogramming might be likened to actually removing a particular transparency, whereas reprogramming would be similar to simply placing another transparency on top of it so that its effect was no longer immediately apparent upon the screen.

Numerous modalities currently used recognize the existence of these so-called programs as a fundamental cause of much suffering. Most modalities, however, go for the quick fix wherein the person is simply reprogrammed in order to eliminate some apparently destructive outer pattern of behavior rather than taking the time to change consciousness as is done when we unprogram ourselves. The results of these two diametrically opposed approaches may appear the same in terms of observable behavior. Indeed, for every truth there is always a counterfeit for truth. However, while the behavior may be the same, the underlying attitude and/or choice (or lack thereof) matters: doing the right thing by our own free choice is different from doing it simply because we are programmed to do it. Not only that, but because the underlying cause remains untransformed, people are certain again to find themselves in difficulty.

While it may take considerable time, patience, and effort to actually unprogram our reactive patterns, it is well worth it. The process of unprogramming leads to an expansion of consciousness, an increase in awareness, greater free agency, and the evolution of the soul. Reprogramming, while it may remove many of our obvious outer symptoms and behaviors and make our existence more comfortable for the moment, results in a contraction of consciousness, diminished awareness, a lessening of free agency, and further movement down the involutionary spiral into identification with matter.

Working from the Bottom Up

In order to get to underlying causes—judgments and resistances which lead to formation of crystals—we must ordinarily begin at the bottom, so to speak. We move from the physical body to the emotional and eventually to the mental in the process of uncreating the self-imposed bondage of our own resistances. We begin by obeying physical laws pertaining to the physical body, which will have the result of dissolving various crystals. Chief among these are various laws of nutrition which will be discussed in Part Two, as well as the appropriate application of certain disciplines (including, but not limited to, Body Electronics covered in Part Three) which will help dissolve the crystals. This, in turn, will yield up the stored suppressed patterns of thought, word, and emotion which have been locked into the crystals. Once released for us to reexperience, they may be transmuted.

Through physical discipline, we access the emotional body from the bottom up as well, meaning that we begin at unconsciousness and move grediently towards enthusiasm. As we move from unconsciousness to apathy to grief and so on, each level is mastered by experiencing it with enthusiasm. Anything less than enthusiasm is rooted in some form of resistance and, after all, what we resist will persist. So the emotional body is transmuted, level by level, by enthusiasm consistently attained and maintained, which we term the Law of Love. This is simple to express in words, yet the sincere seeker must make concerted effort to truly master and understand this principle.

A great challenge to moving through the levels of emotion with enthusiasm involves use of memory. For until we can remember what we have resisted, we will remain incapable of transmuting and releasing it. If we are incapable of remembering the past, then we are also incapable of being in the now, for our resistance will continue to color our perception. "One is condemned to repeat that which one cannot remember."

At level of unconsciousness there is little memory; indeed, there is little awareness in general. We simply do not remember. At the apathy level we still have little memory, for we *can't* remember. Yet this is a slight improvement, for we are now aware that there is something that we cannot remember. At the grief level memory is general in nature: we simply have a general picture which is sufficient to justify our grief. We may think we have specific memory, but that is not yet possible. At the fear level we are closer but still unwilling or unable to see specifics. Only at the anger level do we finally get specific memory, this, however, being one-sided and confined to a single point of view. This point of view is always perfectly justified, and any other point of view is wrong as far as we are concerned. Thus, there is no reason at the anger level. At the pain level we can see things from another point of view, albeit painfully. Here we move through the fire of the kundalini relative to that area of life, thus transmuting the emotional body in this area only.[2] After the pain level is reached and embraced, we can then move on to the level of enthusiasm where we can view the situation with equanimity and impartiality. From here we become capable of entering into the mental body.

At the level of the mental body we are capable of viewing the duality and encompassing both sides of it simultaneously. This resolves the existing resistance and judgment and restores our free agency in this area of life, and we manifest a noticeable absence of restriction and/or limitation in this area. Whereas previously we couldn't perceive clearly and make choices in this area due to our own self-imposed patterns of judgment, these limitations then become conspicuous for their absence.

If we can release one area of judgment, we can let go of others. The process will continually accelerate as our window of free agency expands as each layer of resistance and judgment melts away like dew before the morning sun. The darkness of resistance will fight against the light of awareness and love. This certainly includes the levels of darkness within each of us. Yet light will eventually prevail if we are willing to apply certain basic principles on physical, emotional and mental levels.

The Underlying Pattern of Perfection and How It Is Obscured

ALL DISEASE AND DISCOMFORT ON A PHYSICAL LEVEL STEM FROM RESIS-tance on emotional and mental levels, and over time resistance becomes crystallized, causing reactive patterns of response to life. In addition to those which stem from our resistance to experiences of life, a wide array of reactive patterns are present from birth. These are also based on resistance to experience, but from an earlier time. As any parent can attest, the personality of a child (which has considerable relation to these reactive patterns) is already fairly pronounced at birth.

It is not that we are faulty creatures in some way, for each of us has a blueprint of perfection initially. To go back to our overhead projector analogy, this blueprint might be compared to a transparency with an image upon it of a body free of all imperfections. Yet superimposed over this initial blueprint, there is generally a considerable distortion which obscures this pattern of perfection. These distortions might be compared to transparencies which contain imperfections which are superimposed over the initial perfect transparency. Each of these distortions is related to some sort of resistance.

Given the condition of the physical body in most instances, it may be hard to believe in a pattern of perfection. Faced with the outer evidence of so much imperfection, it is often quite a challenge to recognize the underlying state of perfection, when all outer evidence seems to scream the contrary. The overhead projector again provides a helpful way of understanding how perfection can still be there, even when only imperfection is evident. Suppose an initial transparency with the image of a perfect body is placed upon the projector by itself. The image upon the screen will also appear perfect. When a transparency with an imperfection is placed atop the perfect transparency, the image on the screen will no longer appear perfect. Yet if the imperfection is minor enough, it will not be difficult to see the perfection underneath as we look at the image on the screen. And perhaps as we add a few more transparencies, each with another imperfection, for a certain period we may still be able to see the perfection underneath the increasing imperfection as we continue to gaze at the image on the screen. But sooner or later, when enough imperfection has obscured the underlying perfection, we will no longer be able to see it. Yet no matter how much imperfection is heaped upon it, the initial perfect transparency has never left the projector. In a similar manner, no matter how imperfect our physical body and its state of health may appear, it is important to remember that we always have an underlying pattern of perfection, for after all, each of us was made, "in the image and likeness of God." It is just that there are a few overlays upon this image. So let us consider some of the sources of these overlays.

THE HEREDITARY LEVEL

One major category is the Hereditary Level. This includes but is not limited to those patterns encoded within our DNA. The Hereditary Level includes all those patterns which we have inherited from our parents and other ancestors, whether encoded within the DNA or otherwise. Most people realize that we inherit various physical tendencies from our parents. Yet we may also inherit the resistances of our ancestors, including the memories of events. After all, it is these underlying resistances that lie at the root of the physical tendencies in the first place. In other words, if our image on the screen looks like the images of one or both of our parents to some extent, it is because some of their transparencies have been copied and added to our stack. It makes sense that if we inherited the outer manifestation or effect, it must be because we have also inherited the inner essence or cause, and these patterns, memories and tendencies may be actually encoded in the DNA. Many people have had clear and precise memory of experiences which happened to their parents or other ancestors that no one told them about. These experiences have been experienced from the point of view of the other person, and the memory has been as clear and detailed as that person's own memories. In certain instances, it has been possible to compare notes with our parents and corroborate the accuracy of the recalled event. And in numerous instances, as these inherited memories were recalled and the associated resistances were released, profound physical healing has taken place, for resistance on the Hereditary Level can have as significant an impact upon our health as resistance that originates in our present existence.

THE SOUL LEVEL

Another major category of overlay is from the Soul Level and pertains to our own previous experiences in other incarnations. Not everyone will agree that each of us as an intelligence has experienced previous lifetimes in other bodies. (A debate on this issue at one seminar was brought to a quick end when one gentleman stood up and announced, "I don't believe in past lives, and I didn't believe in them in my last lifetime either.") The experience of many people suggests that the patterns and the memories of these previous experiences are still present, that the Soul Level is as real and as influential on our health as the Hereditary Level.[3] However, the important thing is eventually to be able to recall instances in this lifetime when we have had similar experiences or feelings. We are ultimately here to deal with the situations of this lifetime, and it is unlikely we will have much success resolving anything in a past life if we remain unwilling or unable to deal with the here and now. Also, whether we believe in past lives or not, the suppressed memories which are most crucial and relevant will be those of this lifetime. In other words, if a particular issue then was not successfully resolved, it is doubtless still an issue now, and we have ample opportunities in this current lifetime to deal with it. Hence, whether or not we believe in past lives is ultimately of little concern here. For our plate is probably more than full with the concerns of this lifetime already.

THE ENTITY LEVEL

A third major category of overlay might be termed the Entity Level and pertains to the possibility of entity involvement. Indeed, I have heard that certain psychologists have taken the position, based upon years of experience and observation, that all disease is related to the presence of entities.

The term *entity* refers to either a separate intelligence or a powerful thought form which has virtually taken on a life of its own. In either case, the entity represents an energy overlay which exerts a marked effect on our behavior. Entities often seem an outlandish concept to someone who has not experienced or at least observed them firsthand. Yet I have seen numerous people who, despite heavy initial skepticism regarding entities, have come to regard their existence as quite self-evident.

A number of related situations tend to be referred to as entity involvement. In some cases, the entity is an actual separate human intelligence that is no longer inhabiting a body of its own. Rather, this intelligence is trapped or stuck within the energy field of a living individual. To give an example, suppose a person was put under general anesthetic in order to undergo surgery. States of induced unconsciousness such as general anesthetic tend to leave an individual open to entities. Nearby in the hospital, another individual was in the process of dying. The intelligence of the deceased can be attracted to and trapped in the energy field of the individual under anesthetic. Another possibility is that the entity is a separate intelligence, but not a human intelligence. This has been observed on many occasions as well. In other cases, the entity is not an actual separate intelligence, but what might be termed a thought form. Imagine that if an individual has a sufficiently intense pattern of resistance, this pattern could create a distinct thought form. And while this thought form would not be an independent intelligence in the strictest sense, it might be said to virtually take on a life of its own. Some suggest that Multiple Personality Disorder constitutes an extreme instance of this type of entity, where various patterns of resistance are sufficiently strong as to appear as separate personalities.

It should be clearly understood that an entity is not the cause of any of our resistances, but more of an effect. A particular resistance will create a hole in our energy field or aura. Since nature abhors a vacuum, this hole will soon be filled, and as like attracts like, the hole will be filled with a similar energy to the resistance that created the hole in the first place. Thus, our entities are in many ways a reflection of our own resistances.

LAYERS UPON LAYERS

These three categories of influence, the Hereditary Level, the Soul Level and the Entity Level, may each have a profound influence on our physical, emotional and mental health, providing overlays on top of a basic pattern of perfection. In many seminars on Body Electronics, people have experienced either some type of past life memory or entity involvement during a pointholding session prior to these possibilities even being mentioned in lecture. That is, such things seem to come up whether or not people have any expectation that they might. Indeed, I have seen them come up for people who had previously expressed their utter disbelief in such possibilities.

It is important to note that these three levels may overlap with each other in numerous possible ways. The Hereditary and Soul Levels may overlap if we as a soul were our own ancestor in a genetic sense. To give another example, the Entity Level may overlap with the Hereditary Level such that an entity may be passed down from a parent to a child. The permutations are numerous. Certainly, what came from where may not be obvious when we view the overall pattern as reflected upon the "screen," but in any case the dynamics of healing will be the same.

Resistance, Health, and Consciousness Change

As we have stated already, both health and disease have their origins on the mental level. When resistance exists at this level, we have dropped out of a state of enthusiasm on the emotional level. We might also say that resistance at the mental level warps or distorts the emotional body. If the resistance as well as the distortion are held in a state of creation long enough, the eventual result will be some problem on the physical level. The ensuing physical symptoms are the outer manifestation of the inner condition of resisted thought, word and emotion. The process of restoring health will typically be in reverse order to that of falling from our pattern of perfection and becoming ill. To restore health, we begin at the physical and move up through the emotional and on to the mental level. This may be considered as analogous to the principle of healing crisis (see Chapter Six), wherein we heal in reverse chronological order to the manner in which we developed the complaint. While healing is often initiated with physical steps, including nutrition, in order for it to be complete it must eventually encompass the emotional and the mental levels.

Many people, myself included, have initially been drawn into various healing practices in response to physical complaints. Some have been quite successful in healing their physical problems. Most have ended up with far more than they were initially looking for. While they started out looking for physical improvement, they ended up with considerable emotional, mental and spiritual improvement as well. Many people have been far more impressed with the changes on these other levels, even when the physical changes were beyond what they dreamed of when they began. This has led me to observe that physical healing is a pleasant side effect of consciousness change.

THE HUNDREDTH MONKEY PHENOMENON AND MORPHIC RESONANCE

So far we have looked at how change of consciousness will affect us as individuals. And yet we are all connected such that whatever any of us does will affect everyone else. However, not only our outer actions but also our thoughts or consciousness can have a huge impact upon the universe and all life in it. Ken Keyes calls this the *Hundredth Monkey Phenomenon* and explains how it works:

> ... when a certain critical number achieves an awareness, this new awareness may be communicated from mind to mind. Although the exact number may vary, the Hundredth Monkey Phenomenon means that when only a limited number of people know of a new way, it may remain the consciousness property of these people. But there is a point at which if only one more person tunes-in to a new awareness, a field is strengthened so that its awareness reaches almost everyone![4]

If we read Keyes' account of the hundredth monkey carefully, several key points stand out. First, when these monkeys were learning to wash sweet potatoes before eating them, an innovation by one young monkey that others soon picked up, it seemed most easy for consciousness change to be passed on or made available within a family. Mothers seemed to pick it up from their children. In addition, up to a certain point, the increase in numbers was more or less one monkey at a time. But eventually, after six years, a critical mass was reached, and as soon as this critical mass was reached, the change of consciousness was immediately available all over. Monkeys elsewhere, who had no contact with those on Koshima Island, changed consciousness overnight.

Similar ideas are presented in *A New Science of Life* and other books by the noted biologist Rupert Sheldrake. Sheldrake uses the term *morphogenetic field* to describe a dynamic field that links numerous individuals located all over. Each individual can affect the field, and each is simultaneously influenced by the field. The term *morphic resonance* is used to describe the effects of individual members upon the field and vice versa. Sheldrake also presents much evidence for the idea of critical mass.[5]

I have seen much in the area of healing that corroborates these concepts. Often when one member of a family experiences a consciousness change or healing crisis, other family members reap similar benefits despite no obvious difference in any of their habits. It seems as if one family member changing makes it possible for others to do so more readily. For example, the eyes of participants in Body Electronics sometimes lighten in color, as will be discussed in Chapter Twenty. Yet sometimes their children's or parents' eyes will also get lighter despite no obvious effort or change on their part at the time. Other times, a person will go through an intense healing crisis with specific symptoms, for example, severe back pain. As this happens, their parent or child may inexplicably go through an hour or two of intense back pain, even when the family member is many miles away. Distance seems quite irrelevant to this effect, which is in keeping with Sheldrake's theories of morphic resonance.

Resonance involves two things having an effect upon one another because they vibrate at similar frequencies. The correct note can shatter a champagne glass, for example. Two people who are close genetic relatives will possess many of the same energy patterns; in other words, they will vibrate at similar frequencies. As a result, they are in a good position to exert tremendous influence upon one another by resonance because their DNA patterns are close enough to resonate.[6]

Besides the close effect of one family member upon another, the idea of morphic resonance helps explains the critical mass or hundredth monkey phenomenon. Perhaps if enough members of the morphogenetic field change in a particular way, the entire field will shift, and thus, all its members may change easily. Sheldrake offers much experimental evidence of this phenomena.

All of this suggests that each of us will ultimately affect every other member of the field to some extent. While our effect may be more pronounced on those most closely related to us, we still have an effect on everyone else and vice versa.

WE ARE ALL PART OF THE SAME WHOLE

The implications of these concepts for health and healing are many. One is that as more people are able to overcome a particular problem, it will become easier for all those who follow to do so. As individuals we must, of course, still deal with our own situation as we strive to regain or maintain our health. Yet, we are all in this together. Sometimes in a given area, we might be the first monkey. Other times we might be the hundredth. Or we might be somewhere in between. Or, in many cases, we are one of the many monkeys that benefit after the first hundred. It is not a question of making any "monkey" more important than any other. It is merely understanding that our individual experiences may be taking place in a broader context of unity and connection as opposed to separation and disconnection. For we are all ultimately part of the same whole, all appearances to the contrary.

Chapter Three

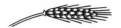

The Great Paradox of Healing

Most people are in a hurry to get better, so they can get back to whatever made them sick in the first place.
John Whitman Ray

That which we obtain too easily, we esteem too lightly. It is dearness only which gives everything its value. Heaven knows how to put a proper price on its goods.
Thomas Paine

If one advances confidently in the direction of his dreams, and endeavors to live the life he has imagined, he will meet with a success unexpected in common hours.
Henry David Thoreau

WHAT KEEPS US FROM PERCEIVING OUR UNITY WITH EACH OTHER and with everything around us is resistance. As we have also said, it is resistance that leads to ill-health. Resistance is an attitude of anything less than unconditional love, and as alluded to earlier, whenever we resist something, one result is to perpetuate the very thing that we are resisting. From this, we can deduce some crucial principles pertaining to healing the body.

The Willingness to Not Heal and the Desire to Heal

LET US CONSIDER HOW THIS RELATES TO THE HEALING OF OUR BODY. Suppose we have a particular physical condition, and we are quite unwilling to have that condition. If we are not willing, we do not have unconditional love for it. In other words, we resist it. The result of this resistance is to perpetuate the very condition that we are resisting, and so long as we keep perpetuating this condition with our continued resistance, no amount of outer effort will bring healing.

If we work this line of reasoning backwards, we may come to a surprising conclusion. Clearly, if our resistance to the condition is helping to perpetuate that condition, we must let go of this resistance. One aspect of letting it go is to be willing for that condition to exist and even continue: an unconditional acceptance. In order for healing to be possible, we must be willing to not heal. One necessary condition for healing is the willingness for it to not take place, and as many can attest, taking this attitude is easier said than done.

However, nothing is brought into outer manifestation without the desire for it to be so. It is imperative that we understand that only through the exercise of desire can anything, including healing, take place. Thus, we come to another important principle: in order for healing to be possible, we must desire this healing.

These two preceding principles, when considered together, present a seeming paradox. It would appear that in order for healing to take place, we must on the one hand desire this healing. On the other hand, and at the same time, we must be willing for it not to take place. This may seem impossible, yet it is not once we understand the crucial difference between desire and attachment.

Desire and Attachment

DESIRE HAS TAKEN ON A NEGATIVE CONNOTATION IN RECENT TIMES, AND to some extent this may be due to how we translate ancient teachings from other languages into modern English usage. We are led to believe that desire is wrong and must be utterly abolished if we are to progress. However, in actuality, desire is necessary in order for anything to be brought into existence. Indeed, nobody would even try to abolish desire unless they first had a desire to abolish it! It is not desire, then, that is interfering with our progress; rather, it is our attachment to its fulfillment, attachment being the unwillingness for the desire not to be fulfilled, a form of resistance.

It is quite possible to have a desire without being attached to its fulfillment. In the absence of this attachment, there is no resistance, for we are willing for the desire to remain unfulfilled. As a matter of fact, the desire is far more likely to be fulfilled when there is no attachment to its fulfillment.

With this understanding of the difference between desire and attachment, the previous paradox is easily resolved. For healing to be possible, we must desire this healing and yet have no attachment to it. We must remain willing to not heal. This principle can be readily understood, yet understanding it intellectually may be far simpler than following it, as many have found.

Commitment

APPLICATION TO OUR OWN SITUATIONS MAY BE EXTREMELY DIFFICULT. Imagine how challenging it would be to have a serious illness and be willing not to recover from it. Imagine how hard it might be to be willing to remain seriously ill indefinitely, perhaps even to die. Imagine applying this principle in an advanced case of cancer, for example.

But there is more. It is not enough merely to be willing to not heal, though that is already challenge enough for most of us. If we are going to heal, we also need to commit our full effort to the process. Now, it might be hard enough to be willing to not heal in a circumstance where we are not required to put out any effort. But I am suggesting something even harder: to put out maximum effort and simultaneously to have no attachment to the outcome. For healing to be possible, we must be willing to put our full effort into the process and yet have no attachment to the outcome of that effort.

The Great Paradox

IF WE PUT IT ALL TOGETHER, WE ARRIVE AT THE FOLLOWING: FOR HEALING to be possible, we must desire this healing and yet have no attachment to it: we must remain willing to not heal. We must be willing to put our full effort into the process and yet have no attachment to the outcome of that effort. Again, intellectual mastery of this complete concept is not enough to heal us; we must be able to put it into practice. It is not enough to "talk the talk." We must also be able to "walk the walk."

Attachment: The Myth of Sisyphus

THE FRENCH EXISTENTIAL PHILOSOPHER ALBERT CAMUS WROTE A FAMOUS essay called "The Myth of Sisyphus" in which he considers the plight of the character Sisyphus from Greek mythology. Sisyphus had angered certain of the gods, and he received a severe punishment. As Camus expressed it, "The gods had condemned Sisyphus to ceaselessly rolling a rock to the top of a mountain, whence the stone would fall back of its own weight. They had thought with some reason that there is no more dreadful punishment than futile and hopeless labor."[1] The punishment of Sisyphus has much to do with the foregoing principles, for it clearly recognizes the human tendency to be attached to the outcome of our efforts. Sisyphus received the "unspeakable penalty in which the whole being is exerted toward accomplishing nothing."[2] I would argue that it is precisely the attachment to the outcome of our efforts that makes such a penalty so difficult.

To leave behind attachment to the outcome of our efforts to heal is to experience the effort itself with nonresistance. Since illness is a result of resistance, when the attachment to a desired outcome is gone (no resistance), only then is the fulfillment of this desire possible. Thus, the trick is to experience the process of working towards our own healing while letting go of having to heal. We enthusiastically engage in pursuing the desired healing, yet let go of all attachment to the healing itself and receive with love whatever may come.

Most writers might focus primarily upon the unending and futile physical efforts of Sisyphus. However, Camus chose to look also at the attitude with which Sisyphus engaged in his efforts: "It is during that return, that pause, that Sisyphus interests me. . . . I see that man going back down with a heavy yet measured step toward the torment of which he will never know the end. . . . At each of these moments when he leaves the heights and gradually sinks toward the lairs of the gods, he is superior to his fate. He is stronger than his rock."[3] It is in his attitude that Camus is able to find a sort of victory for Sisyphus: "I leave Sisyphus at the foot of the mountain. One always finds one's burden again. But Sisyphus teaches the higher fidelity that negates the gods and raises rocks. He too concludes that all is well. . . . Each atom of that stone, each mineral flake of that night-filled mountain, in itself forms a world. The struggle itself towards the heights is enough to fill a man's heart. One must imagine Sisyphus happy."[4]

And so perhaps for each of us as well, the secret is to be happy, regardless of our own burden. The burden or punishment Sisyphus has received may or may not be just or deserved. Yet either way, it is his to carry, it is his to experience. I would suggest that whether we consider our own circumstances just or deserved, they are nonetheless ours to carry, ours to experience. Perhaps it is not the burden we carry that is important, so much as how we carry it. For it is in the manner we choose to carry it that we surmount it in the end. Sisyphus does not overcome his rock by succeeding in getting it to remain at the top. He succeeds by letting his heart fill with the satisfaction of meeting his fate, enjoying the doing rather than fixating upon the outcome. We can make a similar choice to be happy or not, whatever our own "rock" may be, thereby letting go of resistance to our experience.

Chapter Four

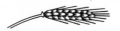

The Nature of Resistance

If you are distressed by anything external, the pain is not due to the thing itself, but to your estimate of it; and this you have the power to revoke at any moment.

Marcus Aurelius

We drag our pasts behind us unaware, and each of us lives with our disinherited selves.

Henri Bergson

Identity precedes activity.

Douglas Morrison

I have sworn upon the altar of God, eternal hostility against every form of tyranny over the mind of man.

Thomas Jefferson

CREATION IS THE PROCESS OF BRINGING SOMETHING INTO OUTER manifestation. The intelligence consciously holds a particular pattern of thought, word, and emotion in a state of creation, and this composite pattern from the inner essence is then brought forth as an outer manifestation. The process of uncreation is the reverse of this. If the intelligence ceases to put forth the creative effort, then the outer manifestation will cease to exist, but only so long as resistance has not entered the picture. For once resistance has entered the picture, it is no longer possible simply to rescind the creative effort. This creative effort is now obscured by the resistance itself, and the resistance must be dealt with appropriately before it is possible to uncreate.

Resistance and Judgment

RESISTANCE CAN BE DEFINED AS AN ATTITUDE OF ANYTHING LESS THAN unconditional love, which embraces all things. In the physical universe, however, there is opposition in all things: everything is defined in terms of numerous pairs of opposites that we refer to as dualities. When we say what something is, we inherently say what it is not, for that is the nature of duality. Neither side of a given duality is inherently right or wrong, for each simply is. Cold is not better than hot any more than hot is better than cold, at least not in any absolute sense. In a given context and for a given purpose, one may be preferable to the other: cold certainly works better for refrigeration, and hot is more effective for cooking. Yet again, neither is inherently better than the other, only better in a particular circumstance and for a particular purpose.

Resistance can be said to originate in judgment, and simply put, a judgment is identifying with one side of a duality to the exclusion of the other. One side is made right or good and the other side is made wrong or bad. And so resistance is set in motion. It is that simple. Judgments seem to serve us well in certain circumstances; after all, even a stopped clock is correct twice a day. And yet they so obviously work against us in other circumstances.

Resistance and Awareness

ONCE WE JUDGE ONE SIDE OF A DUALITY AS GOOD AND THE OTHER AS bad, we tend to close off awareness to some extent. When we have resistance in a given area, we are not capable of seeing things as they actually are. However, the process of creation involves the conscious mind: creation and uncreation both come from the conscious mind. When we resist a particular creation, we start to become unconscious. Resistance holds in the unconscious mind the pattern of thought, word and emotion that is

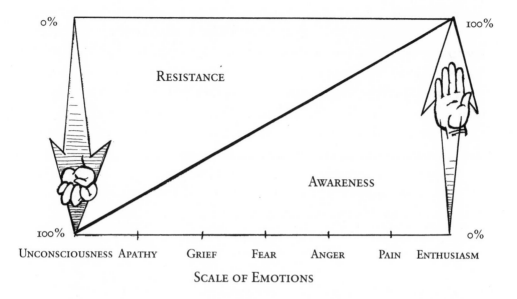

FIGURE 5: RESISTANCE AND AWARENESS

resisted, and so long as this continues, the outer manifestation of that resistance will also persist. The conscious mind is like the tip of the iceberg, the small fraction that can be seen above the surface. The unconscious mind is the much larger fraction that lurks invisibly beneath the surface. I am told that it was not the part of the iceberg above the surface that sank the *Titanic,* but rather the portion beneath the surface. Similarly, the unconscious mind must be addressed if we are to release ourselves from the bondage of our own resistance. We must learn to see beneath the surface, for that is where the real danger lurks.

However, with respect to lack of awareness (unconsciousness) and resistance, it is not all or nothing; we are not completely aware or else completely resistant. There is a gradient scale of resistance and/or awareness, and this scale may be expressed in terms of the Scale of Emotions as presented in Chapter Two.

At the top level, enthusiasm, we are ordinarily free of resistance in a given area of life. As a result, we have complete awareness in this area of life and can see things as they are. Thus, at the level of enthusiasm, we have total awareness and zero resistance. At the opposite end of the scale of emotions, the level of unconsciousness, we ordinarily have the opposite situation. Resistance is typically total at this level. We merely react according to our programming, without even realizing it. Thus, at the unconsciousness level, we have total resistance and zero awareness. As we move from enthusiasm gradually towards unconsciousness on the scale of emotions, awareness will generally decrease and resistance will generally increase. On the other hand, as we move from unconsciousness up towards enthusiasm, awareness will typically increase and resistance will typically decrease.

Resistance and awareness can therefore be seen to have an inverse relationship to one another. The more resistance, the less awareness, and the more awareness, the less resistance. Perfect awareness would therefore require a complete absence of resistance. The degree to which we resist is precisely the degree to which our awareness is impaired.

Freedom and Awareness

PART OF THE DEFINITION OF FREEDOM IS BEING ABLE TO EXERCISE OUR free agency in a given situation; The ability to do so is very much dependent upon having full awareness of the situation. Without full awareness of our choices, we are not capable of choosing. To put it simply: freedom is predicated upon awareness. A lack of awareness implies a lack of freedom, and lack of awareness might also be considered a state of ignorance. Therefore, we might also note that ignorance and freedom are incompatible. It can be inferred from all this that the nature of resistance is to restrict freedom, to enslave us. Since it is we who have set resistance in motion with our judgments, we can conclude that resistance results in a self-imposed state of bondage.

Reactive Mechanisms

THIS SELF-IMPOSED STATE OF BONDAGE TAKES THE FORM OF A VARIETY of reactive patterns that might be termed stimulus-response mechanisms. To a large extent we are each governed by these reactive patterns, though it is difficult to see the truth of this at first. For when our resistance is extreme, our awareness will be correspondingly minimal, and we will not realize how resistant we truly are. As we gradually release some of our resistance, our awareness will correspondingly increase. We will become somewhat more aware of how resistant we truly are. Thus, we have an odd situation: as we become less resistant, we become more aware of how resistant we actually are. Many people who have worked diligently upon the release of their resistances have had the same experience. To begin with, most do not feel that they are especially resistant. Most people sincerely believe that most of what they are doing is free choice. Then as layer after layer of resistance is released, awareness increases. As this happens, it becomes apparent how much of that "freedom" was actually enslavement to reactive patterns.

RESISTANCE SHAPES OUR EXPERIENCE

Reactive patterns will tend to get stronger over time, as a result of continual reinforcement. This can be explained in terms of the Law of Attraction, which states that like attracts like. When we have a given resistance, we are holding what we are resisting in a continual state of creation. This energy pattern acts like a beacon, constantly emitting its energy pattern into the universe. The result is that our resistance tends to draw to us exactly what we already resist. Each time we act out a particular reactive pattern, that pattern is reinforced or strengthened.

The pattern of resistance, reaction, and further resistance is not inevitable but merely likely for a few simple reasons. Suppose we already have a certain degree of resistance in a given area. Anytime a situation arises that is likely to trigger this resistance, we are already starting out with several strikes against us. For as a result of our resistance, our awareness of the situation is diminished and so is our freedom. We are predisposed to resist already. For example, suppose we resist people being rude and tend to take offense whenever we encounter what we perceive as rudeness. As a result, we will tend to have a lower threshold than most for rudeness, and will tend to react to it strongly and rapidly, even when the offense may have been slight. Each time we resist rudeness, our basic pattern of resisting rudeness is reinforced. Thus, it is likely over time for the resistance to get stronger.

Some would suggest that we become what we resist: that by resisting something, we take on that energy and become the very thing we resist.

There is undoubtedly truth in that; yet the very fact that we resist something indicates that it is already within our own nature. In other words, we are simply resisting out there that which already exists in here. We are resisting outside of ourselves that which we are.

RESISTANCE ALSO SHAPES OUR PERCEPTION

While we should understand that our resistances tend to attract to us the very experiences we resist, it is equally important to recognize that resistance also shapes our perception of our experience. This is often expressed in the phrase "we see through a glass darkly." In the example of a person resisting rudeness, we have said that the person would therefore tend to experience rudeness on a regular basis. Resistance would shape their experience. But there is another aspect to consider. When rudeness is resisted, it will tend to be seen by whomever has that resistance, regardless of whether or not it is actually there. We may see rudeness where it truly does not exist, though it is quite real to us. We may find the waitress quite rude, for example, but perhaps nobody else at our table has any idea what we are complaining about. Our resistance to rudeness sufficiently distorts our perception that we see it where nobody else does.

Overcoming Resistance

AS HAS BEEN STATED, ALL RESISTANCE ORIGINATES IN JUDGMENT—IDENtifying with one side of a given duality to the exclusion of the other, entering into a state wherein we are no longer impartial to both sides. The process of overcoming a given resistance will therefore involve returning to a state of impartiality wherein both sides of the duality can be considered without resistance or attachment to either. This is sometimes referred to as encompassing that duality.

Overcoming resistance will also mean focusing on specifics rather than generalizations, for judgments are generalizations about life. It is insisting that things are always a certain way, rather than recognizing the uniqueness of every situation. Judgment might also be considered a flattening of life, wherein we lose the ability to see the exceptions to these generalizations. For example, take the generalization: "Nobody loves me." A basic principle is that one counterexample disproves a generalization. Hence, the recognition of a single person that loves us would be sufficient to disprove the generalization. But if we consider the relationship between judgments, resistances, perception, and belief systems, it may not be so easy as that. We may be unable to see that somebody actually does love us, even if this love is right in front of us continually. We may be surrounded by love, and yet this love may remain invisible to us. For it is indeed difficult to see something we do not believe exists. One reason it will be difficult to see love given a belief that "nobody loves me," is that our resistance to not being loved will tend to trap out attention upon not being loved. Thus, we may be so busy looking at not being loved that we are unable to see that we are.

A given resistance may have played itself out in countless events in our lifetime and beyond. If we are to overcome the judgment or generalization behind it, we will need to recall one or more specific memories wherein the resistance was activated. If we remain at the level of general memory only, we will typically remember only enough to justify our continued resistance. Yet if we can recall specific events, eventually the various resistances are recalled and released, and thus, the underlying judgments will also fall away. For within each specific event there lies the possibility for us to discover the truth and let go of our judgment. In this example of "nobody loves me," remembering an event wherein we felt that to be true, and then within that event discovering it was not really true, will help us overcome this resistance.

BEADS ON A STRING

A helpful analogy is to consider a virtually endless string of beads. Each bead may be likened to a specific event, and each is related by a common pattern of resistance—the string that runs through all of these beads. In examining these events, what we are ultimately after is not any particular one, but the underlying pattern of resistance. If the resistance itself is resolved, then all these various events become irrelevant, at least so far as that resistance is concerned. (Some of these events may remain quite relevant in that they will involve other resistances that have not yet been resolved, for the same bead may have more than one string through it.)

To go through one memory and release our resistance in that event is similar to taking a single bead off the string. Given the virtually infinite length of the string, one bead more or less would appear to make little difference. But it is through a specific memory that the common pattern of resistance can often be encountered. Imagine that the beads are strung quite tightly on the string, tightly enough that the string is neither accessible nor even visible. Yet by removing a single bead, we can grab the string. Once we have the string, we can give a good pull and unstring all of the beads. In a similar fashion, by dealing with one specific memory, we can gain access to the common resistance, and thus have the opportunity to resolve it.

NOT FIRST OR WORST

Because the specific memories with respect to a common resistance occurred in a particular chronological order, some would argue that it is therefore essential to recall the "first" of these events. This assumes that this is where the resistance originated. Others would note that the resistance occurred with various degrees of intensity in the various remembered events. Remembering the "worst" of these memories would seem most useful as the resistance is most intense in these.

Yet if we go back to our string of beads, it is clear that the string can be accessed via any of the beads. This is also true of a given resistance and the many memories in which that resistance has been made manifest. All we need is any one of these specific memories in order to find the common resistance. It need not be the first or the worst.

Layers of Resistance

THE WORK OF OVERCOMING RESISTANCE IN ONE AREA AT A TIME REVEALS that there is considerable interaction between resistances. There are indeed numerous layers of resistance, much like an inverted pyramid. We might begin with a few basic resistances at the bottom. On the basis of these resistances, others are formed. And the process goes on until eventually we have a vast and increasingly interlocked edifice of resistance. Over time, the architecture and complexity of our resistances becomes impressive. Our accumulated resistances form an expanding monument to our self-imposed state of bondage. We bind ourselves with layer upon layer.

The full extent of these layers of resistance is rarely evident when all we

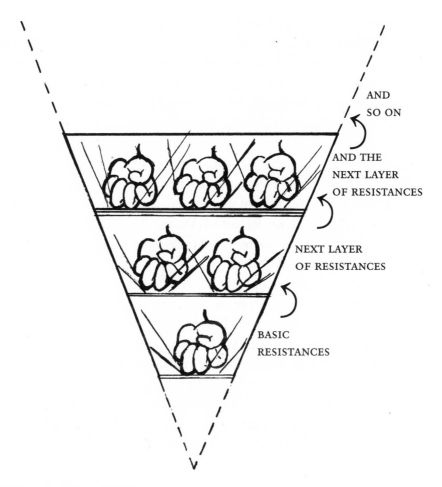

FIGURE 6: LAYERS OF RESISTANCE

can see are the surface ones. But as we start to excavate a bit, we find that there are many levels of resistance within each of us that can be aptly likened to the layers of an onion. As each newly discovered resistance melts away, the opportunity emerges to encounter and transmute deeper and more subtle layers that are then more capable of being worked with. Depending upon our attitude, this tendency to find ever deeper layers may be both frustrating and rewarding: frustrating if we remain attached to an eventual outcome; rewarding if we can be grateful for the opportunity to consider each newly revealed layer as it is gradiently released from the crystals within us.

As we continue to unfold, each of us encounters our own set of challenges or opportunities. At times we may become disheartened because as we peel away a few layers of our resistances, we look at our past and realize how powerful resistance has been to shape our experience. In the present we feel our comfort zones being stretched and have to surmise that even now resistance is a powerful force. For even as one resistance drops away and the universe realigns itself in accordance with our newly emerging state of consciousness, another resistance from within ourselves is revealed along with its expression in the outer world around us. As we look ahead to the future, we may in our impatience wonder if there is any end to our resistances. We may despair of ever reaching the center of the onion. And yet our impatience is simply a not so subtle reminder that we each have much that may still be mastered.

However, nothing is gained by haste. Our resistances are everpresent within us, at least until we transmute them. Thus, they are available for our perception and for us to work with. And they are amply reflected and made manifest in life all around us. Yet the more we hurry, the less clearly are we able to see this. As Dr. John Whitman Ray states most people are in a hurry to get better, so they can get back to doing whatever made them sick in the first place. Let us each learn patience. We have already held ourselves in bondage for a lengthy time with our many resistances, so the process of fully resolving each of them may also be long.

SURFACE AND DEEPER LAYERS

We may take comfort in knowing that once the process of working through resistance has begun, it acquires a momentum that makes working through subsequent layers less difficult. Consider the inverted pyramid. As massive as the top becomes, it has no stability if the pyramid is all above ground level; stability necessitates it being primarily buried underground, therefore as more and more of the top layers are revealed, more will topple away. And so it is with our own layers of resistance. Their only stability lies in remaining essentially buried; they cannot last long once exposed. The deeper layers may be exposed simply by working first through the more superficial layers that hide them.

As we work through to ever deeper layers, there is another obvious

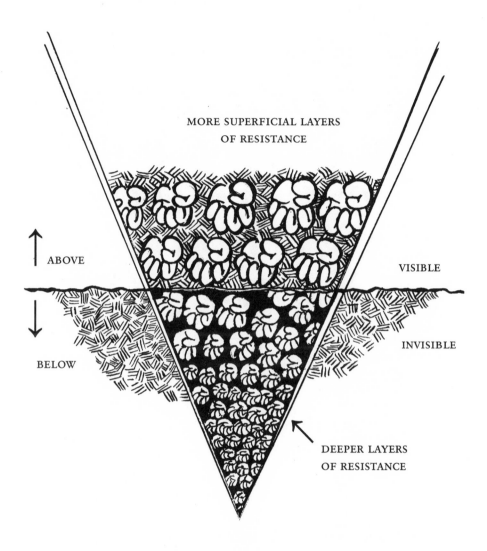

MORE SUPERFICIAL LAYERS
OF RESISTANCE

ABOVE

VISIBLE

BELOW

INVISIBLE

DEEPER LAYERS
OF RESISTANCE

FIGURE 7: SURFACE AND DEEPER LAYERS

bonus. When a surface resistance is resolved, that does not take care of any other resistances, yet it does reveal the next deeper layer of resistance. This deeper resistance may have more than one resistance based upon it. Hence, when it is resolved, other resistances that were based upon it will also drop way, and this is true whether or not they were considered en route to this deeper resistance. Of course as ever deeper layers of resistance are resolved,

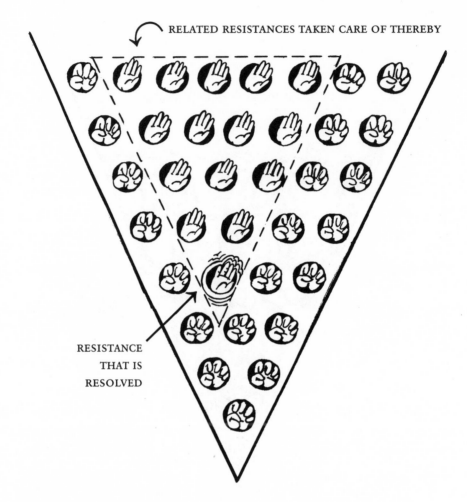

RELATED RESISTANCES TAKEN CARE OF THEREBY

RESISTANCE
THAT IS
RESOLVED

FIGURE 8: RESOLVING DEEPER RESISTANCES RESOLVES RELATED
RESISTANCES

the number of related resistances that will correspondingly drop away will increase geometrically. Hence, the more deeply we excavate, the more the whole process of demolishing the pyramid will accelerate.

RESISTANCE TO RESISTANCE AND METAPHYSICAL ARCHEOLOGY

Resistance cannot be resolved without love or enthusiasm, yet it is important to bear in mind that this must be genuine. It does us little good to fool ourselves that we love something that we do not. Rather, we should recognize that we do have resistance, and we should then determine if we can love this resistance itself. If we can love the resistance, then we have the opportunity to eventually resolve it. Yet often we do not love the resistance either. In fact, we resist this resistance. So, rather than pretend we love the resistance, we may need to see if we can love the resistance to the resistance, for it is simply not possible to resolve the resistance itself if the resistance to the resistance is unresolved. The resistance occurred first, followed by the resistance to the resistance. Hence, we must resolve them in reverse order, dealing with the resistance to the resistance first, then the underlying resistance.

In archeology, as we excavate down through various layers, the more recent material will be nearer the surface and thus will be encountered first, and the less recent material will be further from the surface and therefore encountered subsequently. And so it is with resistance, resistance to the resistance, resistance to the resistance to the resistance, and so on. This process of delving through the various layers of resistance can be considered "metaphysical archeology."

CHANGE OF UNCONSCIOUSNESS?

The goal of such metaphysical archeology is change of consciousness through release of resistance. However, such a change is complicated by multiple layers of resistance. Suppose we work through a particular resistance which has governed our behavior in a given area of life up to now. We begin to experience what appears to be freedom in this area because resistance is gone and our behavior is no longer governed by it. We may certainly call this a *change of consciousness*. Yet more often than not, our behavior will still be governed by various deeper resistances of which at present we are still quite unconscious. So it may be equally fitting to say we have also had a *change of unconsciousness*. For we are probably still bound by deeper resistances that we are not yet able to see. But rather than look at this from a pessimistic viewpoint, please consider that this is often a necessary phase we must pass through en route to resolving these deeper resistances as well.

Freedom from Resistance

WHAT WOULD OUR LIVES BE LIKE IF WE WERE FREE OF RESISTANCE? Again, our resistances are based upon judgments, which involve identifying with one side of a duality to the exclusion of the other. Hence, judgment and resistance involve being locked into a particular state of identity to the exclusion of other possible states of identity. We are identified with one side, and not with the other. We could say then that resistance flows from these states of identity in which we have become fixated or stuck. Resistance has also been shown to govern our behavior or activity to a tremendous extent. While each of us may have a small window of free agency, much of our activity is totally predetermined by our resistance.

If we put these two together, we might say simply that identity precedes activity. Were we free of resistance in a given area, we would be capable of assuming any possible state of identity quite freely. We would not confuse ourselves with our roles or be trapped by them. With this freedom of identity would come the freedom to choose any possible course of action, for the freedom of activity is based upon the freedom of identity. It is not possible to do that which it is not possible to be first.

"Quantum Leap"

A TELEVISION SHOW CALLED "QUANTUM LEAP" SHED SOME INTERESTING light on this idea of playing a role and yet understanding that we are not that role. The protagonist of the show was a scientist named Sam who was stuck in a time travel experiment gone amuck. Each episode he would "leap" into a new circumstance somewhere within the span of years from his own birth to the present, and he apparently had no control over whose life or role he leaped into or when. But each time, he would find himself in the role of this other person. As far as anybody else in that person's life was concerned, he was that person: he looked like them; he sounded like them; and so forth. The other person might be male or female, young or old, black or white, rich or poor. Sam quickly discovered that he had no choice but to make the best of the role he leaped into each time. He knew he was not that person, but as nobody else did there was not much point in saying, "Hey, this isn't my problem." The only way he could leap out of that particular role was to resolve some tricky situation that person was already in before he took on their role. His failure to do so would not only be harmful to them; it would be harmful for himself as well. He could be killed, for example. As soon as he resolved things in a given role, he would leap out of that role and into the next. His hope was that sooner or later he would simply leap back into his own self.

Some might say that Sam was put in an unfair situation where he had to assume responsibility for things that were not his responsibility. However, what fascinated me about the idea was that in the end, his situation was basically the same as yours or mine. We are all in a particular role at a particular moment, and we are all responsible for how we behave in that role. The crucial advantage that Sam had over you and me is that it was obvious to him that he was not really the role he was playing. Most of us, however, are sufficiently identified with our roles that we have long since ceased to understand that we are not the roles we play nor the resistances that define these roles. Perhaps we might have more success resolving the various entanglements we find ourselves in if we could be reminded from time to time that we are not our roles or our resistances. Perhaps we might then resolve these resistances with greater enthusiasm.

Chapter Five

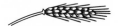

The Requirements of Health and Healing

There is no better way to discover the governing fundamental laws than to apply the ideal of ultimate simplicity.

Max Born

We are free to choose our actions ... but we are not free to choose the consequences of these actions.

Stephen Covey

Bad men cannot make good citizens. It is impossible that a nation of idolaters or infidels should be a nation of free men. It is when a people forget God that tyrants forge their chains. A vitiated state of morals, a corrupt public conscience, are incompatible with freedom.

Patrick Henry

I F OUR INTENTION IS TO REGAIN OUR HEALTH AND/OR TO MAINTAIN IT, our model gives us a number of principles that must be understood and applied.

Love, Which Melts Resistance

I N THE ABSENCE OF LOVE, MOST ANYTHING ELSE THAT WE PUT INTO PRAC-tice will be of little avail to us. When we remain in a state of resistance (which is the absence of love), we will simply continue to perpetuate that which we are resisting. Love is the central teaching of most major religions, however expressed. Jesus, for example, taught as follows: "Thou shalt love the Lord thy God with all thy heart; and with all thy soul; and with all thy mind. This is the first and great commandment. And the second is like unto it, Thou shalt love thy neighbor as thyself. On these two commandments hang all the law and the prophets" (Matthew 22:37–39). Jesus suggested that all other principles depend upon these two. And clearly these two both depend upon love. If we neglect this essential teaching of love, then most all else will be futile.

Dr. Ray uses the phrase "lovingly and willingly endure all things," and it might be wise to amplify this admonition somewhat. The physical universe is the outer manifestation or effect. The cause or inner essence is within. When we do not lovingly and willingly endure all things, we are therefore in a state of resistance towards the outer or the effect and we perpetuate the very thing that we resist. Another effect of our resistance to the outer is that when we resist anything, our attention becomes trapped or fixated upon that which we resist. As such, we remain in a position where it is not possible for us to see the inner or the cause. Thus, by resisting the effect, we not only perpetuate the effect, but we remain incapable of seeing the cause. As we are incapable of seeing the cause, we are certainly incapable of doing anything to remove it.

On the other hand if we can lovingly and willingly endure all things, we have essentially ceased resisting the outer or the effect. By so doing, we are in a position to begin to search for the cause. Thus, lovingly and willingly enduring all things is a necessary step on the path to uncovering and transmuting the cause of illness or unhappiness within ourselves. This makes change possible.

Of Action and Attitude

At first, some people are a bit cloudy on the concept of lovingly and willingly enduring all things. As most of us are focused almost entirely upon the outer, or physical, there is a tendency to view this dictum as a recommendation as to course of action. People conclude, therefore, that we must remain in a situation even if we have resistance to it. For example, if someone is swinging a big stick at our heads, this principle would require us to hold still so they would have an easy target, which is quite absurd. For "lovingly and willingly endure all things" is not a recommendation as to action at all. It is a recommendation as to attitude. It is not about what we do; it is about the attitude with which we do it. It is about doing whatever we do with love.

AN EXAMPLE

A simple example will explain this principle. Imagine yourself walking across a beautiful pasture on a lovely summer day to enjoy a fine lunch in a nearby cafe, wearing some new clothes that you are particularly pleased with. Then, to your surprise and consternation, you inadvertently slip and fall face first into a huge pile of cow manure. It is all over your face and hair, all over your new clothes, in your eyes and ears. You've even managed to swallow a bit.

Now if "lovingly and willingly endure all things" were truly a recommendation as to action, since we doubtless have at least a bit of resistance to the cow manure, we might have to lie there for the rest of our life. Yet it is not a recommendation as to action, but as to attitude. It is not about whether we lie in the cow manure or whether we get up. It is about doing whichever we do with love.

We can do nothing to change the fact that we are now in the cow manure. But as to what will happen to us in the future, not only our actions but our attitudes will have much to say about that. One person might get out of the cow manure in a state of great resistance, and without the slightest bit of love for any aspect of the experience, proceed across the pasture. As their resistance not only remains but has doubtless been reinforced, it is reasonable to assume that another pile of cow manure awaits them in the future as the Law of Attraction predicts. On the other hand, someone else might also get up from the cow manure and proceed across the pasture. But even though their actions are identical to those of the first person, they might do so with an entirely different attitude. They undoubtedly have resistance as well. But if they make the effort, they can master their resistance rather than being mastered by it. If this resistance can be transmuted and released, then there is no need for them to attract a similar experience to themselves in the future. They have let go of the resistance on the inner, so the outer experience is no longer needed by them. Of course in order to be able to let go of the resistance on the inner, we must first of all cease resisting the outer.

Forgiveness

FORGIVENESS IS ANOTHER NECESSARY REQUIREMENT FOR HEALTH AND healing. When we hang on to resentments and grudges, or when we refuse to forgive others or ourselves, healing becomes difficult if not impossible. It is that simple. One of the biggest favors we can bestow upon ourselves and the world in general is to make it our business to practice forgiveness. This is simple to express, but is a challenge at times to put into practice. However, the more we do it, the easier it will become for us. A lack of forgiveness can be a huge obstacle to health and healing.

Gratitude

GRATITUDE ALSO PLAYS A CENTRAL ROLE IN HEALTH, HEALING AND MUCH else. An excellent presentation of the concept of gratitude may be found in *The Celestial Song of Creation* by Annalee Skarin. She notes that gratitude may also be considered "great attitude." She further notes that gratitude is "the principle of increase and multiplication." For when we are grateful for that which we do have, this opens the doors of the heavens to even greater blessings. On the other hand, our lack of gratitude for a small blessing shows that a larger blessing would simply be wasted upon us. Thus, our ingratitude shuts the doors of the heavens so we cannot receive more, and even that which we do have tends to be taken away from us sooner or later.

Consider the relationship between gratitude and health. It is not important really how our current state of health compares to that of anyone else. It is not important whether or not it seems fair to us. Quite simply, we have the health that we have right now. Being grateful for the health that we have opens the door and makes it possible for us to receive an improvement. Yet if we are not grateful for the level of health we do have, no matter how meager it may seem to us, then we are guilty of ingratitude. An improvement in our health is unlikely, for we have shut the door to that possibility through our own ingratitude as well as set the stage for a decline in our health, sooner or later.

GRATITUDE IN ADVANCE

True gratitude, like love or forgiveness, is unconditional. To love somebody only if they love us in return is not truly to love. To forgive somebody only if they forgive us or only if they do as we wish is not truly to forgive. In a similar fashion, to be grateful only if our health improves is not being grateful for the health we have right now. In each case, we are being conditional. Gratitude for our health puts no conditions on what happens to our health in the future. It is not a trick or a technique we do simply in order to get a desired result. That would be manipulation, not gratitude.

If we desire healing, then we can simply feel right now the gratitude we would feel if we were already healed. Some might call this "gratitude in advance." But again, it is not meant to be a trick or a means of manipulating things merely to get the healing we desire. The gratitude must be genuine and without condition. The benefit of this gratitude in advance is that it is simultaneously an expression of faith. In other words, by being as grateful now as we would be if we were already healed, we are exercising faith that on one level it is indeed already so.

Faith

A SCRIPTURAL DEFINITION IS THAT FAITH IS THE ASSURANCE OF THINGS hoped for, the evidence of things not seen. This definition reflects two separate elements of faith. If we are to regain health, we will need to understand and apply each of these aspects. That the cause is on the inner and the effect on the outer has been presented elsewhere in detail. Let us look at faith from the perspective of cause and effect.

When most people think of faith, they generally think of the ability to believe in something they cannot see or which does not yet exist. In the first half of our definition, we see this side of faith as "the assurance of things hoped for," that aspect of faith which moves from cause to effect. We have the assurance, which exists on the inner and is therefore cause. And we have the faith that if this cause exists, then the effect or the things hoped for will eventually come into existence on the outer. This might entail having the faith that our health can improve. This aspect of faith, moving from cause to effect, will certainly play an important role in our journey to greater health. After all, it is unlikely we will move far on such a journey if we lack in faith that it is even possible. The assurance of things hoped for is one aspect of faith.

Yet there is another, equally important, aspect of faith, and it will also play a large role in our journey to greater health. For faith is also "the evidence of things not seen." The evidence would be the effects which are clearly obvious on the outer, and the things not seen would be the causes which exist on the inner and cannot be seen. This aspect of faith is moving from effect back to cause. We see within our own body certain effects, and we have the faith that these effects come from certain causes within us, despite the fact that these causes are unseen at present. These causes would be patterns of thought, word, and emotion that we hold in a continual state of creation through our resistances. To begin with, we do not yet know what these causes may be. Yet we have faith that they are there, for we can see the evidence of these causes in the form of their effects. And in our journey to greater health, this second aspect of faith is as important as the first. We not only have faith that we can regain our health, but we acknowledge that the effects we are currently experiencing have their causes within us. And this is faith as well.

For example, suppose we have a problem with our back. It is faith to believe that it can be corrected. This entails belief in an effect (the healed back) that does not yet exist on the outer. Certainly such faith will help this to happen. Yet it is also faith to believe that the back problem itself is the effect of certain patterns of resistance within us. We do not know what these may be. Yet as a matter of faith, we have only to consider the back problem as an effect to realize that it must have a cause. Faith is knowing with certainty that for every cause there is an effect, and for every effect there is a cause.

Problems and Solutions Are Both Within

It is often more comfortable to consider ourselves an innocent victim of circumstance than to take responsibility for our own circumstances. The idea of exercising faith to acknowledge that the causes are within us for whatever outer effects we are experiencing is uncomfortable for some. Yet if we place the source of our problems outside of ourselves, we are placing the solution outside of ourselves as well. If we are unwilling to acknowledge that we are part of the problem, then we are in all likelihood not truly capable of being part of its solution either.

Invisible Boomerangs

We are often met with circumstances where it is a challenge to acknowledge that the effect that we are now experiencing is the result of any cause on our part. From our limited perspective, these effects seem to have struck us for no apparent reason; we have done nothing to bring them about. Yet it is not simply our actions which have consequences: every thought, word or emotion is a seed we plant, and of course, we reap what we sow. This principle applies over a long period of time, far longer than we can readily recollect.

Through our thoughts, words, emotions, actions, attitudes and otherwise, we have thrown out into the universe a vast number of invisible boomerangs. We typically have little recollection of most of them. We cannot see them as they leave our hand, for they are not physical yet. But they circle around out there gathering form, shape and momentum, and sooner or later they all find their mark and return to us. Those which come back to us quickly enough may jar our memory sufficiently such that we can recall having released them in the first place. But many will take much time to return: perhaps years, perhaps even lifetimes. Some, in the process, will also gather considerable momentum. Because of the timelag and our forgetting, it is easy to believe that we are simply a victim of a boomerang, that somebody else threw it, or that it hit the wrong person.

But if we have faith, we realize that every effect has a cause. We also know that we cannot be part of the solution unless we are willing to recognize our role in the problem. This attitude sets us to looking for ways we can effectively work to improve our own situation. Besides developing attitudes of faith, love, forgiveness, and gratitude, we must make some changes in how we eat and how we live if we want to heal.

Nutrition

NUTRITION PLAYS A SIGNIFICANT ROLE IN REGAINING AS WELL AS MAINtaining health, and without proper nutrition, it is unlikely we will succeed. Yet even with the best of nutrition, there is no guarantee of health, for there are a multitude of other factors, physical and otherwise. However, good nutrition is necessary for health and healing. Principles of nutrition will be presented in Part Two.

Elimination

A HEALTHY BODY REQUIRES GOOD ELIMINATION AS WELL AS GOOD NUTRItion. A body that is supplied with all necessary nutrients and whose wastes are eliminated promptly will generally thrive. Thus, we can see the importance of the various channels of elimination: the colon, the skin, the urinary system, the lymphatic system, and the respiratory system. When one of these systems is inadequate or overloaded, the others must bear the weight as well and the entire body is effected. Various practices help encourage proper elimination through these channels of elimination. The intake of adequate quantities of water is essential for both digestion as well as elimination. Without enough water, our nutrition will be impaired no matter how adequate our diet may be. In a similar fashion, all of our channels of elimination will be greatly hindered in their proper function if we do not consume sufficient water on a daily basis. (See Chapters Seven, Thirteen, and Fourteen for more about the importance of elimination.)

Exercise

THE HUMAN BODY IS DESIGNED TO BE USED. EXERCISE IS ESSENTIAL TO maintain or regain health. The muscles of the body will start to atrophy to some extent even within a few days of not being used. In an earlier day, exercise as such was probably not needed, for life itself was sufficiently demanding physically for most people that this need of the body was readily met. Yet in much of the world today, it is possible to live with little or no physical activity, and the consequences for our health are pretty obvious to most of us. It is important to engage in activities that will promote strength, stamina, speed and flexibility. The fitness of our muscles and bones has a direct effect upon the fitness of our organs, glands and other tissues, not to mention our emotional and mental states. However, most of the adult population is steadily decreasing in both bone and muscle mass from one year to the next. While weight may remain the same, body composition can change significantly as bone and muscle decrease and fat deposits increase. "If we don't use it, we lose it."

There are direct reflex relationships between muscles and corresponding organs and glands. Promoting the health of the muscles provides direct benefit to the organs and glands, and healthy muscles require activity that promotes strength, stamina, speed and flexibility. It was once believed that we cannot increase muscle mass after a certain age, but this has now been thoroughly disproved. Studies with geriatric patients in nursing homes have shown that a moderate program of weight training can increase muscle mass at virtually any age. Furthermore, maintaining or increasing bone mass and density is also dependent upon many of the same sorts of activities as will promote muscle mass. And again, studies have shown that bone mass and density can be increased, even in geriatric patients, with a moderate exercise program.

Exercise has a significant effect upon the immune system as well. Moderate exercise can enhance or improve immune function significantly. There is a caution here, however: if a little of something is good, more is not always better. With respect to exercise and the immune system, it has been shown that excessive levels of training, such as that of competitive endurance athletes, will actually lower immune function. The exact point at which exercise becomes excessive is not precisely defined as far as I am aware. But most of us are unlikely to move beyond it.

An appropriate type, amount, and intensity of exercise can be selected, and the intensity and amount can be suitably increased as appropriate. If a person has followed a particularly inactive lifestyle for years, it may take some time to rise to a healthy level of physical fitness. Obviously, certain physical conditions make most types of exercise out of the question. While it is beyond the scope of this book to address the subject exhaustively, there are forms of exercise such as rebounders or mini-trampolines that can provide some degree of exercise to practically anyone. When in doubt people should seek medical or professional advice.

Sleep

SLEEP IS ONE OF THE MOST BASIC AND OBVIOUS OF HUMAN NEEDS, A significant piece of the puzzle when it comes to maintaining or regaining health. It is also one of the most routinely neglected, a piece that is often absent from most approaches. I strongly recommend *The Promise of Sleep* by Dr. William C. Dement. Dr. Dement began his research on sleep in 1952 during his second year in medical school. At this time, sleep research was very much in its infancy. He began his work under the direction of Professor Nathaniel Kleitman, author of one of the first books on sleep and whose team was at that time in the process of discovering and naming REM or rapid eye movement. Dr. Dement has been at the cutting edge of sleep research ever since that time, and some of his findings are most relevant here.

Almost all adults require between seven and one-half and nine hours of sleep per day, with eight and one-quarter hours being average. There are few people who can truly thrive on less sleep than this, and in such cases it appears to be genetic. There is no evidence to indicate that it is possible to adapt the body to get by on less sleep than this. As Dr. Dement puts it, "there will always be people who think they can handle the effects of fatigue or train themselves to get by with less sleep in order to get more work done. But all available evidence indicates that this isn't so. Every individual needs a specific amount of sleep, and this amount cannot be altered."[1]

When people sleep less than this, they accumulate what is known as *sleep debt*. For example, if a person who requires eight hours sleep per day only sleeps seven hours per day, in one week their sleep debt will increase by seven hours. Ample evidence indicates that this sleep debt needs to be paid back hour by hour with extra sleep. In the above example, the seven hours of sleep debt accumulated in a week of sleeping one hour less per day than needed could be paid off by sleeping an extra hour per day (or nine hours each day) for the next week. The body keeps track of sleep debt for at least the previous two weeks. It may well keep track of it for much longer than two weeks; this is simply the longest period yet studied. And importantly, virtually any daytime drowsiness is a sign of sleep debt.

A number of sleep disorders are quite common, and many people are unaware that they have one. However, most medical doctors have little familiarity with sleep disorders. As a result, it is unlikely they would suspect that a sleep disorder underlies many disease conditions, including but not limited to serious situations such as heart attacks and strokes. In Dr. Dement's hometown of Walla Walla, Washington USA, many of the primary care physicians have been trained to recognize sleep disorders. In numerous cases, patients diagnosed with other conditions had been treated for years without success. Yet when their underlying sleep disorders were recognized and corrected, many of their other health problems readily disappeared, being largely attributable to the sleep problems. Many lives have been saved as a result.[2]

When people are not getting enough sleep, they will be impaired physically, emotionally and mentally in numerous ways. These include lowered vitality, diminished healing ability, compromised immune function, poor intellectual function, diminished coordination, mood swings, emotional instability and more. Sleep debt also significantly increases the effect of alcohol upon coordination and reaction time. Many automobile accidents attributed to alcohol can be partially attributed to fatigue. It has been shown that an amount of alcohol that has no measurable effect when there is sufficient sleep can have a tremendous effect when the person gets even a few hours less sleep the preceding night than they needed. Many accidents (including, but not limited to, motor vehicle accidents) are largely attributable to sleep debt and consequent drowsiness or fatigue. (In this category are a large percentage of industrial accidents, including the Exxon *Valdez* oil spill, the Bhopal chemical spill in India, and the nuclear accidents at Three Mile Island and Chernobyl.)

THE MECHANICS OF SLEEP

The drives to sleep and wakefulness are largely governed by two distinct and overlapping processes, known as the *sleep homeostat* and *clock dependent alerting*. The sleep homeostat works basically as follows: after a certain amount of time awake, the sleep homeostat will bring on the urge to sleep, and after a certain amount of time asleep, when the homeostat gets far enough in the opposite direction, the homeostat will bring on the urge to awaken. If we were solely governed by the sleep homeostat, we would most likely move from being asleep to being awake every few hours in a manner similar to cats. We would most likely also require more than the eight and one-quarter hours of sleep most of us require per day. For such sleep is not as efficient as the longer sleep periods more typical to humans.[3]

But along with the sleep homeostat, we are also governed by clock dependent alerting. Each of us has our own unique circadian or daily cycle. For example, some of us are "morning people," or what Dr. Dement refers to as *larks,* while others are "night people" or *owls.* The exact timing of this cycle varies from one person to the next. In general, each of us has a daily cycle of clock dependent alerting which involves a morning as well as an afternoon/evening peak with a lull in between. It should be noted that the peaks of clock dependent alerting are in general strong enough to overcome the effect of sleep debt upon the sleep homeostat, unless the sleep debt is truly enormous. Thus, the person with an average sleep debt is typically able to awaken in the morning despite the sleep debt. But when the morning peak disappears and the afternoon lull follows, anyone with much of a sleep debt will go through a period of drowsiness. (Many incorrectly attribute this period of drowsiness after lunch to the demands of digestion or to blood sugar swings or various other causes. Yet according to Dr. Dement, in the absence of significant sleep debt, it does not occur.) So fatigue or drowsiness is a sign of a large sleep debt. The late afternoon or evening peak is generally stronger than the morning peak. It needs to be, of course, for by this time of the day we have a greater sleep debt than when we woke up in the morning. In most cases, the afternoon or evening peak is sufficiently strong that the afternoon drowsiness will disappear, unless the sleep debt is enormous. This is why most people experience a "second wind" as the late afternoon or evening peak kicks in, and why many people who are quite tired at a predictable time each afternoon find themselves fairly alert a few hours later.

Again, it must be emphasized that each of us has a unique cycle. Some will have their morning peak quite early, and as a result, will be very early risers. Their afternoon lull may be midday, with their next peak coming in late afternoon. As this wears off, they will tend to go to bed early. Others will have their peaks and lulls several hours later, and as a result will typically be later to rise in the morning, later to bed at night, and their lull may be much later in the afternoon or even the early evening. These unique individual cycles often change over the course of our adult life. One of the most effective ways to do so is simply by exposure to bright light. Over time the cycle can be shifted to an earlier one simply by early morning exposure to bright light each day—watching the sunrise, for example. Or to switch the cycle to a later one, bright light later in the day, such as watching the sunset or bright lights in the evening, will tend to help.

It appears that prior to the advent of the electric light, substantial and detrimental sleep debt was uncommon, as most people slept sufficiently. Prior to the electric light, most people were asleep when it was dark and awake during the day. But with the electric light, many people began to stay awake far into the night and to lose touch with the natural cycle of day and night. The types of lights available prior to the electric light were not sufficiently bright to impact upon the daily cycle of the body. With the advent of the electric light came the possibility of working twenty-four hours a day. Dr. Dement goes into great detail on the many detrimental effects of shift work on our sleep and health. Many accidents occur a few hours after midnight at a time when clock dependent alerting is at a minimum and people are therefore most prone to drowsiness if they have much of a sleep debt.

Prior to modern times, travel was sufficiently slow that it was easy enough for the body to adapt to the gradual changes in longitude as we headed east or west. Only in the modern age has jet lag become possible. Dr. Dement goes into considerable detail on this as well, and explains it in very clear terms with respect to the sleep homeostat and clock dependent alerting. He also offers some very practical suggestions as to how to minimize the problems associated with jet lag.

We must learn to consider sleep an essential need for the body, much like water, air, and food. We neglect sleep at our own peril, and if we choose to operate a motor vehicle when drowsy, we do so at the peril of others as well. There is much more that could be said about sleep, but the most important is that no matter how many positive things we do to bring about better nutrition, water intake, exercise, and of course consciousness change, we are still missing a huge piece of the puzzle if we neglect our need for sleep. As Dr. Dement himself puts it, "The fundamental principle that should guide everyone is this: We are not healthy unless our sleep is healthy."[4]

Light and Darkness

BOTH LIGHT AND DARKNESS ARE ALSO IMPORTANT TO HEALTH AND HEALing. Much of our endocrine activity is greatly influenced by exposure to light and to darkness. For optimum health our bodies are designed for exposure to sunlight through our eyes and on our skin. Our pineal gland, which governs or influences our endocrine system, responds directly to light and to darkness. In order for us to be fully awake, exposure to natural light appears necessary, and without this, our body does not come fully awake but is still half asleep. The effect of a lack of sunlight on our emotional states is also well documented. The term *Seasonally Affected Depression Syndrome* has been coined in recognition of this fact. In more extreme latitudes, during the winter months when sunlight is scarce, depression is far more common. Along with depression come elevated rates of suicide, homicide, alcoholism and a myriad of other problems. With respect to depression in particular, it is worth noting the relationship between the pineal gland and enthusiasm. Perhaps when the pineal is deprived of sunlight, our enthusiasm shuts down to some extent. Language often reflects such things, for a cheerful person is said to have a sunny disposition, and a gloomy person is said to have a cloud over their head.

Those interested in further research on light and its effects upon health should refer to *Light, Radiation, & You* by John Ott. To some extent the benefits of sunlight can be approximated by full spectrum lights. These are special types of light bulbs which have a power distribution across the spectrum of visible and invisible light that is more similar to sunlight than that of conventional light bulbs.

Exposure to sunlight itself is preferable; and for optimum benefit, we need to be outside on a clear day. Receiving sunlight through the eyes, necessary for the pineal gland and the whole endocrine system, is interfered with to varying degree by clouds, sunglasses, eyeglasses, contact lens, and being inside behind windows. For optimum benefit, we need to be outside on a clear day. Exposing the skin to sunlight to an appropriate extent is also necessary to our health. The interaction of sunlight with the oils in our skin produces vitamin D_3, and this vitamin plays a significant role in calcium metabolism. Overexposure to the sun to the point of sunburn is clearly foolish, yet it is equally foolish to avoid the sun entirely, as is often recommended nowadays. The ability of our skin and body to tolerate and benefit from sunlight appears to be related to the presence of certain fatty acids in our diet. (This is addressed in Chapter Ten.)

In addition to sunlight, we also need darkness, for while we may manage to sleep without a dark environment, it appears that we do not fully rest. Without the signal of darkness, the body is not able to fully shut down and recharge its batteries.[5] It is therefore imperative that we sleep in a fairly dark room if we are to become properly rested. While the body does appear capable of adjusting to working the night shift and sleeping during the day, this is not optimal for most of us. Yet if we must follow such a schedule, we must provide ourselves with a sufficiently dark sleep environment. And it is also important that we manage at least a certain amount of exposure to natural light.

Air and Breathing

CLEAN AIR AND PROPER BREATHING ALSO PLAY A SIGNIFICANT ROLE IN promoting health. Some would suggest that regular exposure of the skin to fresh air is also essential to the health of the skin, and hence our health in general. (See Chapter Fourteen for more on the importance of fresh air.)

Water

L IKE SLEEP, BOTH WATER QUANTITY AND WATER QUALITY ARE ESSENTIAL
to health, and like sleep, their crucial roles are frequently neglected. As
the body itself is primarily composed of water, its importance would seem
obvious, yet often the simple things, when ignored or neglected, prove our
undoing when it comes to health.

WATER QUANTITY

The importance of consuming sufficient quantities of water daily is explained
most thoroughly in *Your Body's Many Cries For Water* by F. Batmanghelidj.
Born in Iran, Batmanghelidj received his medical training in London, and he
eventually returned to his native country. After the 1979 revolution, he was
stripped of all his assets and sentenced to death. While in prison, the guards
realized his value to them as a doctor, and he was spared. One of his patients,
who had peptic ulcers, came to him in severe pain one night. Having no medication available, all he could do was suggest the patient drink two glasses
of tap water. The severe pain totally disappeared within eight minutes. And
so began Dr. Batmanghelidj's research on the role of dehydration in a vast
array of health problems and the use of water in their treatment. Eventually
freed from prison, Dr. Batmanghelidj currently resides in the United States.
Despite the success of his theories and extensive clinical evidence of his claims,
for the most part the medical establishment has ignored him. For this reason, he decided to present his findings and theories to the general public, in
the hopes that maybe the message will get out in that manner. While I would
strongly encourage everyone to read *Your Body's Many Cries For Water,*
what follows are a number of conclusions one could draw from reading this
excellent book. The importance of water is aptly summarized by Dr. Batmanghelidj as follows: "Water, the solvent of the body, regulates all functions, including the activity of the solutes it dissolves and circulates."[6]

GETTING OUR DAILY MINIMUM

The majority of people are chronically dehydrated. This state of dehydration tends to increase as we age, that is, our body's percentage of water tends

to diminish with age. Dehydration is among the most significant and severe stresses on the body and its cells. Furthermore, the thirst sensation is an unreliable indicator of dehydration. Dehydration can be quite pronounced despite an absence of thirst. In fact, the thirst mechanism becomes less and less reliable as dehydration increases, and the thirst mechanism also tends to become less reliable with age. One fairly simple and accurate manner to assess the body's relative level of hydration is to note the color of the urine. The urine should be extremely pale yellow in color, almost clear. The urine being typically much darker than this generally indicates dehydration. Salt also plays a key role in the thorough hydration of the body. Most people require a minimum of three grams or a half teaspoon of salt per day. Deficiency in salt contributes to a shortage of water outside the cells.[7]

When we do not provide the body with sufficient amounts of water, the body is forced to enter into what Batmanghelidj terms *drought management* mode. Not all parts of the body will be equally deprived of water: the body has a natural set of priorities as to which tissues and functions are most vital for its survival. Therefore, in chronic states of dehydration, not all parts of the body will be treated equally. For example, roughly sixty-six percent of the shortfall is taken from within the cells themselves, with another twenty-six percent taken from around the cells. The remaining eight percent will come from the blood. For this reason, blood tests are a poor means of assessing dehydration, for the blood will remain within reasonable norms even when other parts of the body are severely dehydrated.[8]

Batmanghelidj suggests as a bare minimum that our daily need for water is at least half an ounce for every pound of body weight. Thus, a person weighing 160 pounds would require a minimum of eighty ounces or two and one-half quarts of water per day. (This translates to roughly thirty-three milliliters per kilogram of body mass. Thus, a person who weighs seventy-five kilos would require a minimum of two and one-half liters of water per day.) It should be noted that this amount is a minimum. Depending upon many factors such as the amount of exercise, time of the year, amount of perspiration, type of diet, and more, the amount of water needed can be substantially more than this. Again, the color of the urine is a fairly good indicator in the long run as to whether or not we are getting enough water.[9]

A longstanding state of dehydration cannot be overcome in a matter of days. Drinking massive amounts of water over a short time will not be effective in reversing dehydration, and it may in fact be dangerous. The best approach is to recognize that being consistent over time will reverse the state of dehydration. In practice, it may take a considerable period of time to bring about a thorough level of hydration in the body: we must be patient and consistent. Also, the daily water intake will have greater benefit when it is spread out throughout the day rather than consumed in a few large batches. The body can only utilize so much water at a given time; the rest is not retained. It is especially important to drink water prior to eating, optimally about thirty minutes prior. As will discussed below, digestion is very much dependent upon full hydration. But in general, it's best to spread the water intake out over the day.

I have found a useful way of explaining why it is best to spread the water out, and why rehydration takes time. Imagine that we have forgotten to water a houseplant such that the soil in the pot is extremely dry and hard. If a large amount of water is poured into the pot all at once, most will simply run straight out the bottom, for the soil can only receive so much water at a time. On the other hand, if one is patient, the same amount of water can be received by the soil. It is simply a matter of giving it in much smaller amounts, spread out over time. And so it is with our own bodies.

If we currently consume far less water than our minimum, how long it will take to reach the necessary amount can vary widely depending upon a multitude of factors. For some it will be a week or two, for others, a few months, and some much longer. And under certain conditions a drastic increase in water intake would not simply be ineffective; it might be extremely dangerous. If the kidneys are not capable of producing more urine to keep up with the extra water, water retention can occur. While for some this might result in a bit of edema around the ankles, for others it might present a dangerous situation in which fluid accumulates around the lungs or heart. There are circumstances in which it would be strongly advisable to increase water intake gradually under proper supervision. While the latter will not be the case for most, it is nonetheless vital that it is understood by all.

As water intake is increased, many people find that their thirst mechanism seems to reactivate and recalibrate. Some who drank little water before and rarely experienced thirst may be in for a surprise. For initially many people find that as they drink more water, they actually get more thirsty. The thirst mechanism is becoming active again, and as it does so, it often becomes more sensitive.

It is crucial to understand also that there is a significant difference between water and other fluids. The body needs water in order to be properly hydrated. Most other fluids will not satisfy the need for water, and in fact, many fluids will actually cause further dehydration even though they appear to satisfy our thirst. Alcohol and any beverage containing caffeine are prime examples of this. Not only does the water within them not serve to hydrate us, but the body actually has to use some of its precious water reserves (along with the water in the beverage) just to get rid of the beverage. So alcohol, coffee, black tea and all beverages containing caffeine (such as many sodas) simply increase our state of dehydration. Or put another way, not only does that cup of coffee not count towards our daily water target, it might be said to count negatively. For we will have to drink another glass of water just to break even on the coffee![10]

CONSEQUENCES OF DEHYDRATION

Proper hydration plays a substantial role in the function of our digestive system, and many problems such as stomach ulcers, heartburn, and other related complaints can result directly from dehydration. However, these can often be reversed quite readily by rehydration. The stomach lining is meant to be protected from the highly acidic contents of the lower stomach by a mucus coating. Without sufficient water, this mucus coating cannot be formed, and in its absence the acid may eat a hole through the stomach lining. This condition is known as a stomach ulcer. If the acidic stomach contents are to pass on into the small intestine without harm, the pancreas must secrete a watery bicarbonate solution into the duodenum or upper portion of the small intestine to raise the pH. Again, in a state of dehydration this is difficult for the body to do, and the body is faced with a difficult choice: it can allow the stomach contents into the duodenum and thereby risk a duodenal ulcer. Or it can reverse peristalsis and send the food back towards the esophagus. Heartburn, reflux, nausea, hiatus hernia and eventually more severe problems such as esophageal cancer may result.[11] Batmanghelidj has demonstrated a clear relationship between dehydration and a staggering number of other complaints, and is able to offer not merely plausible explanations as to why but much clinical evidence and all sorts of testimonial evidence.

Constipation is one such condition. The intestines secrete a substance known as *motilin,* which stimulates peristalsis: the waves of muscular activity that move food through our digestive tract. Motilin is secreted in direct proportion to the amount of water we drink, and hence, a lack of water will slow down peristalsis, leading to constipation. This is quite sensible, in that the less water we drink, the more our body will be required to reabsorb from the large intestine. The diminished peristalsis allows greater reabsorption of water, making bowel movements difficult.

Batmanghelidj suggests that dehydration plays a part in many serious illnesses. For example, he claims that Alzheimer's Disease is primarily a condition of dehydration of the brain cells, and so is insulin-dependent diabetes. He attributes much of the chronic pain in the body to dehydration, and furthermore claims that many essential functions in the body are hindered or diminished by dehydration. These include energy production, neurotransmitter transport, enzyme activity, and use of oxygen by the cells. He relates most heart and lung disease to dehydration, including anginal pain. Migraine headaches, depression, chronic fatigue, fear, anxiety, and insecurity can all also be caused or aggravated by dehydration, and many of these conditions will diminish considerably or disappear entirely with nothing more complicated than rehydration. In addition, multiple sclerosis and other diseases of the nerves can be linked directly to dehydration.

High blood pressure is often caused by dehydration, and then further aggravated by the use of diuretics and the restriction of salt intake. Batmanghelidj not only offers a convincing explanation as to why it is best treated with gradual rehydration and salt; he offers much clinical evidence and many testimonials to that effect. The deposit of cholesterol in the blood vessels he also attributes largely to dehydration, since when introduced into the cell membrane cholesterol retards the passage of water out of the cells, it is a natural response by the cells to prevent further dehydration.

Batmanghelidj also relates rheumatoid joints to dehydration, for it is the water within the cartilage of a joint that provides much of the lubrication that is needed to protect the joint's contact surfaces. Many lower back problems are also linked to dehydration. When we are fully hydrated, the water within the discs will support seventy-five percent of the weight of the upper body. The surrounding connective tissue will account for the remaining twenty-five percent. In the absence of full hydration, the disc is simply not able to perform this function and will shrivel or shrink as it dehydrates. Many cases of low back pain and sciatica are completely resolved with rehydration.

One final example of a common complaint often caused by dehydration is asthma. The lung tissue responds to dehydration by constricting in such a manner as to reduce its surface area. This has the effect of slowing down the rate of water loss. Batmanghelidj likens this to the manner in which leaves will shrivel during a drought as the plant also strives to reduce the amount of water lost through respiration. Many cases of asthma have been totally resolved by rehydration, amply demonstrating Batmanghelidj's theory.

By now it should be clear that something as simple as increasing water intake can provide enormous benefit to our health. It can also prevent many problems from occurring. However, if we remain dehydrated, it will be difficult at best to regain or maintain our health.

Water Quality

Besides drinking enough water, we must drink water of high quality. The water that we use for cooking, bathing, and growing our food should ideally be of high quality as well. Healthy water will contribute to the health and healing of the body in numerous ways. Such water will have a number of characteristics which will be discussed below. These characteristics will include certain physical characteristics, including but not limited to chemical purity, but will also include what may be termed energetic qualities. In contrast, water lacking or deficient in these physical or energetic characteristics for any reason may damage our health and retard or prevent the healing of the body.

A staggering array of basic metabolic processes are dependent upon water, and the quality of the water present determines to a great extent how well or how poorly these processes are performed. For example, the efficiency with which we are able to digest and assimilate nutrients is greatly influenced by water quality and so is our ability to transport these nutrients. The effectiveness of our systems of detoxification and elimination will also depend upon water quality, and our circulatory and lymphatic systems are clearly dependent upon water quality for their proper function. In fact, given that our body is more than seventy percent water, it would be fair to state that all functions and structures within our bodies cannot help but be dependent upon water quality. Our brains, for example, are about ninety percent water.

THE NATURE OF WATER

Most of us have been taught to view water as a very simple substance. We are taught that it is just H_2O, a molecule composed of two hydrogen atoms combined with a single oxygen atom. From this perspective, the highest quality water would be that of greatest chemical purity. Hence, our efforts would be directed towards finding or producing water that was primarily H_2O with as few impurities as possible. Towards this end a great many different sort of filters, distillers, and other devices have indeed been devised.

Yet water is a unique and unusual substance when we consider it more closely. According to noted scientist, inventor and researcher Dr. Patrick Flanagan, "Water is the only substance on earth that is simultaneously available in three distinct states: solid, liquid, and gaseous."[12] Most substances increase in density as temperature drops and they move from gaseous to liquid to solid. That is, they contract as they are cooled and expand as they are heated. Water, however, does not entirely follow this rule. Its maximum density occurs at about 4 degrees C. (At sea level, water ordinarily boils at 100 degrees and freezes at 0 degrees C.) As it freezes, it expands rather than contracts, which is readily apparent if we consider that ice floats rather than sinks. (Were this not the case, ice would form at the bottom first rather than on the surface, and as a result many organisms that spend the winter at the unfrozen bottom of lakes and ponds would not be able to survive.)

While the basic formula for water is H_2O when it is in the form of vapor, once it enters into a liquid form it is no longer so simple. Flanagan estimates that if a liquid molecule of water were indeed mere H_2O, then based upon its molecular weight it should boil at approximately minus 80 degrees C and freeze at minus 100 degrees C.[13] Dr. Horst Felsch, an Austrian civil engineer, gives slightly different estimates, namely a boiling point of minus 100 degrees C and a freezing point of minus 120 degrees C.[14] In either case, however, if water were merely H_2O then it ought to be gaseous rather than liquid in the temperature range at which it is clearly found in a liquid form. Dr. Felsch explains this mystery by noting that at room temperature, normally about 300 to 400 water molecules are linked together by hydrogen bonds. A water molecule at room temperature is therefore not simply H_2O, but 300 to 400 H_2O joined together to form a "grand-molecule." As a result of this greatly increased molecular weight, water has the boiling and freezing points with which we are familiar.[15] He notes further that:

> Water in its liquid state is a super-molecule. And it has a net-like structure and the reason for that is the dipolarity of water and the resulting hydrogen bond. If water were only H_2O, that is, monomolecular, then it would have a gaseous state at room temperature.... It is only because of this hydrogen bond that it is liquid, because it is a giant molecule, and for this reason alone, life has been able to develop on earth. All living structures contain water in some form, but the water has to be liquid. If it were a gas, there would be no life.
>
> So you see how important this special form of water structure is.... These aggregates consist of 300 to 400 water molecules. And the fact that they do exist can be proven with x-ray and neutron diffraction and also with infrared and raman spectroscopy. Ludwig and Kokoschinegg reported on this in the 1980s.[16]

Physical Characteristics of Healthy Water

Water is not such a simple thing after all. There are a number of significant physical properties that may be investigated and related to the quality of that water. While chemical purity is indeed one such property, there are numerous others as well. Professor Vincent was at one time the chief hydrologist in France, responsible for making sure that the best possible water was made available to the various villages, towns, and cities throughout the country. In this capacity, he had the opportunity to compare health statistics from different localities with the quality and characteristics of the local water supply. He found that the effect of water upon health was quite pronounced and highly specific. Health and longevity varied considerably from one locality to the next based upon overall water quality. Mortality was considerably higher in localities with poor water quality than in those with water of high quality. Furthermore, by analyzing a number of different properties of water, he found that different types of water were clearly linked to different types of illnesses. Some types of water would result in a much higher cancer rate, while other types of water would contribute to cardiovascular disease, for example.[17] Based upon his own extensive research, Professor Vincent determined that healthy water must possess at least three qualities to be biologically compatible. This is known as the *Bio-Electronic "Vincent"* method or BEV. The first of these characteristics is a pH range of 5.2 to 6.8. Ideally, water should be slightly acidic. Neutral pH being 7.0, this means that somewhat below 7.0 pH is optimum. The second characteristic is known as rH_2, a measure of oxidation and/or reduction. Oxidation is taking electrons away from a substance, while reduction is giving electrons to that substance. On this scale, a reading of zero would indicate a maximum of electrons or a state of being highly reduced. A reading of 42 would indicate a minimum of electrons or a state of being highly oxidized. A reading of 28 is considered more or less neutral. Ideal water should not be too reduced, but should possess a value between 25 and 29. The third characteristic is R or resistivity, referring to amount of dissolved solids. A high value of resistivity indicates a low level of total dissolved solids. Ideal water has a fairly high resistivity.[18]

Naturally occurring water that possesses these three characteristics is increasingly rare. Water purification units which involve reverse osmosis as well as several other stages are available which will produce water that will satisfy Vincent's three criteria. Ordinary tap water can thus be filtered to where it will possess a suitable pH, be slightly reduced, and have a high resistivity. However, as will be discussed shortly, water filtration itself can greatly damage the quality of water in other ways. This damage can be both physical as well as energetic. So water filtration, at least by itself, is not the solution to the problem of providing healthy water. But before we move on to these other considerations, there are several other physical properties of water that must also be considered with respect to its overall quality. These include molecular cluster size, dissolved oxygen content, and surface tension.

Water responds to various pollutants by encapsulating them. This results in molecular clusters that are larger than would be ideal from a health perspective. When these clusters are too large, water has a lessened ability to help transport nutrients, including oxygen, to our cells, as well as to help eliminate wastes from our cells. All basic metabolic processes which involve water will proceed less effectively for this same reason.

Another physical factor that relates to the quality of water is the dissolved oxygen content. Healthy water will have a relatively high content of dissolved oxygen, which helps contribute to a well-oxygenated body. (As discussed in Chapter Ten, a healthy body is well-oxygenated.) A poorly oxygenated body provides an ideal environment for the proliferation of pathogenic bacteria as well as cancer.

Another index of water quality is its *surface tension,* the force that causes water to adhere to itself. Surface tension can be measured, for it is "the amount of force that is required to break or tear the surface of water apart."[19] As water performs its various functions in the body, it comes into contact with various substances. "All substances have what is known as a wetting index. This index is representative of the surface tension required to wet that substance."[20] Water can only wet a given substance if its own surface tension is sufficiently low. If its surface tension is too high, it is not able to wet that substance, and hence not able to perform its function properly. One simple example is the process of digestion. Food must be wet by our digestive juices in order for proper digestion to take place, and our digestive juices must have quite a low surface tension in order for digestion to proceed properly. The ability of our body to produce digestive juices of suitably low surface tension is greatly influenced by the surface tension of the water we consume. Hence, water with too high of a surface tension will inhibit proper digestion as well as numerous other metabolic processes.

Surface tension can be measured in units known as *dynes per centimeter* or dynes/cm. According to Dr. Patrick Flanagan, most tap water has a surface tension in the vicinity of 73 dynes/cm. Based upon years of extensive research, Dr. Flanagan has concluded that healthy water should have a surface tension somewhere between 55 to 65 dynes/cm.[21] Thus, most drinking water has too high of a surface tension to be considered truly healthy.

Energetic Characteristics of Water

Significant physical properties related to the quality of water include its chemical purity, pH, rH_2, resistivity, molecular cluster size, dissolved oxygen content, and surface tension. There are undoubtedly other physical factors of significance as well. Yet the works of Viktor Schauberger and Johann Grander tell us that the energetic qualities of water may be of even greater importance to our health than these physical factors. We may purify water so that impurities are removed from the water, yet typically the "memory" or "vibration" of these pollutants remains. This memory that is stored in the water does indeed have a detrimental effect upon our health. *Living Water* by Olof Alexandersson is an excellent introduction to the work of Viktor Schauberger, and *On the Track of Water's Secret* by Hans Kronberger and Siegbert Lattacher presents Schauberger as well but with a primary focus on the work of Johann Grander.

According to Schauberger, there is a natural cycle of water in nature which must be allowed to runs its course if we are to have healthy water. Let us follow this cycle beginning at the point of evaporation. From there, the water vapor will end up in clouds, and from the clouds, it will eventually return to earth in the form of precipitation. As it passes through the atmosphere, rain has the job of removing pollutants from the air. Thus, while most people think of rain water as pure, it is far from that, even under the best of circumstances, for it has cleaned the air on its way down. In fact, it has recently been reported in Europe that rain water has much higher levels of many pollutants than are allowable in drinking water. Often, this rain water flows in streams and into lakes or the ocean as surface water before eventually evaporating again. Yet according to Schauberger, this is not the full cycle as nature intended it but only half a cycle. In this half cycle, water never has the opportunity to become reinvigorated to its highest quality, which can only happen in the full cycle.

In the full cycle, ideally water does not flow over the surface after falling, rather, it penetrates into the ground and passes deep below the surface. Deep within the earth, water is purified in a physical sense, as various contaminants are removed. Just as importantly, it is purified in an energetic sense. The negative or harmful information it has picked up is stripped from it, and certain beneficial frequencies or vibrations are imparted to it as well. It then emerges at the surface again as spring water, and is at the peak of its cycle at that point. When we collect surface water, which has not penetrated into the ground, we are using water that is deficient in many regards. According to Schauberger, water that is pumped up from below is immature, not finished yet, not ready for our use.

That water can pick up negative as well as positive information, retain this information as a sort of memory, and then pass this information on to us when we consume this water is at first difficult to accept from the standpoint of orthodox science. Dr. Horst Felsch suggests an interesting scientific explanation of just how this may take place using the example of common table salt dissolved in water. The formula for table salt is NaCl or sodium chloride. Thus, a molecule of table salt is composed of an atom of sodium joined to an atom of chlorine. When dissolved in water, the ion bond joining the sodium and the chlorine is separated. As the sodium and chlorine separate in this manner, the chlorine pulls an electron away from the sodium. The result is a chloride anion, with a negative charge due to the extra electron, and a sodium cation, with a positive charge due to the missing electron.[22] As most are aware, ordinarily opposite charges will attract each other and similar charges will repel one another. However, the negatively charged chloride anion and the positively charged sodium cation are prevented from joining together by an insulating layer of water forming around them, a process known as *hydration.*[23]

A single molecule of H_2O has a neutral charge itself. However, since the bond between the oxygen and the two hydrogen atoms is closer to the oxygen than to the two hydrogen atoms, the oxygen end will have a somewhat negative charge whereas the hydrogen end will have a somewhat positive charge. Water is termed a *dipole* for this reason, which means it has a negative and a positive pole. (The oxygen would be the negative pole, and the two hydrogen atoms would be the positive pole.) For this reason, individual water molecules do not orient to one another in a haphazard fashion; rather the positive pole of one will be attracted to the negative pole of the next. The formation of these *hydrogen bonds* results in molecular clusters of 300 to 400 individual water molecules.[24]

Now, in the example above, when table salt is dissolved in water, we end up with sodium cations and chloride anions which are prevented from joining one another by an insulating layer of water known as a *hydration envelope*. Naturally, the positively charged sodium ions will attract the negative pole, or oxygen end, of the water molecule. And the negatively charged chloride ions will attract the positive pole, or hydrogen end, of the water molecule. The exact nature of this hydration envelope will vary from one ionic substance to the next. The sodium ion will be surrounded by precisely eight water molecules, with the oxygen end of the water molecules facing the sodium ion. The chloride ion will be surrounded by three water molecules, with the hydrogen end of the water molecules facing the chloride ion. The number of water molecules that will surround a particular ion is known as its *hydration number*.[25]

Once this first layer of dipolar water molecules surrounds a given ion, this determines in turn the structure of the next layer. For example, around the sodium ion will be found eight water molecules with the oxygen next to the sodium and the hydrogen away from it. Since like charges repel and unlike charges attract, the next layer of water molecules will inevitably follow the same pattern. As Felsch notes, "An ion ... determines through its charge and the size of its surface the way the water molecules have to arrange themselves. When the first hydration envelope is already occupied, then all the other water molecules have to keep to the same order or arrangement. This order is carried on further for many, many steps."[26]

Thus, each ionic substance dissolved in water will have its own unique hydration envelope, which will determine the structure of the water in its vicinity. We may think of this hydration envelope as the signature of that substance. We might also think of this as *information*. Dr. Felsch proposes that it is this information that affects us rather than the substance itself:

Around each ion dissolved in the water, there is a water envelope that is very specific for this ion, and it consists of water dipole molecules. Because of the hydrogen bonds, the shape these water molecules take around the ion has a lattice-like structure. The living organism, for example a human being, is trained to be able to recognize such water structures. And he knows, therefore, that when the water structure has a particular make-up, it means that a sodium ion or a chloride ion is dissolved in it. Because each of these ions have a specific hydration structure. And if we spin this thread further, then it is enough for the body alone to be able to recognize the water structure and it does not have to penetrate the center to make certain that there is really a sodium ion or a chloride ion present.[27]

If our bodies respond to the information rather than the substance itself, then we can see that water is indeed capable of picking up and passing on information. Water can also retain this information as a memory for long periods of time. And interestingly enough, water's capacity to do all of these things seems to be optimized at a temperature only slightly above human body temperature. As noted by Felsch:

According to tests made by Engler and Kokoschinegg in 1988, water has a structural memory and a structural variability, and because of this it can store acquired information over a long period of time and hand it over to the body. One aspect of this is very astonishing indeed: at 37.5 degrees Celsius, that is the human body's operating temperature, water has the minimum specific warmth and the maximum structural possibilities through a practically infinite number of structural combinations.[28]

What this means in practical terms is that water is a highly efficient carrier of information, which it picks up wherever it goes, and in turn passes on to us when we consume it. This may comprise positive information which will benefit us as well as negative information which will be harmful to us. If we recall the full cycle of water proposed by Schauberger, in an ideal world rain water would penetrate deep into the earth where it would be purified both physically as well as energetically. Any harmful information that it had acquired would be removed from it in the process. Additionally, it would be imprinted with beneficial information. This water, pure both physically and energetically, would then rise to the surface and emerge in a pristine spring. In the modern world, however, water is recycled over and again, becoming more and more polluted with harmful information or memory.

Water retains the memory of whatever impurities it has picked up, unless this memory is erased as Schauberger suggests it would be were water allowed to complete its full cycle. If we simply remove these impurities, their memory or energy pattern remains in the water. Thus, water filtration does not remove this information or memory. Some research suggests an even more surprising situation: removing impurities through filtration may actually increase their detrimental effect upon us. It appears that filtration actually amplifies the energy pattern of the impurity, even though the impurity itself is no longer physically present. For as a solution becomes more and more dilute, not only is the hydration envelope preserved, it is actually made more and more uniform.[29] And as the hydration envelope becomes more clear, the information is not erased but is actually strengthened. (This might be compared to a homeopathic remedy, where the remedy becomes more and more potent at higher dilutions.) Thus, while water filtration can do much to remove physical contaminants from water, it not only does not remove the harmful information but reinforces it. As a result, many researchers are suggesting that water filtration alone may actually do more harm than good if we consider that it is the information, not the substance, that may have the greatest impact upon our bodies.

Unhealthy Water Defined

A wide range of toxic substances are routinely found in most drinking water. Many of these substances are absorbed by the body in large amounts by bathing or showering. While it is beyond the scope of this book to itemize all of the possible contaminants found in our water, a few of the more prominent can be listed.

Chlorine is found in virtually all municipal water. Chemical reactions between chlorine and various organic compounds produce a group of potent carcinogens known as trihalomethanes. For optimum health chlorine must be removed from drinking and bathing water. A staggering number of pesticides, fertilizers, herbicides, and other chemicals have also been found in water samples from around the world. Many are known or suspected carcinogens. The majority have never been adequately tested to determine their possible impact on our health. We can only speculate as to the possible health risks involved from the ingestion of these untested chemicals, either alone or in combination with one another. Many believe that these unknown health risks may be at least as formidable as those already known. Contamination with human or animal waste matter is another concern. The presence of parasites, viruses, and bacteria in the water is a potential health risk. Inorganic minerals, commonly found in well water, are a health risk, as these nonchelated minerals have a tendency to settle in the tissues of greatest weakness. Also commonly found in our water are high levels of toxic heavy metals. These include lead from many of the lead pipes still in use, as well as cadmium, which leaches out of most types of pipes with the exception of brass. And finally, much of the water in certain countries is deliberately contaminated with sodium fluoride, an extremely toxic waste product of the aluminum and fertilizer industries and also commonly used as rat poison. There is much controversy as to whether or not sodium fluoride has any beneficial effects on the teeth. (See Chapter Fourteen for a fuller discussion of sodium fluoride.)

With respect to all of the above physical contaminants, many are harmful in themselves. Others are harmful because of the information they impart to the water. Whether through their actual presence in the water, through this information, or both, these contaminants result in unhealthy water.

There are a number of other influences that cause damage to water, primarily through the information they impart to water. These include electromagnetic pollution (see Chapter Fourteen), microwave ovens (see Chapter Eleven), radiation, ozone and ultraviolet sterilization, distillation, reverse osmosis filtration, as well as frictional damage from water being forced through pipes. Many people make considerable effort to procure what they consider to be healthy water for drinking and cooking yet continue to bathe and shower in ordinary tap water. Some assume that since they are not drinking the water in the bath or shower, its effect upon them is minimal. Sadly, this is not the case:

A spokesperson for the EPA's Office of Drinking Water said in 1986: "We have become more concerned with the inhalation exposure from volatile chemicals in the water, particularly for the shower. We've done some rough calculations which suggest that the risk of exposure from taking a shower is roughly equivalent to (the exposure from) drinking two litres of water a day."[30]

Naturally occurring healthy water is increasingly rare. Most water contains numerous physical contaminants, as well as a tremendous amount of detrimental information. And all known forms of water purification or filtration not only do not remove this negative information, they actually strengthen it. Putting all that together, we could conclude that the situation is bleak. In principle, the solution to this predicament must go beyond traditional means of water treatment to include the removal of the negative information from our water and its reinvigoration with beneficial information. Enter Johann Grander.

Grander Water

Johann Grander, an Austrian naturalist, has succeeded in producing devices that remove the negative memory or information from water and also impart certain beneficial energy patterns to the water at the same time. In so doing, ordinary tap water is transformed into water of very high quality. This is extensively documented in *On the Track of Water's Secret*. Indeed, there are over 100,000 users of Grander technology worldwide as of this writing.[31] The Grander Water Units have been subjected to much scientific scrutiny, and while scientists are often at a loss to explain how or why these devices work, they are nonetheless forced to acknowledge that they produce measurable and consistent alterations in many properties of the water that passes through them.

The Russian Academy of Natural Sciences conducted their own extensive research of the Grander units for over three years. A particular concern of theirs was finding a technology that could help to deal with radioactivity. They were sufficiently impressed that in September 2000 they conferred upon Johann Grander their Silver Honorary Award for developing the Grander technology. They concluded based upon their exhaustive research that it was "scientifically proved that Grander water lowers radioactivity." They noted also that "through Grander's method it becomes possible to strengthen the energy and information characteristics of the water, thereby making it more valuable. His discovery is for science of worldwide significance."[32]

The Grander Water Units are not filters, and they do not physically remove impurities from the water. Instead, they remove the negative information found in the water or erase the memory of any contaminants that water has contacted previously. As a result, the water molecules will form smaller clusters of a more ideal healthy size. The Grander units not only remove the negative information found in the water, they imprint the water with beneficial frequencies which help it to maintain a beneficial structure including molecular cluster size. There are many benefits of such treatment. Granderized water will have a greater amount of dissolved oxygen, thus helping us to establish and maintain a properly oxygenated body as well as providing many other health benefits. Our own bodily fluids will also transport other nutrients more readily to our cells as well as remove waste materials more easily.

The Grander Water Units significantly reduce the surface tension of water, which makes water far healthier and more biologically available. Basically, with a lower surface tension, the water is "wetter" and thus a more effective solvent. While the physical contaminants are not actually removed by the Grander units, the water itself is altered so that these impurities are suspended and not absorbed by the body. This was demonstrated in an interesting manner: First, a bath was filled with ordinary tap water, and the levels of various impurities in the water were noted. Then, a person bathed in this water. After the bath, the levels of these impurities were measured once again, and they were found to have decreased. This indicates that the body had absorbed a substantial quantity of toxins from bathing in the tap water. Another way to express this would be say that the human body had filtered or cleaned the bath water. No wonder we so often feel tired after a long bath, for it is tough work cleaning the water! The same experiment was repeated with water from the same tap, only this time the water was run through a Grander Water Unit first. When measured after the bath, the levels of impurities in the water were now found to have increased. This indicates that rather than toxins passing from the water to the person, the reverse happened. Toxins were actually removed from the body by the Granderized tap water. In other words, the water could clean us, which is, after all, the object of a bath. Many people report subjectively that after bathing in Granderized water they feel refreshed rather than tired, and perhaps this experiment shows part of the reason for this.

Water treated with a Grander Water Unit also appears to inhibit the growth of unhealthy bacteria, and to virtually wipe it out over time. While unhealthy bacteria are inhibited, healthy bacteria are encouraged and dissolved oxygen is increased. As a result, septic and sewage systems operate far more effectively, with much less odor, and with better aerobic functioning and more rapid bio-degradation of waste matter.

Another benefit when a Grander Water Unit is installed on a household's water supply is that it obviously and rapidly removes scale or other deposits within the plumbing lines and prevents any further deposits. Bacterial and other corrosion is also removed and prevented. As a result, pipes, hot water tanks, dishwashers, pumps, air conditioners, heating and cooling systems, radiators, washing machines, boilers, and other equipment will last far longer and with much less frequent maintenance.

Besides the health benefits of lower surface tension discussed earlier, such water is more effective for cleaning dishes, laundry, etc. This means that detergent use can be greatly reduced, and the temperature on the hot water heater can also be reduced. In addition, significantly less chlorine will be needed in swimming pools. Similarly, the use of chemicals in boilers and cooling towers will also be greatly reduced. All of these mean not only significant cost savings, but more importantly substantial environmental benefits through the use of the Grander technology. Plants and animals also benefit from the use of Grander water. Crops grown with Grander water are healthier and with biomass increased typically between twenty-seven to forty percent. Livestock and pets will also benefit, of course.

The Grander devices do not require maintenance, electricity, or chemicals. Properly installed, they are built to last a lifetime, with no parts to replace. They do not produce any detrimental byproducts. In fact, with a Grander unit installed on a home, waste water will actually benefit the environment as it will act upon the other water it comes into contact with to help revitalize it as well.

For those who are still concerned about any physical contaminants found in their water, it may be wise to filter their water first, then run it through a Grander unit. While a filter will remove some or most of the contaminants from the water, it will not remove the negative information and the filter itself will also damage the water. For this reason, the Grander unit is best used after the filter, for by so doing not only is the initial negative information removed but also the damage from the filter itself can be corrected.

In Conclusion: Taking Individual Responsibility

AS WE HAVE SEEN, THE REQUIREMENTS FOR HEALING INCLUDE WILLingness to work on the mental and emotional levels to dissolve resistance through love, forgiveness, gratitude, and faith. We also set the stage for healing by attention to the physical level, working with nutrition, elimination, exercise, sleep, light and darkness, air, and water quantity and quality.

The foundation for work in these areas, and thus requisite for healing, is an attitude of individual responsibility. However, our habit, encouraged by many of our healing and spiritual institutions, is to look outside ourselves. There is an attitude which I have dubbed "I'm broken, please fix me," and it is characterized by the idea that somebody else will heal us. We do not see ourselves as capable. Sometimes we start out with conventional medicine. If we do not get the results we are hoping for, we may eventually resort to alternative methods and/or some form of natural healing. Perhaps we may even attempt some fairly unusual or radical methods. We may go to various gurus and/or faith healers. And yet, if we still carry the "I'm broken, please fix me" attitude along with us as we move from one thing to the next, chances are we will never quite get the desired results. The problem may not be the methods we are attempting but in our continued tendency to place all responsibility for our healing upon other people. Certainly others can be of great benefit in our healing. Yet we must also take a large measure of individual responsibility as well. It is our health.

Prayer

MUCH ASSISTANCE IS AVAILABLE TO US FROM HIGHER LEVELS: IT IS freely available. There is one prerequisite, however: we must ask for it. Whether our asking is done through prayer or otherwise, it is important to recognize that whatever blessings come our way are indeed from above, and that we need to remember to ask for them in order to receive them. However, "God helps those who help themselves," so once we have put out our prayers, rather than simply waiting for God to do the job, let us be God in action and do whatever is necessary and appropriate to bring about that for which we have prayed.

Chapter Six

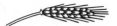

The Healing Crisis

Man alone, of all creatures on earth, can change his own pattern. Man alone is the architect of his destiny.
William James

The great revolution in our generation is the discovery that human beings, by changing the inner attitudes of their minds, can change the outer aspects of their lives.
William James

We are born to succeed not to fail.
Henry David Thoreau

BEFORE ANYONE EMBARKS UPON A HEALING PROGRAM THEY SHOULD have a basic understanding of the *healing crisis.* A healing crisis can be described as a period of imbalance and discomfort as the body heals: we experience adverse symptomology similar to what has been suppressed and/or experienced in the past. These symptoms are among those typically considered to be the signs of disease in conventional approaches, but here they are recognized as an indication that we are actually improving. The feelings of discomfort are due to the toxic burden which had accumulated in the past and which the body is now actively eliminating during the healing crisis. In simple terms, we will often feel worse as we are actually getting better. This concept is recognized and widely applied in many modalities of holistic health. Other names for the same basic phenomena include *tracing, reversal, cleansing,* and *cure.*

What to Expect

THE IMPORTANCE OF THIS CONCEPT CANNOT BE OVERSTRESSED. ITS IMPLI-cations for nutrition are immediate, for improving our nutritional state may precipitate a healing crisis. It's beneficial to recognize what is happening. Most of us have been conditioned to interpret any sign of discomfort as a negative sign. Hence, when the healing crisis appears as a result of a positive dietary change, it may be seen as a sign that the new diet is not helpful, and it will be abandoned. For this reason alone, it is essential that we understand this important concept.

The relative severity of the healing crisis will be related to the degree of improvement in our nutritional state. Therefore, any radical improvement in diet may lead to a healing crisis of substantial proportions. This underscores the need for advising all patients about what they may expect in the way of physical symptoms as they clean up their diet.[1]

In my own experience, significant dietary improvements were accompanied by severe symptoms of healing crisis. I did not understand these at the time, as I had naively assumed that I would feel better if I ate better. In my efforts to comprehend this apparent contradiction, I consulted several different holistic professionals. Each considered the symptoms I was experiencing to be a negative result of items still in my diet; none even considered the possibility that these symptoms were a positive sign. In hindsight, I later realized that none of these professionals had any understanding of the healing crisis. Had I understood what was going on, I would have been far better equipped to deal with the intense symptoms, both physical and emotional, that I experienced. It would have made quite a difference to have known that these symptoms were a positive sign as opposed to a negative indication. While the symptoms would have been much the same, my attitude would have been much more positive. For this reason I make a point of counseling every individual I see as to what they may possibly expect to experience as their diet improves.

An excellent description of some of the symptoms we might expect during a healing crisis is found in *The Essene Gospel of Peace, Book One*:

> And the breath of some became as stinking as that which is loosed
> from the bowels, and some had an issue of spittle, and evil-smelling
> and unclean vomit rose from their inward parts. All these unclean-
> nesses flowed by their mouths. In some, by the nose, in others
> by the eyes and ears. And many did have a noisome and abom-
> inable sweat come from all their body, over all their skin. And
> on many limbs great hot boils broke forth, from which came out
> uncleannesses with an evil smell, and urine flowed abundantly
> from their body; and in many their urine was all but dried up
> and became thick as the honey of bees; that of others was almost
> red or black, and as hard almost as the sand of rivers. And many
> belched stinking gases from their bowels, like the breath of dev-
> ils. And their stench became so great that none could bear it.[2]

In addition to the physical symptomology, emotional and/or psychological aspects may be involved in the healing crisis. Suppressed emotions
will come to the surface, and along with these will come memories. All
manner of old emotional trauma and painful memories can be part of the
healing crisis, and events and emotions which had been entirely forgotten
may rise to the surface with alarming intensity and rapidity. We will have
a much greater chance of successfully weathering the emotional as well as
the physical aspects of the healing crisis if these basic concepts are thoroughly understood before we find themselves in the middle of such experiences. It should also be understood that there is a wide range of intensity
possible. Most of us will experience relatively minor physical discomfort,
if any, and little emotional distress in the event of routine and minor dietary
improvements. However, in the event of radical dietary changes, the healing crisis may be quite intense. In such cases, it is imperative that the nature
of the healing crisis be well understood in advance.

Besides nutrition, many things can precipitate a healing crisis. Some are
physical, but many are otherwise. Something as simple as the practice of
love or nonresistance can bring on a healing crisis. Forgiveness can do the
same. Or gratitude. And so on. Anything of an uplifting nature can potentially help bring on a healing crisis.

Balance, Regeneration, and Degeneration

ON THE PHYSICAL LEVEL, HEALING MAY BE INDICATED IN SEVERAL WAYS. The presence or absence of symptoms is not always a reliable indicator of health improvement, for symptoms may become more pronounced due to a decrease in health, but they may also become more severe as we improve in a healing crisis. Symptoms may disappear eventually as we improve in health. Yet they may also disappear simply because they have been suppressed. Hence, keeping track of symptoms is not the surest way of determining in which direction we are moving. Why this is so can be explained if we consider the concept of balance and the successive levels of balance we reach in a healing process.

Consider a building with many floors. Leading from each floor to the floors immediately above and below will be stairs. Exactly halfway along each set of stairs there is a landing. Each floor may be considered a relative level of balance. Each set of stairs will represent the transition or state of imbalance that exists between the relative levels of balance. One can move up a set of stairs, and thus to a higher level of balance, as well as down a set of stairs to a lower level of balance. In either case a state of imbalance or transition occurs as we move from one level of balance to another. At each of these respective levels of balance, a relative state of equilibrium and an absence of unpleasant symptoms is experienced. While balance is present at each of these levels, a higher level of health is enjoyed at successively higher levels of balance.

When we move from one level of balance to another, we must move out of balance to get there. These intermediate states of imbalance are known as either *healing crises* or *disease crises*. If we are moving from a lower to a higher level of balance, we move through a healing crisis en route. If we are moving from a higher to a lower level of balance, instead we move through a disease crisis, with resulting degeneration of the body. Thus, a healing crisis would involve moving up a flight of stairs, while a disease crisis would involve moving down a flight of stairs.

True healing of the physical body involves moving up through a series of healing crises as successively higher levels of balance are reached. Symptoms will appear and disappear with regularity in accordance with Hering's Law of Cure: "All cure starts from within out and from the head down and in reverse order as the symptoms have appeared."

Those familiar with kinesiology or muscle testing, should note that results can vary in accordance with where we are with respect to balance and imbalance. Traditionally, it has often been assumed that if we test "strong" on a given item, it is "good" for us, and that if we test "weak," it is "bad" for us. Yet in reality a "strong" test shows that this item will bring us back towards the closest level of balance within our current position, while a "weak" test shows that this item will bring us away from the closest level of balance. This means that if the closest level of balance is above us, then a "strong" test does show that something is "good" while a "weak" test shows that something is "bad" for us. Yet if the closest level of balance were below us, the exact opposite would be true. A "strong" test would show that something was "bad" for us, and a "weak" test would show that something was "good" for us. Thus, for muscle testing to be of much use, we must know where we are relatively on the scale. We can do this by testing an item which we already know is good or bad for us. Testing such an item will show more or less where we are on the chart.

How this works can be readily seen in the diagram. If we are on a flight of stairs and above the landing, then the nearest level of balance is the floor above us. Therefore, anything beneficial to us will pull us up or closer to this nearest level of balance: what is "good" will test "strong" if we are on any flight of stairs and above the landing. Anything that is detrimental to us will pull us away from the nearest balance; therefore, what is "bad" will test "weak" when we are on the stairs and above the landing. However, let us now consider a position that is on the stairs but below the landing. The nearest level of balance is now the floor beneath us. Thus, what is beneficial to us will pull us up, away from the nearest balance. What is "good" will test "weak" when we are on the flight of stairs and below the landing. And what is detrimental to us will pull us down to the nearest balance; therefore, what is "bad" will test "strong" when we are on the stairs but below the landing. So we can see that muscle testing might get completely opposite results when we are on a given flight of stairs, depending upon whether we are above or below the landing. This suggests that to move

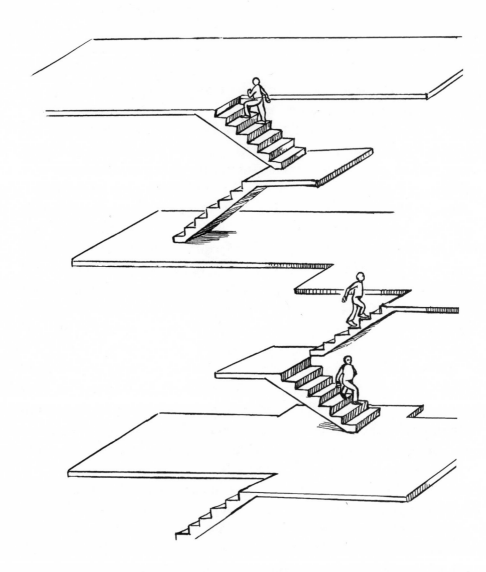

toward health is not always to move toward balance.

    Muscle testing when we are on any of the floors (where we at the peak of balance) can be inconsistent as slight changes in position can move us from above to below balance or vice-versa. Similarly, when we are on any of the landings (where we are at the peak of imbalance), muscle testing can be inconsistent since slight movement in one direction or another can change which is our nearest level of balance. A more detailed discussion of this entire concept can be found in *The Healing Crisis* by John Whitman Ray.[3]

This discussion of muscle testing should suggest that a fundamental distinction must be made between *balancing* the body as opposed to *regenerating* the body. The former is the removal of symptoms until a state of relative balance is attained, followed by the maintenance of this state by whatever means necessary. This is at best a modest level of healing. Regeneration of the body involves moving up from one level of balance to succeeding levels of balance through a series of healing crises (states of imbalance.) This is necessary for true healing.

The absence of symptoms should not be confused with true health or healing. It is a shame that so many define health as merely the absence of sickness. If the concept of the healing crisis were better understood, symptoms could be seen as indications that we are moving toward better health when proper remedies are being applied.

Going through the Healing Crisis

EXPERIENCING A HEALING CRISIS CAN BE MOST UNCOMFORTABLE, AND often there is a part of us that will unconsciously seek to stop the healing crisis and its attendant discomforts. This might take the form of an urge for certain foods that are not especially uplifting for us, which if consumed might end the healing crisis and bring us swiftly back down into balance. I have seen quite intense healing crises ended effectively by this means. For example, the discomfort of withdrawal from alcohol can be ended by taking a drink. Alternately, we may get the urge to avoid eating the very foods that brought us into the healing crisis in the first place. However, to keep moving toward health we must go through the healing crisis. The basic rule is pretty simple: whatever gets us into healing crisis will help get us through it. We need to keep doing whatever got us into the healing crisis if we want to make it through, and if not doing certain things helped get us into the healing crisis, we need to keep not doing the same things.

Thought, Energy, and Matter

IN RECENT TIMES, DISCUSSIONS OF HEALING AND THE HEALING CRISIS ARE found in works within the emerging field of energy medicine. And so it might be asked what role energy plays in the model we are developing here. So, in addition to the mental, emotional and physical levels, we might also consider levels of thought, energy and matter.

The level of matter is familiar to us all, and most conventional healing techniques, including many natural ones, focus entirely on the physical level. That the structure of matter is to a great extent influenced by the level of energy has long been recognized in certain fields such as acupuncture, and we have abundant evidence that the structure of matter may be altered by manipulating the underlying pattern of energy.

However, while matter will indeed follow energy, it is important to understand that energy in turn will follow thought. That is, both energy and matter may be altered through changing the underlying pattern of thought. Thus, thought or consciousness is the level which must be reached for permanent change to occur. Intervention at the physical level, for example, surgery to remove a tumor, does not change the underlying causes of the condition. If the underlying pattern of thought, word, and emotion remains held in a continual state of creation through continued resistance, then it is only a matter of time before the outer manifestation reappears in some form. This will also be true of intervention at the level of energy. It is indeed possible to remove physical symptoms through some form of manipulation at the energy level, for example, through removing blockages to energy flow. However, if there is no corresponding change of consciousness at the level of thought, then the underlying cause remains unchanged and blockages will again occur. Effect must always follow cause, and if underlying causes remain unaltered then the effects must eventually reappear. Hence, a change of thought or consciousness is necessary for permanent healing.

PART TWO

Nutrition

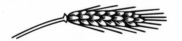

FOR MANY OF US, THE PROCESS OF CONSCIOUSNESS CHANGE (LEADING to healing) is best begun through work on the physical level, bringing our bodies to a state of *nutrient saturation,* defined as the state wherein the body is supplied with sufficient amounts of all essential nutrients (including minerals, enzymes, essential amino acids, vitamins, essential fatty acids, as well as any as yet unknown essential nutrients), while at the same time making certain that these nutrients are properly digested and assimilated by the body. Nutrient saturation can be seen as a necessary foundation of health as well as healing. In a state of nutrient saturation, a person is abundantly supplied with all the necessary nutrients to enter into and successfully pass through a healing crisis so that the regeneration of the body may take place.

As discussed extensively in Part One, there is far more to healing than physical factors such as nutrition. Emotional, mental, and spiritual factors are also intrinsic to the process, and a major part of healing involves resolving our resistances. Clearly, then, nutrient saturation all by itself is not sufficient to guarantee our healing. Yet it certainly makes the likelihood of healing far greater.

The process of working with and eventually resolving our resistances involves attaining and maintaining attitudes of love, forgiveness, and gratitude. A poor state of nutrition tends to affect our emotional state in a negative manner, while a good state of nutrition tends to affect our emotions in a positive manner. Thus, a state of nutrient saturation (or the lack thereof) may have a significant impact upon whether or not we manage to master our resistances rather than being mastered by them. It's not that we cannot master our resistances when on a poor diet; rather it is more difficult to do so. As discussed in Chapter Two, each emotion is mastered by experiencing it with enthusiasm. Most of us will find this easier to do when full of energy as a result of proper nutrition. In contrast, when our bodies are lacking in essential nutrients as a result of deficient diet or when we are poisoned by all sorts of unnatural foods, we may find it much more difficult to feel a given resistance with enthusiasm. We may remain trapped by a given resistance pattern.

The process of resolving our resistances also involves much energy and effort on our part. When properly nourished we are far more likely to have the surplus energy needed to heal on all levels. When undernourished and toxic, we are unlikely to have the extra energy needed to heal on any level. Nutrient saturation and other physical factors set the stage for mastery of the emotional body, which in turn sets the stage for mastery of the mental body.

Yet just as poor nutrition can adversely affect our emotions, so too can poor attitudes adversely affect our nutrition. For when we remain stuck in various levels of emotional resistance, often we are drawn to poor food choices which only serve to reinforce the negative emotions we are already enmeshed within. Conversely, just as proper nutrition can positively affect our emotions, so too can a positive attitude affect our nutrition positively. For when we are able to maintain attitudes of love, forgiveness, and gratitude, we naturally tend to be drawn toward better food choices and digest this food more optimally.

Viewed from a higher level, it can be seen that an interdependence exists between physical factors such as nutrition, emotional factors such as enthusiasm or unconditional love, and mental factors such as encompassing duality. Proper nutrition sets the stage for mastery of our emotions so that we can experience each in turn with enthusiasm. This in turn sets the stage for the eventual encompassment of duality. And as resistance is resolved in this manner, it becomes easier to continue on a course of proper nutrition, thus continuing the upwards spiral toward improvement on all levels. For many of us the most effective starting point onto this upwards spiral is proper nutrition.

Chapter Seven

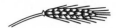

Dietary Reform:
Some Basic Concepts to Master

Teach correct principles and let people govern themselves.
Anonymous

Prove all things; hold fast that which is good.
I Thessalonians 5:21

Therefore, I am firmly convinced that those who really have something to say that is of concern to us all, can express it in a manner that everyone can understand.
Dr. Johanna Budwig

NUTRITION IS THE FOUNDATION UPON WHICH HEALTH OR DISEASE are constructed. Nutrition sets the stage upon which our state of health is determined. However, the importance of nutrition should be neither overestimated nor underestimated. It is as much a mistake to inflate its value as it is to disparage its importance. While nutrition plays a major role in many health conditions, there are other factors. Our state of consciousness (in particular our patterns of thought, word and emotion) is the underlying factor in all outer manifestation. Nutrition and other physical factors mediate the outer expression of this underlying inner essence: our diet can have an enormous effect upon our physical, emotional and mental states. However, nutrition by itself is not the answer for every problem, as there are many other factors. Inherited or genetic tendencies (which may be considered to be patterns of thought, word and emotion as perpetuated through the DNA matrix) will, of course, be another significant factor in determining our health. Different individuals may eat identical diets over many years or even an entire lifetime and yet enjoy widely varying states of health. Clearly there is more to consider here than just nutrition.

For many people, nutrition is primarily about *what to eat* and *what not to eat*. However, while that is certainly part of the picture, *how* we eat is also important, as is our attitude toward dietary reform. In this chapter let us consider some attitudes and principles that underlie a program of good nutrition. Besides the ones discussed in Part One—having faith, letting go of resistance, and being prepared for the healing crisis—some others are worth mention.

Attitude toward Dietary Reform

SELF-RESPONSIBILITY

The ultimate responsibility for our nutrition is in our own hands. It is up to us to determine what sort of diet we will follow. Certainly parents will choose the diet of their children to a considerable extent, but as time goes by, children will assume more responsibility for their own food choices. In the end, each of us is responsible for our own nutrition.

FAITH

Without faith that we can indeed improve our health and overcome whatever problems we face, improvement is unlikely. Some say that all things are possible to those who have faith. Equally true is that a lack of faith may render many things impossible.

OBEDIENCE TO LAW

As in all things, if we wish to achieve a certain result we must obey the particular law or laws pertaining to its accomplishment. This includes relatively simple laws such as those of nutrition as well as progressively higher levels of law. While "faith without works is dead," faith makes possible that which may be realized through attaining and maintaining the appropriate discipline.

PATIENCE

Discipline brings results when it is attained and maintained. In this era of instant gratification, the temptation exists to expect immediate results and to be disappointed if these do not happen. Many people are unwilling to both attain and maintain the required level of discipline to bring about that which they wish. A particular dietary regimen is unlikely to completely undo in a short time that which has resulted from many years of improper living. The race goes not to the swift but to those who persevere until the end.

Principles for Success in Dietary Reform

PREFER CHANGE IN MODEST INCREMENTS

In certain extreme cases, making swift and radical dietary changes is appropriate. Yet in most situations a gradual transition will be much more effective in both the short and the long run. Changing too quickly can precipitate a healing crisis which is too much to handle. Then we abandon any further effort to change. However, if we imagine ourselves ten or fifteen years from now, in much improved health and eating an extremely high quality diet, it will probably not make much difference whether this improved diet was attained in a week or in a year or more. The important thing is that we have been able to both attain and maintain this level, not necessarily how long it may have taken us to get there.

The best way to get where we're going is to determine and enact modest increments of change. A radical transition can be effectively accomplished by a series of simple steps. The overall scope of change desired may appear daunting or hopeless when viewed in its entirety. However, a big change is more readily accomplished by breaking the task up into small steps. "The journey of a thousand miles begins with a single step." Successfully completing a small and simple task builds both the aptitude and the confidence to complete larger and more complex tasks. As we succeed in each gradient step of dietary reform, we will gather increasing momentum for the bigger steps ahead. This is another great advantage of moving in a step by step fashion.

GET RID OF THE WORST FIRST

In improving the diet it is often appropriate to eliminate or reduce the most detrimental items first rather than focusing on less significant hazards in the current diet. Once the worst items have been eliminated, we may then continue on with the process of fine tuning the diet.

PROMOTE GOOD DIGESTION

It's not what we eat that nourishes us, but what we digest and assimilate. The nutrients in food are available to nourish us only after the food has been broken down and its nutrients assimilated. Therefore, it is beneficial to do everything we can to promote the efficiency of digestion.

It's not just what we eat, but how much. Gluttony is a health destroyer. When consumed in excess, even the best of foods can harm us. Digestion does not function efficiently when too much food is consumed or when food is consumed too frequently. It is better to consume a moderate amount of food and digest it efficiently than to overeat and thus hinder digestion. Moderation is the key here.

TREAT, DON'T CHEAT

While the ideal is to adhere to our diet, people do occasionally lapse and then feel guilty. However, our guilt will insure that the food in question is poorly digested. It is far better if we occasionally go off our diet, that we do so with an attitude free of guilt. Treat, don't cheat! If we are going to have the occasional indulgence, we might as well eat it with love in our heart and truly enjoy it rather than consume it with fear and guilt. It is not what we eat on rare occasions that will bring us down, but rather what we eat everyday.

EAT WHILE FEELING GOOD

An attitude of gratitude for the experiences of life sets the stage for all good things to come our way. It is extremely important to maintain a positive attitude while eating, for even the best of foods will provide poor nourishment when eaten in a state of negativity. It is often best not to eat when we are upset. Rather, it is best to eat with love in our hearts and gratitude for whatever meal is before us. Food should be prepared as well as eaten with a positive attitude.

Not only that, but if the diet we are attempting to follow is not enjoyable to us, then it is probably not going to be of much value to us in the long run. We may have changed too rapidly. Or the diet itself may be faulty. Or maybe our attitude needs adjustment. But for the most part, eating should be an enjoyable experience, not a form of self-inflicted torture.

Promote Good Elimination

A body that is supplied with all necessary nutrients and whose wastes are eliminated promptly will generally thrive. Thus the importance of the various channels of elimination: the colon, the skin, the urinary system, the lymphatic system, and the respiratory system. When one of these systems is inadequate or overloaded, the others must bear the weight and the entire body is affected. A good diet will encourage improved colon function which will in turn benefit the other systems of elimination as well as the entire body.

Don't Just Cleanse: Build

There is much emphasis upon the use of certain diets for cleansing or detoxifying the body. Certainly many people are quite toxic, and the elimination of these toxins from the body can result in substantial improvements in health. Simply put, cleansing is important.

Yet building the body is equally important. In the zeal to cleanse, many people put all their emphasis upon cleansing and ignore or neglect building the body as well. Certain types of diets will result in substantial cleansing of the body, yet many are quite deficient in necessary nutrients to build the body. While there may be short term benefit in the form of detoxification, such diets will sooner or later result in a diminishment of health.

Cleansing and building are both important, and in fact, in the long run one will not succeed if the other is neglected. It is not possible to build healthy tissue in a body that remains toxic. And neither is it possible for a body that is deficient in building materials to detoxify, for the organs of elimination will function quite poorly in the absence of necessary nutrients. It is shortsighted to focus upon either cleansing or building to the neglect of the other.

CHEW FOOD THOROUGHLY

Good digestion begins in the mouth with complete mastication of the food. This is especially important with raw fruits and vegetables, as many of the nutrients are made available through the rupturing of the cell wall by mastication. Chewing also provides the opportunity for salivary amylase to mix with the food and initiate carbohydrate digestion. It also liberates the enzymes present in the food so that they may perform their function in the upper or food enzyme portion of the stomach. An additional benefit of chewing is that it provides benefit to the entire body due to the reflex relationship between each tooth and particular organs, glands and other body parts.

INDIVIDUALIZE THE DIET

Many people assume that the same diet would be ideal for all of us. Yet given the vast array of factors involved, this is a dubious assumption. "One man's meat is another man's poison." Our genetic and/or ethnic backgrounds may vary widely. The types of foods that our ancestors have consumed over many generations influences what sort of food is suitable for us. Our blood type (O, A, B or AB) also appears to influence the effect of various foods upon us.[1] There is a growing body of modern research that strongly suggests that each of these four blood types has a distinct diet that is most suitable. Certain foods that may be beneficial to those of one type may be detrimental to those of another. And it is not only modern science that suggests that the ideal may vary from one person to the next, for many ancient traditions say this as well. Ayurvedic medicine has a successful track record going back at least five thousand years in India. In Ayurvedic tradition, there are said to be three basic body types (vata, pitta and kapha) as well as various combinations. Each body type is said to have its own most suitable diet, and what is beneficial for one type may be detrimental for another.[2] Numerous other traditions from around the world make similar observations and categorize people in various ways. Western science has shown that individual needs for most essential nutrients can vary by a factor of at least ten. In the case of many nutrients, variation has been shown to be much greater than this. The best diet for one person is not always the best diet for somebody else.

There is a vast difference between a diet that allows survival versus a diet on which we truly thrive. The fact that we can continue to exist on a given diet, even for years at a time, is no indication that this diet is optimal. We need to find the diet that suits us, that allows us to thrive.

Chapter Eight

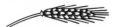

Passing the Test of Reality:
The Work of Dr. Weston A. Price, D.D.S.

Life in all its fullness is Mother Nature obeyed.
Weston A. Price

However convincing or sensible a theory may seem, it really is of little value to us if it fails the test of reality.
Douglas Morrison

Introduction

MANY OF US HAVE A SINCERE DESIRE TO KNOW WHICH FOODS WILL be best for us. To some this may seem a straightforward question. After the first year or two of study, many people conclude that they have a pretty fair understanding of nutrition. Yet many serious students of nutrition eventually come to a point of wondering if they really understand anything at all. For the more we investigate the field of nutrition, the more contradictions are uncovered. The more we understand, the more we discover how much we do not understand.

Controversy and differing opinions abound in the field of nutrition. Sometimes opposite viewpoints seem equally sensible. But in the end, however convincing or sensible a theory may seem, it really is of little value to us if it fails the test of reality.

Sometimes when the answers seem confusing to us, it is good to reconsider the questions. On the one hand, we desire to know what foods are best for us. Yet at the next level we might ask: best for what purpose? This question itself must be broken down: numerous physical considerations must be made.

- How does a particular diet affect our physical body in the short term and in the long term?
- Is it sufficient to maintain a good state of health?
- Is it sufficient to prevent degenerative illness?
- Is it sufficient to support the regeneration of the body?
- Is it sufficient to aid in the recovery from a degenerative illness?
- Is it suitable for a particular lifestyle (e.g. heavy physical labor, intense mental exertion, etc.)?
- How suitable is it at various stages of our life: infancy, childhood, adolescence, early adulthood, middle age, and beyond?
- Is it suitable for a pregnant woman or a lactating mother?
- Is it suitable for parents preparing to conceive children?
- How will such a diet on our part affect future generations?

Besides these physical considerations, there may be other factors for some people:

- How will a particular diet affect our emotions and our emotional development?
- How will it affect our mind and our mental and intellectual development?
- How will it affect our spiritual development?
- What are the ethical considerations of a particular diet?
- What are the karmic consequences of a particular diet?

Numerous other relevant considerations may exist: the question of what foods are best is not so simple after all. A particular diet may be excellent in certain of these respects and yet quite poor in others. Depending upon the unique considerations of a given individual, it may be possible that no diet satisfies all of them. Perhaps the answers are not easy because the questions are not easy either.

Sometimes the best beginning for each of us is to reconsider our priorities. To help with this, the work of Weston Price will be highlighted in this chapter. It may help us to answer our questions and set our priorities. Just as importantly, it may help us to see a few questions we might otherwise have neglected to ask. I strongly advocate that all serious students of nutrition obtain the book *Nutrition and Physical Degeneration* by Weston A. Price, D.D.S.[1] who has become known to many in recent years for his pioneering research in the early decades of the twentieth century on the disastrous health consequences of root canals.[2]

In his later years, Weston Price devoted much time to travel and research into the cause of dental caries. He and his wife spent much of the 1930s traveling to remote areas of the globe and investigating the dental as well as the overall health of various populations sufficiently isolated so as to be eating a diet free of all modern processed foods such as white flour, white sugar, canned foods, vegetable fats, and so on. These included Swiss villagers high in the Alps; Gaelic peoples inhabiting remote islands off the coast of Scotland; Eskimos; North American Indians in various parts of the contiguous United States, Alaska, and Canada; Melanesian and Polynesian Islanders; various African tribes; Australian Aborigines; Torres Strait Islanders; New Zealand Maori; and Peruvian Indians. Although his purpose was to study how diet influences dental health, his findings have a great deal to tell us about nutrition and health overall.

Dental Caries, Other Degeneration, and Nutrition

IN MANY OF THE AREAS HE VISITED, PRICE WAS ABLE TO COMPARE PEOPLE still on their native diets with people of the same stock who had shifted or were in the process of shifting over to a diet containing modern processed foods, the foods of "commerce" and "civilization." In several of these areas, Price had access to skulls that were hundreds and even thousands of years old, and these skulls provided the opportunity to compare the dental health and cranial structures of these modern populations with that of their ancestors. Price recounts a great deal of this work in *Nutrition and Physical*

Degeneration, a work meticulously researched and full of hundreds of photographs and a large amount of data from Price's own research.

In Price's day there was vigorous debate on the cause of dental caries. Price's position was if we want to understand what causes dental caries, we need first to find populations among whom dental caries are virtually absent. Then we determine what they are doing and identify what those with caries are doing that differs. However convincing or sensible a theory may seem, it really is of little value to us if it fails the test of reality. Reading Price's book, one cannot help but be struck that Price does not present idle theories, but rather a tremendous amount of reality. In village after village around the globe, Price would painstakingly examine all the teeth of large numbers of people. He would check for any evidence of dental decay, past or present, as well as any sign of abnormality in the dental arches or cranial structure. The typical diet of each community was also studied in detail and samples of the various foodstuffs were taken for analysis. The sheer volume of data that he collected in his travels is staggering.

Price found that in the modernized populations just the odd individual was free of dental caries. But with great consistency in the isolated populations, dental caries were the exception rather than the rule in those still adhering to their traditional diet. The diets of these populations were as varied as their geographical settings might suggest. But what was consistent was that so long as they remained on traditional diets that were free of "modern" imported foods, they remained virtually free of dental caries. (This was generally accomplished without a toothbrush or any attempt at dental hygiene. Price typically had to clean the debris off the teeth before he could examine them for any dental decay.) In addition, members of these groups continued to produce healthy offspring with properly formed dental arches with ample space for all thirty-two adult teeth, and with proper cranial structures, including in particular the facial structure. Among people on such a diet, there was little evidence of insanity, mental retardation, criminal behavior, delinquency, and many other all too common aspects of "civilization." Birth complications were also rare, as women conceived in these conditions would typically have pelvic structures more than adequate for birthing their own children. Degenerative illnesses such as cancer, diabetes, heart disease, arthritis, and osteoporosis were quite rare or even entirely absent.

A short time after these populations turned away from their native diet and began eating processed foods, all of the above factors shifted in a most detrimental fashion: dental caries rapidly became prevalent; degenerative diseases appeared with great frequency; and insanity, mental retardation, criminal behavior, and delinquency all became commonplace. The first generation of females conceived under these conditions routinely experienced complications when giving birth to their children due to a decided narrowing of the pelvic structure—a situation almost completely unknown to their female ancestors. These negative traits which were all once the exception rapidly became the rule under the influence of modern foods.

Nutrition and Future Generations—Intercepted Heredity

IN ADDITION, PRICE CONSISTENTLY OBSERVED ANOTHER TREND. IN THESE cultures, generation after generation of individuals with fine dental arches and excellent cranial structures had been produced for thousands of years. Yet as soon as one or both parents shifted over to a modern diet and away from their native foodstuffs, changes were observed in their offspring. Children conceived subsequent to this change were typically born with inadequate dental arches as well as deformed cranial structures. The dental arches were often of insufficient size to allow space for all of the teeth, resulting in crowding of the wisdom teeth, crooked teeth and various other abnormalities. Typical cranial deformities included a narrowing and overall underdevelopment of the face, often in particular of the middle third or maxillary portion of the face. Such cranial and dental deformities are shown in numerous photographs in Price's book *Nutrition and Physical Degeneration*.

Besides the obvious physical deformities in the offspring that resulted from their parents making the transition away from their native diet to a civilized diet, it was clear also that these children were damaged in many other ways, not the least of which was in their level of intelligence or mental capacity. Price noted a few of the injuries that in his view were typically "associated with prenatal injuries, caused by parental vitamin and mineral deficiencies, before and at the time of fertilization. These affect the germ cells, thereby producing a defective fertilized ovum and defective fetus. In this group are hare-lip, cleft palate, narrow hips, narrow face, constricted nostrils, mental backwardness, juvenile delinquency, skull defects of the face and the floor of the brain, brain defects, mongoloidism, idiocy, etc."[3]

This suggests that maternal nutrition during both pregnancy and lactation is important, as many have rightly emphasized. Yet if we ignore the tremendous influence of maternal and paternal nutrition prior to conception, it is the equivalent of shutting the barn door after the horse has bolted. It is too late to prevent the damage that has already taken place. The child is already injured at this point due to the defective egg and/or sperm resulting from the faulty nutrition of parents. The previously fine constitution of the parents is not passed on to the child intact, but is distorted through their nutritional transgressions: the sins of the parents are indeed visited unto the children.[4] Price used the term *intercepted heredity* to describe this situation.[5]

More on Dental Caries and Nutrition

PROPER NUTRITION PROVIDES PROTECTION

Price made some interesting observations concerning tooth decay and nutrition. Firstly, sufficient nutritional improvement will typically arrest all dental decay. Improved nutrition will result in improved quality of the saliva itself, and so long as the saliva also has access to the cavity, no further decay takes place. Secondly, under the same circumstances, the decayed dentine will be remineralized via the saliva to a point of becoming quite hard or petrified. In other words, not only is further deterioration of the teeth halted, but the teeth will begin to regenerate. These first two observations are certainly impressive enough. Yet Price's next two observations are positively astounding. When dental pulp is exposed, this normally results in infection since the oral bacteria now have access to the interior of that tooth. Yet Price observed on many occasions teeth which were worn down to the gums, such that one would have expected exposed dental pulp. Yet the pulp in most cases had never been exposed, for even as the teeth were worn down, they were continually remineralized such that the dental pulp remained protected. Furthermore, Price also noted instances where people with exposed dental pulp caused by their adoption of processed foods reversed this situation with a return to their natural diet and preserved those teeth that had been in jeopardy. Price also reports having achieved this same result among some of his own patients in the United States through improving their nutrition sufficiently.[6] Thus, according to the detailed research of Dr. Price, a proper state of nutrition is not only sufficient to prevent or eliminate dental decay, it is also sufficient to bring about quite impressive regeneration of the teeth themselves from a pre-existing state of deterioration.

DENTAL DECAY PRECEDES PHYSICAL DEGENERATION

Dental decay does not merely accompany physical degeneration: it quite clearly precedes it. Dental decay is like the proverbial "canary in the coal mine." The canary will succumb to the poisons in the air before the miners do. Thus, the canary serves as a warning to the miners to get out before they succumb as well. In a similar manner, the teeth will tend to succumb to our poor dietary habits in advance of the rest of the body. Thus, we have our own canary in the form of our teeth. As noted by the dentist Melvin Page in *Degeneration—Regeneration* "dental caries is possibly the most prevalent degenerative disease. It affects 98.5% of the people of the USA. Dental caries is relatively easy to prevent, not reduced 30% but by 100%. One must correct the body chemistry to do so and instruct the patient so that the efficiency of body chemistry can be maintained. When we do this we automatically prevent other degenerative diseases which require greater inefficiency of the body chemistry for their inception."[7]

Towards a Sufficient Diet

WE CAN NOW SEE THAT A TRULY SUFFICIENT DIET WOULD HAVE CERtain consistent consequences as a bare minimum:

1. A relative freedom from all tooth decay so long as such a sufficient diet is followed.

2. Should tooth decay exist as a result of a prior insufficient diet, a return to the sufficient diet would arrest all such decay.

3. Any decayed dentine would mineralize or harden up with return to the sufficient diet.

4. Tooth pulp, no matter how much wear the teeth sustain, would typ-

ically not be exposed as long as this sufficient diet was adhered to.

5. If tooth pulp were exposed due to a prior insufficient diet, then return to a truly sufficient diet would result in the formation of new vital dentine to seal off the pulp.

6. Offspring from parents on a sufficient diet would be typically vigorous in all regards, and in particular would have adequate dental arches to allow the proper eruption of all thirty-two adult teeth, as well as proper cranial structures, including full development of the facial structure.

7. The following defects would be rare or absent in offspring when both parents were following a sufficient diet: "hare-lip, cleft palate, narrow hips, narrow face, constricted nostrils, mental backwardness, juvenile delinquency, skull defects of the face and the floor of the brain, brain defects, mongoloidism and idiocy."

8. In individuals on a sufficient diet, degenerative diseases such as cancer, diabetes, arthritis, and cardiovascular disease would be rare or absent.

9. For females who had been conceived by parents on a sufficient diet, complications while giving birth to their own children would also be rare or absent.

Certainly there are many more criteria we might consider for a truly sufficient diet. Yet these nine would all be true of a sufficient diet. Price himself observed many such sufficient diets around the world in various populations. In his own clinics in the United States, he was frequently able to bring about radical improvements in patients' dental problems simply through having them make certain dietary modifications. The improvements included the complete arrest of all dental decay as well as the gradual restoration of the teeth through adequate saliva (which of course, is only possible with adequate nutrition.) In short, he was able to alter his patients' diets sufficiently to meet at least the first five of the above criteria, those pertaining to the teeth themselves.[8]

Common Factors in the Sufficient Diet

The Vegan Diet

Many authors and lecturers, myself included, have advocated and followed a vegan diet. Many of us have felt quite strongly that a pure vegan diet was the pinnacle of human nutrition. Some have believed it best to go straight to a vegan diet. Others have felt we might need to move towards a vegan diet through a series of transition diets. But in either case, the vegan diet was considered the ideal. However, with regard to a vegan diet (that is, one free of all animal products), Price made note of the following:

> As yet I have not found a single group of primitive racial stock which was building and maintaining excellent bodies by living entirely on plant foods. I have found in many parts of the world most devout representatives of modern ethical systems advocating the restriction of foods to the vegetable products. In every instance where the groups involved had been long under this teaching, I found evidence of degeneration in the form of dental caries, and in the new generation in the form of abnormal dental arches to an extent very much higher than in the primitive groups who were not under this influence.[9]

That is, Price himself *never* once observed a pure vegan diet to be effective in preventing dental decay, and he did observe consistently that people who followed such a diet produced offspring with typical deformities of the dental arches and the overall cranial structure, as well as extensive tooth decay. It may well be possible for a vegan diet to meet the above criteria for a sufficient diet, but it has not to my knowledge ever been accomplished by any known culture. On the one hand, we might consider that the fact that something has not been observed does not automatically imply that it is impossible. Yet we might also consider that it may not be so simple to devise a truly sufficient vegan diet.

Sally Fallon provides another piece of evidence in her excellent book *Nourishing Traditions:*

The Anasazi Indians, builders of the famous cliff dwellings in Mesa Verde, Colorado, flourished from 650 to 1300 A.D. and then died out "mysteriously." In the early days of their civilization, they had plenty of game but archeologists find no animal bones in the trash heaps during the final century or so. Late human skeletal remains show bone deformities, rickets, rampant tooth decay and arthritis in individuals as young as 20 years old. The Anasazi ate corn, beans, pine nuts, yucca, herbs and berries. Their diet contained complete protein, essential fatty acids, minerals and vitamins including lots of carotene. Their life-style gave them abundant exposure to sunlight. But in the final years, the Anasazi lacked animal products, particularly vitamin A and D. They died out and we will too if we eliminate animal fats from the diet.[10]

In light of this and of Price's findings, I must now seriously question the ultimate wisdom of following a vegan diet. It would appear plausible that there are certain crucial nutritional factors, whether known or otherwise, that it is either impossible or at the least extremely difficult for humans in our current state to obtain in adequate amounts (as per the above nine criteria) from a vegan diet. If we desire to regenerate our own bodies and minds, if we desire perhaps to produce healthy well-formed offspring, then we must consider that a diet that meets the above nine criteria is advisable.

This brings us back to the basic principle for choosing the best diet. No matter how good our own diet seems in theory, how is it surviving the test of reality? One way we can tell is to ask are our teeth continuing to deteriorate, or are they regenerating? Many people on strict vegan diets have been observed by this author to experience considerable degeneration and eventual loss of their teeth. While numerous other factors may be involved, nevertheless, does such a diet bode well for the long term health of the body? For the production of healthy offspring?

THE SUFFICIENT DIET ACROSS CULTURES

Price made note of a few of the common factors that he observed in all of the sufficient primitive diets that he studied.

It is significant that I have as yet found no group that was building and maintaining good bodies exclusively on plant foods. A
number of groups are endeavoring to do so with marked evidence of failure. The variety of animal foods available has varied widely in some groups, and been limited among others.

In the preceding chapter we have seen that the successful
dietaries included in addition to a liberal source of minerals, carbohydrates, fats, proteins, and water-soluble vitamins, a source
of fat-soluble vitamins.

Vitamin D is not found in plants, but must be sought in animal food. The dietaries of the efficient primitive racial stocks may
be divided into groups on this basis: in the first place those obtaining their fat-soluble activators, which include the known fat-soluble vitamins, from efficient dairy products. This includes the
Swiss in the high Alps, the Arabs (using camel's milk), and the
Asiatic races (using milk of sheep and musk ox). In the second
place there are those using liberally the organs of animals, and
the eggs of birds, wild and domesticated. These include the Indians of the far North, the buffalo hunting Plains Indians and the
Andean tribes. In the third place there are those using liberally
animal life of the sea. These include Pacific Islanders and coastal
tribes throughout the world. In the fourth place there are those
using small animals and insects. These include the Australian
Aborigines in the interior, and the African tribes in the interior.[11]

As mentioned above, nutritional factors difficult or even impossible to
obtain in adequate amounts on a vegan diet may include known factors as
well as unknown factors. Price looked at vitamins A and D, both of which
can only be found in animal foods. Beta carotene is found in many plants
foods and can be converted to vitamin A to some extent. Yet due to a variety of factors, it appears that human needs for vitamin A cannot be fully
met through beta carotene consumption. Price also emphasized that the
fraction of the vitamin D complex that humans produce themselves (vitamin D_3) via the interaction of sunlight and the oils in their skin will not
arrest dental decay, unlike proper vitamin D which can if the other neces-

sary factors are present. Price also looked at another fat soluble factor which was distinct from these, and as of then, unknown: Price used the term *activator X* for this substance. In Price's lifetime, the essential fatty acids had not yet been isolated or named, but later researchers have suggested that activator X may possibly be the essential fatty acids or something related to them. As noted by the Price-Pottenger Foundation, the traditional diets studied by Price "contain at least four times the calcium and other minerals and *ten* times the fat soluble vitamins from animal fats (vitamin A, vitamin D and the Price Factor) as the average American diet."[12]

Modern medical researchers of nutrition like to isolate and name essential nutritional factors. From an intellectual point of view, a given diet is considered acceptable because it contains sufficient amounts of all known nutritional factors. Yet somehow the fact that people existing on such a diet are in an obvious and consistent state of degeneration does not enter into the discussion. However, the cultures Price studied were not concerned with modern science and isolated nutritional factors. As the inheritors of a long cultural tradition, they were simply taught which foods to eat and how and when to gather, catch, hunt and prepare these foods. And if any specific problems did arise, generally these were addressed with the appropriate foods. Special foods were often provided to couples prior to conception as well as to expecting mothers. Perhaps modern medical nutrition is falling short because its methods are fundamentally flawed from the start. If we wish to learn about health, let us study healthy people. We will not really understand much about life and health if we focus primarily upon death, disease and degeneration. To seek out and study characteristics and diets of the healthy rather than the diseased was the technique Weston Price himself utilized.

VARIATIONS IN FOOD QUALITY

Healthy people eat high quality foods, and the quality of foods can vary tremendously depending upon many factors. Price made extensive studies of the nutritional content of dairy products, for example. He had samples of butter and other dairy products from various locations around the world sent to him several times monthly for many years, and he analyzed them. Price found that the best quality dairy products were only possible when the cows had access to rapidly growing grass or hay of a very high chlorophyll content. Even under the best possible circumstances, where the pastures for the animals were ideal, there was still a significant difference in the quality of the butter throughout the year. Chlorophyll content of the livestock's food seemed to be of particular importance. Cows fed on grains and hay of low chlorophyll content are simply not capable of producing adequately nutritious dairy products. (Indeed, on certain diets, their own calves would die if fed only milk.) It was noted, by the way, that butter of the highest quality was a conspicuously darker yellow than the pale butter of poor quality. Some have suggested a similar situation with egg yolks: when the hens have access to grass and other greenery, they produce quite dark yellow to orange yolks, and when denied grass, the yolks are a pale yellow, and thus presumably of inferior quality. Price also noted that butter of higher nutritional quality had a lower melting point and was therefore more readily spreadable or softer than poorer quality butter.

In considering food quality, Price observed quite obvious correlations not just between time of year and amount of sunlight, but also with respect to soil quality. In particular, much evidence was presented that soil quality, and hence food quality, were at their worst in those areas of the United States that had been farmed the longest. It was clear to Price that the mineral content of soil was rapidly depleted by most farming practices. It might be noted here that many of the cultures Price studied relied upon the sea for much of their nutrition. A tremendous advantage of this is the high mineral content of the sea, and hence of most sea food.[13]

Making Use of Price's Ideas

SOME IMPLICATIONS OF PRICE'S IDEAS MUST BE CONSIDERED IF WE ARE to make use of them for dietary reform. A diet that is adequate for mere survival is clearly not the same as a sufficient diet meeting the above nine criteria. People can maintain life (albeit in a state of gradual deterioration) for extended periods of time on many types of diets. They may even feel reasonably well as their bodies slowly decline. But a truly sufficient diet would certainly as a bare minimum meet the aforementioned nine criteria.

It should also be noted that the nutritional demands upon the human body are not constant throughout our life. During periods of growth these demands are greatly increased, and in particular an extremely heavy nutritional demand is placed upon mothers during pregnancy as well as lactation. Thus, a diet that may be sufficient to arrest tooth decay at some point may no longer do so, for example, during pregnancy, lactation, or any period of considerable physical growth on the part of the individual. Many people observe an increase in dental caries at such times, clear evidence of the added nutritional demands.

Please also consider that an individual on a typically insufficient modern diet may change to a different diet, for example a vegan diet, and in the short run may observe many obvious improvements in their health. Yet it is possible that this new diet is not providing certain nutritional factors in adequate amounts or at all. If so, then sooner or later the body's own stores of these nutrients will be exhausted and the process of degeneration inevitable. Thus, we must consider a distinct possibility: a diet which may lead to some improvement in the short term may nevertheless lead to degeneration in the long term. For the black and white mind, this is difficult to grasp.

Many people are not simply interested in the health and development of the physical body, but in their progression on other levels: emotional, mental, and/or spiritual. A crucial question to consider: is a diet that consistently leads to physical degeneration compatible with emotional, mental and/or spiritual progression? Certainly Price noted that the introduction of modern processed and devitalized foods led to physical degeneration. Just as importantly, Price noted that it led to an obvious increase in crime, juvenile delinquency, insanity, poor intellectual development and moral breakdown in general.[14]

Many of the cultures which Price studied had not the luxury of eating more than they needed to survive. However, in modern Western culture, many people apparently operate on the faulty premise that if a little is good, more is better. Based on this, people may harm themselves with excessive amounts of things that would have been fine for them in more moderate quantities. Overconsumption of the given item may be harmful itself, but just as importantly, its overconsumption may lead to inadequate consumption of other essential factors. A person might benefit, for example, from a daily glass of fresh organic carrot juice. Yet if they consume five liters per day on a long term basis, they may cause damage to themselves in several ways. The excessive amounts of sugar may be far more than their adrenals and pancreas can handle without damage. And as a consequence of drinking all the carrot juice they may simply not consume enough other food to meet their other numerous nutritional needs.

Many people operate on the equally faulty premise that if an excess is bad, none is better. Based on this, people may harm themselves by completely avoiding foods that, although detrimental in excess, are fine and indeed necessary in moderate amounts. For instance, a person might understand that excessive quantities of protein, when poorly digested due to weak digestion, can lead to various difficulties. One of these would be a tendency towards the body becoming quite toxic as well as poorly nourished at the cellular level. With this basic understanding, a person might start to see protein as the problem, rather than recognizing that the true problem is poor protein digestion. As such, they might severely restrict their protein intake, in the hopes of avoiding higher levels of toxicity. One likely result of such an approach is protein deficiency. And in this state of protein deficiency, their body's systems of elimination will function even more poorly, resulting in an even higher level of toxicity. Both of these faulty premises are commonly found at the level where we can only perceive things in black and white terms—everything must be either good or bad. We therefore eat large amounts of whatever is good and avoid whatever is bad.

If we move beyond such black and white thinking, we may instead consider protein as a powerful and necessary component of our diets, to be taken in moderate amounts. (See Chapter Nine.) The same applies to *source* of protein. Price's work provides convincing evidence for the benefits of animal protein (as well as animal fats), yet much available evidence suggests that excessive consumption of animal products is detrimental to our health in numerous ways. As such, protein from animal products should be consumed in small quantities only.

Price's findings also suggest that when we make modifications in our own diet, it would be wise and prudent not simply to observe the results of such changes over the first few days, weeks or months, but to consider a much longer time frame. What are the consequences of a particular diet over a period of years or decades? If we are to have children, what are the consequences for these as yet unconceived children? If a particular diet seems to work over the short run for an adult, does that mean that it is adequate for a growing child or for a pregnant and/or lactating mother?[15] These questions are not always easily answered, and yet the consequences of proceeding in ignorance may be enormous and enduring for all concerned.

The Choice to Follow a Vegan Diet

THE LONG-TERM CONSEQUENCES OF DIETARY CHOICES MUST BE CARE-fully considered, even when we have the best of reasons, such as when we believe a vegan diet to be best. Some have suggested that it may be necessary to make the transition to a vegan diet over a period of several years. But perhaps even several years is far too much, too soon. In most cases, our ancestors have been eating animal products for thousands of years or more. It may take many generations (or longer) to make a successful transition to a vegan diet. Edmond B. Szekely is known to many as the translator of the *Essene Gospel of Peace* and the founder of the International Biogenic Society. In his book *Medicine Tomorrow,* Szekely makes the following comment that we might well consider in this regard.

> The older the phase of our ancestor's life the weaker is its influence on our life, while the nearer it is to us in time, the greater is the force which it exercises upon us.
>
> Present man is carnivorous, having eaten cooked foods for the last few thousand years. Our ancestors have transmitted these habits to us and so they exercise a hereditary reflex on our nervous and muscular systems. On the other hand, the structure of our teeth and the digestive system have a close affinity with the fruit-eating simian races and are totally different from those of carnivorous animals. These hereditary factors always have a great force or influence in our organism. We can say that the *structure* of our organism is inherited by us from remote ancestors who were fruit-eating and living in forests; while the *functional* activ-

ity of these organs is inherited from our ancestors of the last few thousand years who had the custom of eating meat and cooked food.

So there is a contradiction in the present human organism. Structurally we are vegetarians, while functionally we are carnivorous and omnivorous. This contradiction in the human organism necessitates a solution. For contradictions in the human organism destroy life just as contradictions in human society cannot continue for long without causing the destruction of the social organism. There are therefore serious biological reasons and facts which necessitate that we should solve the grave biological and physiological contradiction in our organism—the contradiction between its structure and function.[16]

Many of us have aspired or adhered to a diet free of animal products. Some of us have done this in the belief that this was ideal from a health perspective. Others have done this for ethical or spiritual reasons, whether individual or the tenets of a particular faith. Many have done it for both of these reasons, and perhaps others that do not fit neatly into either category. For some it is difficult to separate the two—health and spirituality are perceived as part of the same package. Many, myself included, have at one time been quite adamant that we would never eat flesh foods again.

Yet is it possible to produce ideally healthy offspring on a vegan diet? I once thought so, but Price's work calls this into question. For many, the issue goes far beyond health and goes to the very core of their spiritual beliefs as to the sanctity of all life, and principles of nonviolence. Yet as my friend Kyle Grimshaw-Jones N.D. has noted, is it not violence to our own offspring to provide them with bodies of an inferior quality due to our own inadequate nutrition prior to their conception, gestation and birth? (As Kyle correctly points out, the baby's body is made from the mother's blood, and her blood in turn is made from the food she herself consumes both prior to conception and throughout the pregnancy.) Is it not also violence to raise them on a diet that is not adequate for their bodies and minds to develop to their full capacity? Consider again the list of defects that according to Price are typically due to inadequate parental nutrition: hare-lip, cleft palate, narrow hips, narrow face, constricted nostrils, mental backwardness, juvenile delinquency, skull defects of the face and the floor of the brain, brain defects, mongoloidism, idiocy, etc.[17]

Some who weigh all of the above questions and more might consider that the ideal diet for them may vary over the course of their life. They may choose a vegan diet after their own children have been conceived, born, and nursed. Some parents may then follow a vegan diet, while raising their children on a diet containing some animal products. This is one option of many.

Perhaps a particular type of diet is helpful and even necessary up to a certain level of progression, whether physically or spiritually. Yet this same diet might eventually impede further progression. As noted by my friend Graham Bennett (in a personal letter), "it is well worth considering that any diet may be uplifting to a point but then it may also become limiting, holding us to the level of progression we have reached. It would then be necessary to change the diet to continue evolving or moving in an evolutionary direction."

We might further consider that it is not simply what we do that is important, but the attitude with which we do it. That is, our attitudes are at least as important as our actions. One person might be completely unwilling, from a standpoint of intense resistance, to consume any animal products. Another person, from an equally intense level of resistance, might be totally unwilling to abstain from animal products. In these two extreme cases, what might be most uplifting for each one might be the exact opposite of what might be best for the other. Another individual, after many years of strict veganism, might feel very proud of this, quite attached to it, and devastated by inadvertently consuming some animal product. This person might feel superior to people who are not vegan, and look down upon them. A vegan individual might have a huge resistance to their friends and loved ones not being vegan. Or a person who consumes animal products might feel threatened or upset if those around them choose to be vegan. Many married couples have experienced considerable strain, for example, when one of the two decides to be a vegan and other does not. There are numerous other examples of the resistances we might have with regard to our own choices or the choices others make in this area.

Are we perfectly willing to be vegan? Are we perfectly willing to not be vegan? Are we perfectly willing for others to be vegan? Are we perfectly willing for others to consume animal products? I would suggest that unless we can answer yes to each of these four questions, then we are not really capable of free agency in this matter ourselves. And as a result, whatever choices we sincerely believe we are making in this area are simply reactions born of resistance, however well justified they may appear to us.

What is the path of wisdom in this matter? I think each of us must find it for ourselves, yet we may have an easier time in doing so when we are endowed with a wealth of knowledge. Certainly there is much to be gained from the experiences of others. It is difficult to refute the research of Weston Price. And to ignore this monumental contribution merely because it does not fit neatly into the comfort zones we have created with various nutritional and/or ethical dogmas would be mere foolishness. Weston Price's work is deserving of our sincere and prayerful consideration as we chart the course not just for our own life but perhaps for that of future generations.

Conclusion

Nutrition and Physical Degeneration IS TIMELESS IN THAT EVEN SIXTY years after publication it remains an enduring classic. It is also timely in that Price's message to modern man on the catastrophic effects of a "civilized" or processed food diet on our own health and that of future generations is of increasing relevance to our present circumstances. The average civilized diet of the 1930s, as poor as Price's research showed it to be when compared to the diets of various isolated groups of that time, was still probably vastly superior to that of our own time. For despite the extensive consumption of white flour, white sugar, vegetable fats, canned foods, etc. of that time, many more nutritional nightmares have come on the scene since Price's time. This actually makes his research ever more relevant and crucial if we as a race are to avoid extinction simply through infertility alone. Since Price's time, chemical farming has become the rule rather than the exception; atomic weapons and nuclear power have contaminated the food chain; fast foods and convenience foods of all sorts have largely replaced meals prepared at home from whole ingredients in most households; microwaved foods are consumed widely; food irradiation has come on the scene; numerous toxic food additives have been introduced and are used extensively; many new and deleterious food processing techniques have come into usage; genetically modified foods are now a fact of life; and on and on.

To conclude with some of Price's own thoughts on the matter: "My studies of the primitive races in various stages of modernization show that the causes of our degeneration are due to our failure to obey nature's fundamental laws of life and that all our qualities, physical, mental and moral are primarily determined by the adequateness of our nutrition. This means that the parents must have proper preconception nutrition, the mother adequate prenatal nutrition to be followed, of course, by correct nutrition for the entire family. Our modern degenerative diseases are both an expression of and a measure for our dilemma."[18]

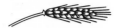

Chapter Nine

Getting the Most Out of Our Food

*Well done thou good and faithful servant: thou hast been faith-
    ful over a few things,
I will make thee ruler over many things: enter thou into the joy
    of thy lord.*

Matthew 25:21

O NE OF THE MORE OBVIOUS PURPOSES OF FOOD CONSUMPTION IS
to meet the body's needs for essential nutrients as well as its energy
requirements. What these essential nutrients are will be discussed
in the next chapter. Yet four areas of concern need to be addressed first
because each has quite an influence upon whether or not the foods we eat
actually meet the body's needs for essential nutrients as well as energy.

The first concern is the *quality* of the food. Many people are familiar
with tables listing the nutrients contained in various common foods. Yet
for any given food item, there can be great variation in quality from one
source to the next. The nutrient values in these tables may bear little relation to the foods actually consumed. Plants will vary greatly in nutrient
content according to the soil they are grown in as well as many other factors. Animal products will vary considerably in quality depending upon
what the animal has been fed. And even a highly nutritious food may not
be of high quality after it has been subjected to various modern techniques
of food processing. The transportation and storage of foods raise addi-

tional concerns related to the quality of what we end up eating.

The second concern is the *quantity* of food we consume at a given time. Health and longevity are influenced to a substantial degree not just by food quality but by food quantity.

The third concern is the *timing and frequency of our food consumption* as well as the *combinations of foods* we consume at a given meal. The amount of time we allow between meals can have a significant impact upon our digestion and various other body functions. And the value and impact of different foods can be influenced by their combination with other foods. When we eat during the day can also have a big impact upon our digestion and elimination.

The fourth concern is the *assimilation* of food. It is not, after all, what we ingest that will nourish us, but what we actually manage to assimilate. Each of these four concerns plays an important role in our health.

Food Quality

Soil Quality

One major influence upon the nutrient quality of most plant foods is the quality of the soil in which it is grown. The nutrients found in most animal products are also derived from plant sources if we consider the food chain, which means that the nutrient quality of most animal products also depends upon soil quality. So it is safe to say that soil quality plays a substantial role in the quality of most plant and animal foods we consume.

Mineral Content

Deficient soil cannot help but produce deficient plants as well as deficient animals. Unlike marine plants and animals, which come from a mineral rich environment, land plants and land animals produced on mineral deficient soil will tend to be mineral deficient.[1]

A major obstacle to obtaining adequate levels of minerals from the food we eat is that most of our modern food supply is grown in mineral-depleted soil. One way to substantially elevate the quantity of minerals occurring in the diet without resorting to mineral supplements is to consume large quantities of sea vegetables as well as other sea foods. Another is to grow much

---

of our own food in soil that has been remineralized using extremely fine rock dust as taught by John Hamaker and Don Weaver in *The Survival of Civilization*. They conducted an experiment comparing the mineral contents of corn grown with conventional methods versus food grown on freshly mineralized soil. Results indicate that conventional methods were producing mineral deficient crops, with the mineralized corn being richer in phosphorous, potassium, calcium, and magnesium.[2]

Results of a more extensive experiment by another team showed that conventional chemical methods diminished mineral content.

> ... in a four year study in which 1,000 crop samples were taken from farms in eleven midwestern states, samples were analyzed for their levels of calcium, phosphorous, potassium, sodium, magnesium, iron, copper, zinc and manganese. The following year, 1,000 new crop samples were taken and analyzed. This procedure was repeated again for the next two years. When the data from the four year study were tabulated, there was an unmistakable decline in the trace mineral contents. To illustrate, in corn, calcium dropped 41%, phosphorous 8%, potassium 28%, sodium 55%, magnesium 22%, iron 26%, copper 68%, zinc 10% and manganese 34%.
>
> Frequently the loss of these minerals in the soil and plants can be related to health problems in man as indicated by the United States Department of Agriculture.[3]

Weston Price also provides some interesting data on the mineral deficiencies of agricultural soil and the adverse impact this has upon our health. In *Nutrition and Physical Degeneration* Price made a particular study of the quality of butter, and he was able to demonstrate a clear difference in the nutrient quality of butter at various times of the year. In particular, nutrient quality of the butter was strongly influenced by sunlight because as chlorophyll content peaked in the grass the cows were eating, the nutrient quantity of their milk also markedly increased.

Different theories explain why our agricultural soils are so mineral deficient. Some place the primary blame upon modern farming practices and consequent soil erosion. Others suggest that the gradual exhaustion of soil fertility is an inevitable consequence of agriculture. While modern farming methods may speed up the process of soil depletion, throughout known human history the fall of most civilizations has closely paralleled the destruction of their topsoil. There are few civilizations in human history which appear to have succeeded in maintaining their soil fertility for more than a few centuries.

SUSCEPTIBILITY TO PESTS

Plants grown in mineral deficient soil will not simply be deficient in minerals, but also less vital than plants grown in healthy soils, and as such, deficient in many other nutrients as well. One sign of this lack of vitality will be their increased susceptibility to pests. This is illustrated by the relationship of wolves and caribou. The caribou are preyed upon by the wolves. It is clear how the wolves benefit from this, for they get to eat. Yet the caribou also benefit as a species, for the wolves will catch the slowest and least fit of the caribou, and this means the more fit are more likely to survive and reproduce. Thus, the long term vitality of the caribou as a species benefits from the predation by the wolves.[4]

A similar relationship exists between plants and their pests. The pests will tend to consume those plants of a given species that are of lowest vitality. While plants cannot run from their pests as the more fit caribou run from the wolves, a healthy plant has mechanisms for defending itself from insects. For instance, sugar content of a plant is somewhat proportional to mineral content of the soil in which it is grown. The plant grown in better soil will have a higher mineral content than a similar plant grown in poorer soil. An insect may be able to eat the plant of lower sugar content without harm. Yet if it eats the plant with higher sugar content, digesting it can produce high enough alcohol levels to kill the insect. Healthy plants can also produce sufficient amounts of substances that serve as natural pesticides. For these reasons, the pests will tend to devour the less vital plants of a given species. It can be argued that the insect pests thereby serve the plants in much the same way as the wolves serve the caribou.

We could learn a bit from these insect pests. If our food crops are being decimated by pests year after year, such that we must depend upon heavy and continued use of pesticides, we are being given a clear message. These crops are of poor quality and low vitality: weaklings, unfit for human consumption. If we had a bit of sense, we might consider thanking the pests for alerting us to this calamity. But instead, we simply shoot (or poison) the messenger. If we improved the health of our soil, the vast majority of our crops would survive. And that small portion of the crop that went to the bugs would simply be the least vital, the portion we would be better off not eating anyway. Our health would be benefited by the pests consuming these weaklings, and the health of subsequent crops would also benefit, as these less vital plants would not bear seed.

Soil Microbes

Soil quality is not simply a question of its mineral content and ability to produce vital plants. Another factor is the presence of soil microbes. Healthy soil has an abundance of beneficial soil microbes in much the same manner as a healthy digestive tract has an abundance of beneficial microbes which play a huge and vital role in human nutrition in terms of our digestion, assimilation and elimination. In a similar fashion, soil microbes play a vital role in maintaining the health of the soil and in making many of the nutrients in the soil available to the plants. It is not enough for the minerals to be present in the soil. They must be taken up by the plants. In the absence of soil microbes, this process is greatly hindered.

Our own friendly microbes are often destroyed through the use of antibiotics and other pharmaceutical (petrochemical) medications, and when these microbes are not present in sufficient quantities, our own nutrition can suffer greatly. In a similar manner, beneficial microbes in the soil may be destroyed by petrochemical fertilizers, pesticides and herbicides.[5] As a result of the decimation of the soil microbe population, what mineral content is still found in the soil may be unavailable to the plants. Hence, mineral deficient crops can result not just from soil deficient in minerals, but also from soil lacking in microbes. The enzyme activity of beneficial microbes plays a tremendous role in nourishing plants as well as humans and animals.

Elimination, of course, is also hindered in humans and animals as a result of the destruction of beneficial microbes. An analogous situation exists in the soil with plants. Many toxins of various sorts end up in the soil, probably more so now than in the past. One of the primary mechanisms of soil detoxification is the activity of the soil microbes and their enzymes, whereby many toxins are broken down into harmless substances. The soil is purified in this manner, and the plants grown in it will not absorb these toxins. On the other hand, the destruction of the soil microbes leaves these toxins in the soil, and hence that much more likely to end up in the crops grown in that soil or in our water supply.

FOOD PROCESSING

Another significant factor related to food quality is various modern food processing techniques. In the interest of extending shelf life, whole foods are processed in all sorts of ways which result in the stripping away of much of the nutrient value of the original whole food. The end result of many of these processes is foods that are variously described as *skeletonized, devitalized, empty* or *foodless* foods. Modern food processing techniques are fantastic at extending shelf life, but unfortunately, shelf life and human life are not always compatible in foods. As the Price-Pottenger Nutrition Foundation suggests, eat only foods that will spoil, but eat them before they do.[6]

HARVESTING, TRANSPORT, AND STORAGE

Certainly it would be best to consume whole foods. Whole foods have undergone little or no food processing, and as such, we are getting the complete package of nutrients as nature intended. Yet even in the case of whole foods, there are some concerns. Some whole foods store well, and much or all of their nutritional value may be maintained for extended periods. Yet many other whole foods must be fresh or there is considerable nutrient loss. Once most people primarily ate locally produced food in season. Nowadays, we expect to eat the same fruits and vegetables throughout the entire year, and pay little attention to their origin. But much of this food is coming from great distances and is far from fresh after such a long journey. To guard against spoilage, it is often picked at a less than optimum state of ripeness from a nutritional standpoint. With fruits in particular, it is essential that they be "finished by the sun" or allowed to ripen while still on the plant if they are to have their peak of nutrient value. When picked at earlier stages for commercial reasons, their ultimate nutrient value to the consumer is often greatly reduced. The end result of these and other considerations is that even our whole foods may not be all that they appear to be.

Food Quantity

WITH THE POOR QUALITY OF MUCH OF THE FOOD AVAILABLE TODAY, many people are simultaneously overfed and undernourished. When our available food has only a small fraction of the nutrient value that food ought to have, it is entirely possible to consume far too much food and still not manage to obtain enough nutrients. Some might argue that overeating is related to the body's drive to obtain adequate nutrients from food that is so conspicuously lacking in these nutrients. Back in the 1930s, Weston Price compared the nutrient value of the typical Western diet with the diets of various isolated and healthy peoples around the world. "When Price analyzed the foods used by isolated primitive peoples, he found that they contained at least four times the water soluble vitamins, calcium and other minerals, and at least *ten* times the fat soluble vitamins from animal foods such as butter, fish, eggs, shellfish and organ meats."[7] When our foods are so low in nutrient levels, it may be difficult to obtain enough nutrients from them no matter how much we eat.

Food quantity has a significant relationship to health and longevity. Experiments have been done with many animal species (from fruit flies to water fleas to trout to rats) relating the amount of food they consume with their longevity and health. A given species of animal is typically divided into different groups, with each group fed identical food and only the quantity of food varying between groups. One group is typically allowed to eat as much as it likes, while other groups are restricted in their food intake. The results are unambiguous: the groups that are allowed to eat the most will have the shortest life spans and the most health problems. And when there are several groups that are restricted in their food intake to varying degrees, typically the group that has the longest life span and the best health will be the group that receives the bare minimum of food necessary. In short, it would appear that from a health perspective we may be far better off eating relatively lesser quantities of food: "Eat to live, rather than live to eat."

The Right Amount of Protein

While it is imperative that we consume adequate amounts of protein and digest it properly, excessive consumption of protein has many detrimental effects upon our health. Excess protein must be broken down in the liver then excreted via the kidneys. Hence both the liver and kidneys are forced to work harder when excess protein is conserved, placing unnecessary strain on these vital organs.[8] Perhaps this is why people with kidney or liver failure often experience tremendous improvement on a diet low in protein.[9] The excess protein is excreted as urea. As urea has a diuretic action, excess protein consumption contributes to dehydration and all those problems associated with it.[10] (See Chapter Five for further discussion on some of the consequences of dehydration.) It is not simply water that is lost in this manner, but many minerals are lost as well, in particular, calcium.[11] Much research shows that even at protein intakes as low as seventy-five grams per day, there is a net loss of calcium daily even when as much as 1400 grams per day of calcium is consumed.[12] The inevitable result of an ongoing daily net loss of calcium is osteoporosis, for the body makes up the deficit by removing calcium from the bones.[13] Dr. McDougall notes that "lowering the protein content of the diet is the most effective means of restoring a positive calcium balance" and thereby preventing osteoporosis.[14]

The excess calcium passing through the kidneys also contributes to the formation of calcium kidney stones.[15] McDougall also notes that "protein consumed in excess of our needs causes destruction of kidney tissue and progressive deterioration of kidney function."[16] High protein foods may lead to the accumulation of uric acid in the joints, known as gout, as well as uric acid kidney stones.[17]

Given much existing research, it may well be wise to consume somewhere in the vicinity of fifty grams per day of protein, which is about half the amount typically consumed in the Western world. Whether the source of protein is animal or vegetable, excess protein is still a hazard. Total protein intake should be adequate but not excessive, and high protein foods should be consumed in moderation.

Moderate Quantity and High Quality

If our food were of optimum quality, it would be fairly safe to recommend that we eat in moderate quantity. Yet the quality of our food puts us in a bit of a dilemma. For if we can be undernourished and overfed, we will probably remain undernourished if we diminish our food quantity while doing nothing to improve its quality. So the most practical recommendation is to eat moderate quantities of high quality food.

Frequency, Timing, and Food Combinations

Frequency

How well we digest, assimilate and eliminate can be influenced in a highly individual manner by how often we eat each day as well as the amount of time between meals. Remember, "the same shoe does not fit all feet." Some people will do best eating frequently throughout the day, eating five or six small meals, because for them it is quite difficult to go even three or four hours without eating. Yet others might need to eat less often each day, and to allow ample time between meals. While these patterns and tendencies may change over a period of years, most of us probably have a reasonably good idea of our optimal pattern. And it may be a good idea to pay attention to the not so subtle signals our body may send us when we deviate from this pattern.

Timing

In addition to how often we eat, the time of day we eat can affect our digestion, assimilation and elimination quite a bit as well, and again, people vary. Some people greatly prefer a substantial breakfast, and find that they run out of energy by the middle of the morning without it. Yet others prefer to eat very little until the middle of the day, and find that if they do eat a substantial breakfast, they will feel sluggish all morning. Some will have a morning bowel movement like clockwork, but only after they first eat a big breakfast. If they skip breakfast, their elimination may be delayed for hours. Others will have a morning bowel movement like clockwork, but only if they drink lots of water and eat little or nothing for the first few hours after arising. If they do eat a big breakfast, their elimination may be delayed until afternoon or evening. Again, while these patterns may vary over the years, we should heed the signals our body provides us.

However, in general, most people will find that their digestive fire is at its peak during the middle of the day, when the sun is near its zenith. For this reason, it makes sense for our largest meal to be in the middle of the day, though many people's schedule does not permit the time to enjoy an unhurried meal at this time. Most people should avoid heavy meals within a few hours of bedtime.

Many people notice that their digestion, assimilation and elimination are greatly influenced by when they arise and when they go to bed. Some people's digestive system will function far better when they are "early to bed and early to rise." Yet others will notice a different pattern: if they get out of bed early it may actually hinder their digestion and elimination. Unfortunately, not everybody's natural pattern of arising and going to bed will be a good fit with the pattern they must actually follow to meet the demands of their lifestyle.

FOOD COMBINING

Many foods which are excellent when consumed separately do not combine properly. When consumed together they interfere with the efficient digestion of the other. For proper digestion requires that some precepts of proper food combining be followed.[18]

The fundamental concept of food combining is quite simple. Since certain foods require different pH conditions in the stomach to digest, to consume incompatible foods simultaneously will hinder or prevent the proper digestion of all the foods involved. In general, fruits require a more alkaline pH for digestion, while vegetables require a more acid pH. Hence, when fruits and vegetables are consumed together, neither tends to be digested well. While we can be extremely elaborate about food combining, and while there are many exceptions and subtleties with regard to certain foods, eating fruits and vegetables separately is the most basic principle. If fruits and vegetables are to be eaten at the same sitting, it is advised to eat the fruits first and then try and wait about thirty minutes or so before eating anything else. On an empty stomach, most fruits will pass through the stomach rapidly. If consumed on a stomach full of vegetables or other heavier foods, the fruits will be held up in the stomach and will most likely cause needless digestive distress. Watermelon provides a simple example of this principle. Many people have experienced a bellyache as a result of having watermelon for dessert. Yet eaten before the rest of the meal, the watermelon would be digested with ease.

There are many other combinations which might be avoided. Those with strong digestion may be able to consume these combinations with little or no apparent difficulty, but certainly those with weak digestion can benefit by avoiding or limiting such poor combinations. These include combining acids with starches, combining protein and starches, combining different protein sources, combining acids with proteins, combining sugar with protein, combining sugar with starch, and combining milk with anything else.

When acids are combined with starches, the acids may destroy the amylase enzyme necessary for the digestion of the starch.[19] When proteins and starches are combined, the more acidic pH necessary for protein digestion may also destroy the amylase, again hindering starch digestion.[20] As for combining different proteins, each protein may require quite different conditions within the digestive system for efficient digestion. And given that most people digest protein poorly, it is probably optimal not to combine different proteins at the same meal.[21] As for combining protein and acids, the pepsin necessary for protein digestion requires hydrochloric acid in order to be activated, and different acids may hinder the activity of the pepsin. Also, fruits that are consumed along with protein will typically remain in the stomach far too long with consequent fermentation.[22] Combining sugars with protein will hinder protein digestion, and will also lead to fermentation.[23] When sugars and starches are combined, starch digestion is typically impaired, and the sugar will typically ferment.[24] When milk is consumed, it tends to form curds in the stomach. And these curds typically interfere with the digestion of any other foods present. Hence, milk is best consumed on its own.[25] In summary, while it is wise to consume a variety of foods, it is best to eat only a few different items at a time.

Assimilation of Nutrients

IT BEARS MENTION AGAIN THAT IT IS NOT WHAT WE INGEST THAT NOUR-ishes us, but what we actually manage to assimilate. Whatever the nutrient content of our food, it will be of little avail to us if it is not properly broken down in the first place so that it may eventually be transported to our cells. We can do a number of things to improve the availability of nutrients from our food. These include having an abundance of raw foods in the diet, using food enzyme supplements, consuming fermented foods, and maintaining the beneficial microbes in our digestive system.

FRESH AND RAW FOODS

We should eat an abundance of fresh and raw foods. Enzymes and other nutrients are destroyed by cooking, even at low temperatures. Thus, in general a raw food will have more nutritional value than the same food when it is cooked. (There are exceptions to this rule, wherein certain foods are preferable when cooked.) Some excellent work on this subject is presented in *Food Enzymes for Health and Longevity* as well as *Enzyme Nutrition*, both by Dr. Edward Howell. Enzyme destruction can begin at temperatures as low as 112 degrees Fahrenheit, or just over 44 degrees Celsius. According to Dr. John Whitman Ray, denaturing of two essential amino acids (lysine and tryptophan) can occur at temperatures as low as 110 degrees Fahrenheit or about 43 degrees Celsius. Thus, eating foods raw rather than cooked preserves enzymes. Enzymes naturally present in raw food aid in digestion and hence in our overall assimilation of nutrients. However, not all raw foods are equal in their enzyme levels. Some raw foods have only minimal enzyme levels in the first place. Yet others are quite enzyme rich, with a surplus of enzymes that will actually assist in the digestion of others foods consumed at the same time.

TYPES OF ENZYMES

Assimilation and elimination can both be improved substantially through the ingestion of high quality food enzyme supplements (along with our food) in addition to the ingestion of foods that are already rich in enzymes.

Enzymes are primarily proteins, and they are necessary in order for a staggering array of bodily processes to take place. We can separate them into three categories: food enzymes, digestive enzymes, and metabolic enzymes. Enzymes may also be distinguished as either being *exogenous* or *endogenous*. Exogenous enzymes are those which come from outside the body. Endogenous enzymes are those that are produced within the body itself.

Food enzymes occur naturally in all raw foods as well as in fermented foods. And unless they are destroyed first, they are generally available to us to assist with the digestion of our food. They may also come to us in the form of a food enzyme supplement. Whether they come in the form of food or as a supplement, food enzymes are exogenous and they are initially used for digestive purposes.

Digestive enzymes are also, as their name suggests, used for digestive purposes. However, unlike food enzymes, they are endogenous: they are produced within our own body. Basically, digestive enzymes are the endogenous enzymes that are used within the digestive system.

All other endogenous enzymes fit into the category of metabolic enzymes. Thus, our body produces both digestive and metabolic enzymes, while food enzymes come from outside. What digestive enzymes have in common with food enzymes is that they both primarily serve a digestive purpose. What digestive enzymes have in common with metabolic enzymes is that they both are produced within the body. And as will be discussed below, the body produces enzymes at a cost.

When we speak of food as well as digestive enzymes, another means of categorizing these enzymes is in terms of what they act upon. *Proteases* are those enzymes which act upon proteins. This includes breaking protein down into amino acids. A protein is a combination of amino acids; thus, a protease can reduce a protein to its building blocks, the amino acids. *Lipases* are those enzymes which act upon fats, including oils. This includes reducing fats and oils to their building blocks, known as fatty acids. And *amylases* are those enzymes which act upon carbohydrates. This includes the breakdown of complex carbohydrates into simple sugars. Since we typically ingest complex proteins, fats, and carbohydrates, these all need to be broken down into amino acids, fatty acids and sugars in order for our body to utilize them. And these amino acids, fatty acids, and sugars are also subject to additional processing by enzymes in order to meet the body's various needs.

EXOGENOUS ENZYMES FIRST

Foods are broken down in the body by enzymes (both food and digestive). In order to break down food the body will first utilize exogenous enzymes, those found in the food (or taken along with the food as supplements), rather than producing any of its own. The body will not waste its own precious enzymes for digestion unless it is forced to. This is demonstrated in numerous experiments and is well documented in the excellent works of Dr. Edward Howell. One of the main effects of a diet of cooked food, beyond the fact that cooking destroys many other nutritional factors, is that the enzyme deficient food puts a tremendous strain on the body. It tends to deplete the body's enzyme potential by greatly overworking the digestive system to the detriment of the entire body. Raw food, on the other hand, is not only generally higher in nutrients but is also much more readily digested as the body can make use of the enzyme content of the food itself. This greatly reduces the burden on the digestive system and, by extension, the entire body.

The more of the body's enzyme potential has to be used for the manufacture of digestive enzymes, the less is available for metabolic purposes. Thus, the consumption of a diet deficient in enzymes not only results in a poor digestive system, but the entire body suffers. For with a shortage of metabolic enzymes as a result of the heavy demand for digestive enzymes, most other bodily processes will also be greatly hindered.

MORE ON ENZYMES

Enzymes are present in every cell of the body. In order for them to perform their numerous functions properly, they must also be found in conjunction with various other nutrients known as *coenzymes*. Coenzymes include vitamins, minerals, amino acids, and fatty acids. Hormones (which are derived from amino acids and other nutrients) as well as prostaglandins (which are derived from fatty acids as well as from other nutrients) also will influence the activity of enzymes greatly. Hence, a deficiency of any of the coenzymes can result in a functional enzyme deficiency, for without the necessary coenzymes present, the enzymes cannot perform their job. The importance of enzymes can scarcely be exaggerated, for little can happen in the body without them.

As Dr. Howell points out, enzymes are not a catalyst in that their mere presence causes something to happen; they are used up in the process as well. If we are using up enzymes for digestive and metabolic purposes at a greater rate than we are replenishing them, then clearly our own enzyme potential will be declining. A decline in enzyme potential is parallel to what we ordinarily term aging or degeneration. As our enzyme levels dwindle, so does our health and vitality. Dr. Howell suggests that enzyme levels may be the nearest tangible quality to what we term "life force."[26]

Enzymes cannot perform their functions properly without such other factors as amino acids, minerals, fatty acids, vitamins, hormones, and prostaglandins. Yet it is equally important to note that none of these can perform their functions properly without the presence and activity of necessary enzymes. The simple amino acids and fatty acids would not even be available to the body in the first place were the proteins and fats we consume in our food not first broken down by enzymes. Minerals from food are similarly made available for use through the activity of enzymes. And the formation of hormones and prostaglandins in turn is also dependent upon enzymes.

A useful analogy with respect to enzymes and other nutrients such as minerals, amino acids, vitamins, and fatty acids would be as follows: if we wish to build a house, we need building materials. Yet an abundant pile of building materials is not a house, for these building materials still need to be assembled in a meaningful fashion by an intelligent work force. Similarly, if we wish to be properly nourished, it is not enough merely to ingest sufficient nutrients. These nutrients still need to be utilized by our own intelligent work force, our body's enzymes.

ENZYMES AND DIGESTION

Food enzymes insure prompt and full primary digestion of proteins, fats, and carbohydrates in the upper portions of the stomach. This is where the initial phases of digestion occur, as documented in the works of Dr. Edward Howell.[27] The stomach is divided into three portions: cardiac, fundic and pyloric, from top to bottom. Dr. Howell terms the upper two portions the *Food Enzyme Stomach,* for it is here that during the first fifteen to forty-five minutes after eating food enzymes, whether found in raw food or introduced as supplements, will be active and will begin the digestion of proteins, fats, and carbohydrates. Beneficial microbes, whether found in the food or already present in the upper stomach, may also play a role here. Starches may be acted upon in the mouth and upper stomach by an amylase normally found in the saliva and known as ptyalin. Otherwise, all of the digestion in the upper stomach is performed by exogenous enzymes. In other words, digestion at this point is not costing the body anything.

After this initial stage, the food will reach the pyloric portion of the stomach. Here the pH will normally drop down sufficiently to activate the enzyme pepsin to continue protein digestion. This lower pH in the pyloric portion of the stomach may deactivate or slow down the activity of the remaining food enzymes considerably. These may be reactivated as the food then passes into the small intestine with its higher pH.

Enzymes will continue to perform various functions throughout the digestive system. It is also suggested that excess food enzymes above and beyond what is needed for digestive purposes may be absorbed into the body and used in other ways. Thus, a diet rich in enzymes can do more than simply lessen the rate of enzyme loss. It can actually increase the body's enzyme potential.

INCREASING THE BODY'S ENZYME POTENTIAL

If we are to regain health, our enzyme potential must not only be maintained, but it must be augmented. Certainly a raw food diet will do much to slow down the rate at which enzymes are expended by the body. However, it is unlikely that even with an absolutely raw food diet the deficit already accumulated can actually be reversed. Raw foods provide valuable food enzymes that will assist in their own digestion. Yet most do little to correct the already existing enzyme deficiency that has accrued as a result of many years of enzymeless fare. For this reason, certain special foods especially abundant in enzymes, fermented foods, and/or food enzyme supplements are strongly urged for all who desire to increase their health.

PROTEIN DIGESTION

One area of digestion where nearly everyone is deficient is in protein digestion. In addition to various supplements that are designed to assist protein digestion, there are at least four fruits that are especially high in natural proteases. Inclusion of these fruits at meal time is therefore a tremendous boost to protein digestion. And given their abundant levels of enzymes, these four fruits can be considered to be exceptions to the earlier recommendation of consuming fruits separately from more concentrated foods. Not only can these four be consumed with other more concentrated foods, it is highly beneficial to do so. These four are the papaya (or pawpaw), kiwi fruit, figs, and pineapple.[28] The papaya contains an extremely powerful protease known as *papain*. The kiwi fruit also contains a powerful protease known as *actinidin*. The fig contains a protease known as *ficin*. And the pineapple contains a protease known as *bromelain*.

Papain is a powerful enzyme which has the unique capability of digesting protein in any pH whatsoever, thus making it superior to any other enzyme currently known as an aid for protein digestion. Most enzymes work effectively only within certain pH ranges. Given the variation in pH throughout the digestive tract, this means some enzymes will work only in certain parts of the digestive system. Papain will work everywhere. Not only will it digest food in the upper stomach, but it will continue in the lower stomach and on into the small and large intestines. Papain also seems to have the ability to digest abnormal tissue, without damaging healthy tissue in any way. Thus the benefits of papain will extend well beyond its benefits to the digestion of protein.

The late Dr. Kurt Koesel spent many decades researching the papaya in Maui, Hawaii and elsewhere. Besides discovering much about the properties of papain, he was also highly successful in developing a number of supplements which would have a high concentration of papain. In particular, he formulated these products from the mature green papaya. "Mature green" is the stage when the papaya is still green with just a hint of yellow or orange on the skin. It might also be defined as the earliest stage of maturity, where the fruit will continue to ripen off the tree. (If it were picked at an immature stage, it would never ripen.) This is the stage when there is the absolute peak concentration of the enzyme known as papain. The flesh of the papaya is quite hard at this stage, and many find it somewhat unpalatable. A good way to consume mature green papaya is to make a smoothie with bananas and other fruit. A small amount of mature green papaya can be quite powerful, so excessive quantities are not needed. The flesh and skin can all be used by most people. Many people also use the seeds in their smoothies. (There is an extremely important contraindication here: Papaya seeds are a natural abortive. It is best for any woman who is pregnant, might be pregnant, or is trying to get pregnant to refrain from papaya seeds for this reason.)[29]

The actinidin found in the kiwi fruit is also a potent protease. It appears that the peak concentration of actinidin is when the kiwi fruit is fully ripe. It can then be readily cut in half and eaten with a spoon. Some people will experience cracking around the corners of their mouth if they eat more than a few kiwi fruit per day. The reason for this is not clear to me, although I have observed it with organic kiwi fruits that were peeled, so I would assume that it is neither a result of pesticides nor something in the skin itself. Kiwi fruit, like papaya, is used as a meat tenderizer, which is a pretty good indication of its potency in digesting protein. Kiwi fruit supplements with high concentrations of actinidin are also available and seem to work well.

Figs contain ficin. I have not seen much research on the ficin. However, I would guess that the peak concentration of ficin is likely to be when the fig is at its earliest stage of maturity, rather than when it is fully ripe. Like a papaya in the early stages of maturity, a fig at this stage has a milky white sap or latex which presumably has high levels of ficin in it just as the papaya latex has lots of papain. The ripe fig, like the ripe papaya, presumably also has a fair bit of enzyme activity. I would suggest, however, that there would be more at earlier stages of maturity. Pineapples contain bromelain. I am uncertain as to when its peak concentration is reached. I suspect that the pineapple has less enzyme potency than the papaya, kiwi fruit or fig.

Much valuable information on enzymes and raw foods is summarized in "On Enzymes: Condensed Summary and Conclusions" from *Food Enzymes for Health and Longevity* by Dr. Edward Howell, reprinted in Appendix One.

Fermented Foods

Lactic acid fermentation is a process in which bacteria known as Lactobacilli ferment carbohydrates, producing lactic acid in the process. The use of fermented foods has a long history in numerous cultures because of their advantages. The lactic acid is a natural preservative that hinders or prevents the activity of other bacteria that would cause spoilage. Thus, fermented foods can be stored without refrigeration for substantial periods of time. The nutrient content of fermented foods greatly exceeds that of the food prior to fermentation because vitamins are produced in the process, as well as other nutrients. Hence, fermented foods are typically highly nutritious. In addition, the nutrients within the fermented foods are typically more readily available. Fermented foods are to some extent predigested by the activity of the microbes, and this conserves our body's own enzyme supply.

In addition, consumption of fermented foods provides our body with a rich source of beneficial microbes and their enzymes. These will further assist digestion. The beneficial microbes will help to establish and/or maintain our own colonies of friendly microbes, and the lactic acid consumed along with the fermented food will also help to rid us of unfriendly microbes. So we benefit in many ways from the qualities of fermented foods: higher nutrient content, greater ease of assimilation, some degree of predigestion resulting in enzyme conservation, and a source of enzymes, friendly microbes and lactic acid.

Friendly Microbes

The process of digestion is a cooperative effort between ourselves and the various beneficial microbes which exist within our digestive system. Under the best of circumstances, we provide them with food and habitat, and in exchange they help us greatly with digestion, assimilation and elimination as well as maintaining a digestive tract that is relatively free of harmful microbes. Friendly microbes not only help break down our food; they also manufacture certain vitamins and nutrients that were not actually present in the food.

Friendly bacteria can be destroyed in a number of ways. Alcohol in concentrations in excess of fifteen percent can destroy friendly bacteria. Antibiotics can wipe out our friendly flora as well. Many other prescription medications will also kill our beneficial microbes. Birth control pills will definitely destroy our friendly microbes. Therefore, it is a good idea for most of us to replenish our supply of beneficial microbes on a regular basis to assure that we maintain adequate amounts to assure our continued health. This can be done through the consumption of fermented foods and/or supplements which will also supply these beneficial microbes.

A Surprise about Synthetic Vitamin C

Here is a fact that may surprise many people. Synthetic vitamin C, or ascorbic acid, will kill friendly microbes. This was noticed and repeatedly verified by Alan Meyer, the founder of AGM Foods near Brisbane, Australia and a noted authority on microbes. Alan was following an old recipe to produce some sort of fermented apple concoction. The recipe called for apple juice, so Alan purchased a bottle of organic apple juice, and according to the label, there was nothing in it but organic apples. Yet it killed the microbes. Several times this happened. Alan then called the manufacturer, and after questioning he discovered that ascorbic acid had been added to the organic apple juice as a preservative because it kills bacteria and is cheap. Unfortunately, it does not simply kill "bad" bacteria, for it gets the good, the bad and the ugly. Since that time, Alan has repeatedly verified that sufficient concentrations of synthetic vitamin C will kill our beneficial bacteria. There has been considerable controversy over the years as to whether synthetic vitamin C is a blessing or a curse. Its proponents claim all sorts of benefits from its use, while its critics attribute all sorts of damage to its use. Both sides can produce apparently sensible arguments. But based on the one fact that synthetic vitamin C will kill our friendly microbes, it would seem to me that the entire debate becomes quite pointless. Whether or not it is doing any direct harm to our own tissues, the fact that it is destroying our gut flora makes it indisputably detrimental to our health.

The Nose Knows

To be healthy we must maintain a robust colony of beneficial intestinal microbes. We can tell whether or not this has been accomplished through a fairly simple means. Those bacteria which are beneficial to humans will typically have a pleasant or at least an inoffensive smell to the human nose. Those bacteria which are detrimental to our health will tend to have a strongly unpleasant smell to us. So the test as to whether we have succeeded is pretty straightforward. If our gut is primarily populated with beneficial microbes, then our feces as well as any flatulence will not have a strongly unpleasant odor. On the other hand, if our system is primarily populated with bad bacteria, then we typically have a strongly unpleasant odor. Please bear in mind that this is not all or nothing. There are degrees of odor ranging from one extreme to the other.

Many people find this concept hard to imagine or understand; the idea that their feces and flatulence could have little or no odor is surprising. Yet I have known hundreds of people who have improved their diet and taken measures to establish and maintain a good population of friendly bacteria, and then found the odor diminish quite markedly and in many cases become almost entirely absent.

Conclusion

IN THIS CHAPTER, WE HAVE EXAMINED A NUMBER OF IMPORTANT FACTORS for optimizing our nutrient status or getting the most out of our food. Food quality is important and inextricably related to both soil quality and the mineral content of the soil. In addition, the role of soil microbes in the production of foods of high quality has been examined. Beyond these concerns, food processing, harvesting, transport and storage have all been considered insofar as they impact food quality.

The effect of the quantity of food that we consume upon our nutritional status has also been explored. It has been shown that the best approach is that of moderate quantity but high quality of food consumed. In addition, the effect of when and how often we eat upon our nutrient status has been considered. Food combining has also been discussed.

It has been clearly established that we are not nourished merely by what we ingest, but rather by what we actually manage to assimilate. Numerous factors related to optimal assimilation, such as the role of enzymes in health and nutrition, have been presented in great detail. The benefits of raw foods and fermented foods have also been explored. Finally, the necessity of friendly microbes in our digestive tract for optimum health and nutrition has been highlighted.

All of these above factors can be seen to play highly significant roles in understanding as well as attaining proper nutrition. And all of them will have an impact on whether or not we can assimilate the essential nutrients we need for health and healing.

Chapter Ten

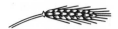

Essential Nutrients and Their Sources

Trifles make perfection but perfection is no trifle.
Michelangelo

On Humankind's Natural Diet

IN THE FIELD OF NUTRITION THERE IS NO SHORTAGE OF OPINIONS OFFERED as to what constitutes the "natural" diet of humankind. Udo Erasmus offers a significant insight into this discussion in his excellent book *Fats that Heal, Fats that Kill.*[1]

> Some nutrition writers suggest that by nature man is a hunter who, since the dawn of our species, has lived on a diet high in animal proteins and fats. These writers, mostly North American or European and affluent, cite evidence of primitive hunting spears, arrows, animal bones, and other artifacts of the hunt found around remnants of fire pits in archaeological sites on all continents. They use historical records of the past to confirm their personal preference for diets high in meats.
>
> Equally vociferous, and marshalling a similarly impressive set of evidence, are writers who claim that man was always a gatherer of seeds, grains, roots, nuts, berries and herbs. Seeds and implements for crushing and preparing seeds have also been found

in archaeological digs. Three-quarters of the world's present population lives on a diet based around vegetables and grains (including rice, millet, corn and beans, buckwheat, wheat, rye, oats, barley, spelt, triticale, sorghum, quinoa and amaranth.) These people consume few animal products. Eggs, meat, blood or milk products are special treats for festive or religious occasions.

It is not clear why these two sets of writers insist that man should have been rigidly one or the other. Survival is a practical matter, and it makes sense that during millions of years of history, climactic changes, and migrations, our ancestors ate whatever they found in their environment and climate. In a state of affluence, we can afford to speculate. In a state of hunger, we eat what we can find and catch.

A third set of writer considers man's original foods to have consisted mainly of raw fresh greens, with some flowers, fruits and roots, and an occasional inadvertent supplement of underleaf insect eggs or worm. Gorillas, chimpanzees, and orangutans live on such foods. This kind of diet required no tools or fire, and would have left little archaeological evidence of its existence.[2]

Rather than spend time speculating as to the natural or ideal diet of mankind, it may be more appropriate to consider what nutrients we require and what are some of the best sources of these nutrients. In addition, we can consider some basic guidelines as to what sorts of "foods" to avoid. Within these general parameters, each of us will eventually work out a diet that works well for us given our own unique needs.

Nutrition and Elimination

AS MOST PEOPLE REALIZE, THE VAST MAJORITY OF PEOPLE IN "CIVILIZED" nations these days eventually develop some type of degenerative disease such as cancer, cardiovascular disease, arthritis, diabetes, osteoporosis, and others. Such diseases are so prevalent that many have concluded that they are virtually inevitable. Many supposedly intelligent people have been heard by this author to make such comments as, "Well, we have to die of something, don't we?" It is clear that most people expect to deteriorate into a state of decrepitude, senility, and eventual demise. Yet is this truly unavoidable? An intriguing experiment was conducted last century that concerned these very questions.

> Dr. Alexis Carrell, at the Rockefeller Institute for Medical Research, took small pieces of heart tissue from a chicken embryo to produce one of the most remarkable experiments in medical history. He attempted to demonstrate that under suitable conditions, the living cell could live a very long time, perhaps indefinitely.
>
> The heart tissue was immersed in a nutrient solution from which it obtained its food. Likewise, waste material was secreted into this same solution. Everyday the solution was changed, taking away waste substances and providing fresh nutrients. It is amazing to report that this chicken heart tissue lived for 29 years in this fashion. It died one day when the assistant forgot to change the metabolized polluted fluid! In other words, autointoxication claimed this great masterpiece of experimental scientific investigation.
>
> Said Carrell of this experience, "The cell is immortal. It is merely the fluid in which it floats which degenerates. Renew this fluid at intervals, give the cell something upon which to feed and, so far as we know, the pulsation of life may go on forever."[3]

This experiment suggests that the cell has an extraordinary ability to continually renew and repair itself under the right conditions. Among these conditions two are fundamental: supply of nutrients must be continually assured, and wastes must be removed. When we extend these basic concepts to embrace the greater organism, we see that this simplicity is ever-present: we must have adequate and proper nutrition, and we must have proper elimination. Whether we are capable of immortality is open to speculation. Yet clearly we need not degenerate as inevitably or as rapidly as is typical today. If we can nourish our bodies and eliminate our wastes, then a much longer and healthier lifespan will be the result.[4]

Essential Nutrients

TWO BASIC CRITERIA DEFINE A PARTICULAR NUTRIENT AS ESSENTIAL. THE FIRST is that the body requires this nutrient for the maintenance of health and for its proper function. The second is that the body cannot make this nutrient itself. (Some will modify this second criterion to include nutrients that the body can manufacture, but not in sufficient quantities to meet its own needs.) Simply put, an essential nutrient is needed by the body, and must ordinarily be supplied from without. (Some might also note that essential nutrients may be supplied from within by our microbes.)

At least forty-five to fifty essential nutrients are currently known. These include eight to ten amino acids, two essential fatty acids, twenty or more minerals, and fifteen or more vitamins, with the possibility that nutritional factors as yet unknown may also be essential.[5] The absence of one particular essential nutrient may also interfere with the utilization and effectiveness of other essential nutrients which are present. Thus, it is imperative that no essential nutrient be lacking if we are to attain and maintain good health.

As stated previously, *nutrient saturation* can be defined as the state wherein the body is supplied with sufficient amounts of all essential nutrients (including minerals, enzymes, essential amino acids, vitamins, essential fatty acids as well as any as yet unknown essential nutrients) while at the same time making certain that these nutrients are properly digested and assimilated by the body. Nutrient saturation can be seen as a necessary foundation of health as well as healing. In a state of nutrient saturation, a person is abundantly supplied with all the necessary nutrients to enter into and successfully pass through a healing crisis. Let us discuss these essential nutrients, which can be broken into six categories: minerals; amino acids; essential fatty acids; oil and protein together; vitamins; light, oxygen, and electrons.

MINERALS

The human body requires numerous minerals for health and proper function. Only about twenty to thirty minerals have been verified to be essential though a great many more elements may later be found to be essential. It is entirely possible that we require at least trace amounts of virtually every element. Minerals play significant roles in virtually every metabolic process occurring within the body.[6] And as mentioned in Chapter Nine, for a variety of reasons, including mineral deficient soil, many people have significant mineral deficiencies.

Without the presence of all necessary minerals, none of the other nutrients can perform their vital functions in the body. Not only are minerals needed in order for these other nutrients to do us any good, certain minerals are also necessary in order for other minerals to benefit us. There is a vastly intricate and synergistic relationship between all essential nutrients such that the absence or shortage of any mineral can hinder the effectiveness of an amazing array of bodily processes too vast to enumerate here.

Minerals can exist in a number of distinct forms, some of which are of greater use to the human body, and others less useful or even harmful. Two forms of particular relevance are *chelated* and *colloidal*. These are distinct forms, and a mineral may be either, neither, or both. A chelated mineral may be said to be organic. An inorganic mineral is rendered organic by plants through the process of chelation. This means that the mineral is surrounded by a ring of hydrolyzed protein. In this organic or chelated form, it may be highly useful to the body. These chelated minerals are then made available to the body through the process of digestion.

A mineral that has been naturally chelated by a plant is highly beneficial to the body, but a mineral that has been chelated synthetically is a different matter. These appear to be useless and perhaps even detrimental to the body, despite their widespread use today. The human body may have some ability to chelate minerals itself. Yet it does not appear that the human body can meet its need for chelated minerals in this fashion. We need to ingest naturally chelated minerals from our food. A few mineral supplements have been developed wherein the minerals are naturally chelated, and these can be used with great benefit.

A colloidal mineral is a mineral with particle size so minute that it will remain in suspension in water. Typically this amounts to a diameter of less than a half micron. If larger mineral particles are stirred into a glass of water, they will eventually settle at the bottom of the glass. A colloidal particle is small enough that it may remain in suspension indefinitely. A huge advantage of a colloidal mineral is that it is highly available to the body, for its minute particle size allows it to effectively bypass the digestive mechanism and move out readily to the cellular level. Unless it is sufficiently small to be colloidal, an inorganic or elemental form of most minerals is of little value to the body. According to many, such an inorganic and noncolloidal mineral can be detrimental.

The human body appears to require many of its minerals in a chelated form, and ideally, a mineral might be both chelated and colloidal and therefore immediately available to the body. If we are looking for a suitable mineral supplement, a chelated and colloidal one has these two distinct advantages when compared to the chelated minerals found in a whole food source such as a fruit or vegetable. First, a colloidal and chelated mineral supplement is readily assimilated by the body for immediate use without the necessity of passing through the digestive mechanism. These minerals are available without the expenditure of the energy required for digestion. This helps to preserve the body's vital force and its enzyme potential. A chelated colloidal mineral in a liquid, when we dip a finger in it, can be tasted in the mouth in under thirty seconds. This demonstrates its almost immediate availability to the body. These colloidal chelated minerals are assimilated much more efficiently, and a much higher percentage will actually be made available for the body. Given the widespread mineral deficiencies in most soil, and hence, most food, a suitable mineral supplement is probably a good recommendation for everyone.[7]

Amino Acids

Amino acids are one of the primary building blocks of the body. They are essential for a vast number of structures and functions in our bodies. One of the most crucial of all body systems is our endocrine system. Endocrine glands secrete hormones into our bloodstream. In addition to being structural elements of the body, amino acids are a component of and a necessary precursor for the formation of all our hormones. Hormones are involved in virtually every bodily processes, and these processes may be initiated, regulated, or arrested by the appropriate hormonal secretions of the endocrine glands. In the absence of the amino acids needed for the formation of a given hormone, that hormone will not be present. As a result, the associated bodily processes will break down. Therefore, all essential amino acids are needed to preserve, attain or maintain health. In some cases, a particular hormone may require all ten essential amino acids for its formation. Clearly the diet must contain all essential amino acids in order for our endocrine system to function optimally. It has also been observed that amino acids are used up at a more rapid rate as the body heals, perhaps due to the increased activity of the endocrine system during regeneration.

There are eight to ten essential amino acids, depending upon our definition of essential. There are twenty to twenty-two amino acids which make up the proteins that exist in our bodies, depending upon what source we believe. We need all of these. Those we cannot make ourselves are known as essential, and those we can make ourselves are called nonessential. However, despite what their name suggests, we very much need the nonessential as well as the essential. The eight amino acids that we do not appear capable of making ourselves are (in rough descending order as to how much of each we require) leucine, lysine and valine, isoleucine, threonine, phenylalanine, tryptophan, and methionine. In addition, both arginine and histidine are often classed as essential amino acids for humans, for there is evidence that while we can make each of these, we may not make sufficient amounts of either to meet our needs. Therefore our diet should contain sufficient amounts of these ten amino acids. And as noted elsewhere, since protein digestion is often poor, we must also take appropriate steps to assure that we not only ingest enough protein but that we actually digest and assimilate it. Evidence suggests that overconsumption of protein, when combined with inadequate protein digestion, can lead to a multitude of health problems.

There is considerable controversy in nutritional circles over differences between animal and vegetable proteins. In theory, while all amino acids can be found in plant foods, and with proper combining of various plant sources we can consume sufficient quantities of them, animal protein should not be necessary. But as we know, however convincing or sensible a theory may seem, it is of little value to us if it fails the test of reality. As mentioned in Chapter Eight, Weston Price noted that without exception all the isolated peoples he located around the world who enjoyed relative freedom from degenerative disease consumed animal protein of some sort. So, while in theory we may not need animal protein, in practice it would certainly appear that we do.

It is also highly recommended that we consume an adequate amount of our protein raw. Two of the essential amino acids, lysine and trypto-phan, are degraded such that they are no longer useful to the body at the very low temperature of only 110 degrees Fahrenheit or about forty-three degrees Celsius.[8] On a diet where most or all of the protein comes from cooked food, lysine and tryptophan might still be in short supply despite an enormous consumption of protein. Thus, those who want to be certain that all essential amino acids are supplied in adequate amounts must include one or more good sources of raw protein in their diet.

Unheated bee pollen can be an excellent source of raw protein. The bee pollen must be dried without allowing it to approach the temperature of 110 degrees Fahrenheit. Such bee pollen is available, generally in a loose form. (Given the temperatures normally involved in putting something into tablets, it should not be assumed that a bee pollen in tablet form is unheated.) Bee pollen which has been collected away from population centers and agricultural chemicals is best, in order to ensure purity.

Another excellent source of raw protein is nuts and seeds. All seeds and nuts should be soaked for about twenty-four hours prior to eating. The exact amount of time required can vary with the type of nut or seed as well as the temperature. There are substances known as enzyme inhibitors in all nuts, seeds, grains, and beans when in a raw but unsoaked state. These enzyme inhibitors allow the nuts, seeds, grains, and beans to remain in a dormant or inactive state for long periods of time and prevent them from germinating in situations where they would have little chance of survival. When the nuts, seeds, grains, and beans are subjected to appropriate con-ditions, including sustained moisture and appropriate temperature, these enzyme inhibitors are deactivated so that germination may commence. If still present, enzyme inhibitors will greatly interfere with digestion. How-ever, digestion may proceed more effectively when seeds, nuts, grains, and beans are soaked, and also, this process will liberate the enzymes found within them. The germination process will also change the nutrient profile in other ways, including increasing the relative levels of various minerals.

There are many sources of raw animal protein as well. Raw fish can be made quite palatable as well as fairly safe from parasites through marination in fresh lemon juice. Udo Erasmus points out that only certain types of fish contain human parasites. "Such fish include cod and other bottom-feeding fish that live close to the shoreline, where both hosts in whom the parasites grow—fish and humans—have regular contact. Open ocean fish that have no contact with humans can be eaten raw because they do not carry parasites active in humans."[9] There are also safe and palatable ways to prepare various raw meat dishes, and raw dairy products from cows, goats, sheep, and other animals will also be an excellent source of raw protein.[10]

ESSENTIAL FATTY ACIDS

There is no better or more complete source of information on essential fatty acids than *Fats that Heal, Fats that Kill* by Udo Erasmus, which is a revision of his original *Fats and Oils: The Complete Guide to Fats and Oils in Health and Nutrition*. Most of the following information comes from these books, yet what I will present here barely scratches the surface of what Erasmus presents.

There are two essential fatty acids. All others can be synthesized by the body if these two are present. These essential nutrients have been shown by leading researchers to be necessary for both the optimum health of the body and for freedom from degenerative disease. They are known as omega-3 (alpha-linolenic acid, or ALNA) and omega-6 (linoleic acid, or LA). Along with proteins, essential fatty acids, or EFAs, are the building blocks of cell membranes and various internal cell structures. They are necessary for the metabolism and transportation of triglycerides and cholesterol and for the development and the function of the human brain. EFAs are also necessary for proper function of the vision, nervous system, adrenal glands, and testes, playing a vital role in sperm formation and conception. They boost metabolism, metabolic rate, energy production, and oxygen uptake. EFAs, particularly omega-3, have been shown to decrease growth of cancer cells, candida, and various anaerobic organisms destructive to the health of the body.

Essential fatty acids are precursors to hormonelike substances known as the prostaglandins. There are three main groups of these, known as PG_1s, PG_2s, and PG_3s. Prostaglandins govern platelet stickiness in the blood, arterial muscle tone, inflammatory response, sodium excretion through the kidneys, and immune function. PG_1s and PG_2s are derived from omega-6, while the PG_3s come from omega-3. PG_2s are triggered by stress and they will increase platelet stickiness, constrict arteries, increase inflammation, decrease sodium excretion, and inhibit immune function. Under normal circumstances the PG_3s would keep the PG_2s in check. Yet were the production of PG_2s to go unchecked, serious consequences could result. A lack or deficiency of omega-3 will result in a lack or deficiency of PG_3s. The ratio of omega-6 to omega-3 is also crucial, as excess omega-6 as compared to omega-3 promotes tumor formation. Research suggests that the ratio of omega-6 to omega-3 should be no greater than 5:1 and more ideally in the vicinity of 3:1. A typical ratio in most people's diets is in excess of 20:1.

Excess nonessential fatty acids compete for a vital enzyme known as D-6-D; thus, an excess of nonessential fatty acids can result in a functional deficiency of EFAs. Research indicates the ratio of nonessential to essential fatty acids should be no more than 1:1. A typical ratio for most people is in excess of 10:1, with almost all of the essential fatty acids being omega-6.

Research reported in the November 1986 *Journal of the National Cancer Institute* indicated that omega-3 and one of its derivatives, as well as three of the derivatives of omega-6, were seen to selectively destroy human cancer cells in tissue culture without damaging normal cells. Dr. Johanna Budwig, a German biochemist, discovered that the blood of cancer patients was deficient in EFAs. A yellow-green pigment was found in place of the normal red blood pigment or hemoglobin. Along with certain dietary improvements, she gave her patients three or more tablespoons of fresh flax oil as a means of getting EFAs into the body. Flax oil is 55–65% omega-3 and 15–25% omega-6. On this program, which included no other supplements, she found that within three months the yellow-green was replaced by red, and the cancer disappeared.

Omega-6 is contained in many vegetable seed oils and seeds, the best sources being safflower (75%), sunflower (65%), corn (54%), and sesame (45%). These oils contain only small amounts of omega-3, however: less than 1%. There are few good dietary sources of omega-3. Pumpkin seed oil (0–15%), soy bean oil (7–9%), and walnut oil (3–11%) all contain omega-3. By far the best source of omega-3 is flax oil, which is 55–65% omega-3 as well as 15–25% omega-6. Bear in mind that the ratio of omega-6 to omega-3 is crucial. Most people have a ratio of 20:1 or more, whereas a healthy ratio would be in the vicinity of 3:1. The ratio of nonessential to essential fatty acids is also critical. And again, most people have a ratio in excess of 10:1 whereas a healthy ratio would be no more than 1:1. For this reason it is important to obtain a source high in essential fatty acids as well as being high in omega-3 in particular. Flax oil meets both of these requirements quite well.

There are few substantial dietary sources of omega-3 other than flax itself, as well as a few others such as pumpkin seeds and English walnuts. Including these items in the diet will certainly help to alleviate the need for flax oil as a supplement. Flax seeds, walnuts, and pumpkin seeds should all be soaked prior to consumption. Many people take soaked flax seeds and run them through a blender by themselves or as part of a salad dressing, as they are difficult to chew sufficiently.

Given the relative scarcity of omega-3 in most foods and oils, most people are far more likely to have excess omega-6 compared to omega-3, and the typical problems which result from this imbalance. However, since flax oil actually has far more omega-3 than omega-6, it should be borne in mind that if flax oil is consumed in sufficient quantities in order to obtain omega-3, and we do not consume much omega-6 from other sources, eventually the opposite imbalance will result. In response to this, various oil blends have been created, which by combining flax oil with other oils give a better balance of EFAs. Interestingly enough, Udo Erasmus notes in *Fats that Heal, Fats that Kill* that the most perfectly balanced oil he has come across is hemp oil. Hemp oil is rich in both EFAs, and has about three parts omega-6 to one part omega-3.[11]

Both omega-3 and omega-6 are extremely sensitive to deterioration in the presence of light, oxygen, and heat. Any or all of these will cause oil to go rancid, and thus, of no benefit and, in fact, detrimental to the health of our bodies. Therefore, oil must be manufactured, processed, stored, and shipped in the absence of light, oxygen, and heat. Flax oil that meets these exacting standards has become widely available in many countries since about the early 1990s. Certified organic flax seeds are processed, bottled, and stored in the absence of light, oxygen, and heat using a technology developed especially for this purpose. Inert black plastic bottles which will not react with the oil are typically used. Any type of glass container, even dark brown glass, allows enough light in to cause rancidity. Indeed, of the three factors mentioned, light is by far the most detrimental, causing rancidity over one thousand times as rapidly as the next worse, which is oxygen. Inert gas is often utilized during manufacture and bottling to insure the absence of oxygen. A special technology is utilized to maintain low temperatures (generally below 96 degrees Fahrenheit) during processing. (Most so-called "cold-pressed" oils have reached temperatures of 160 degrees Fahrenheit or more as a result of friction during the extraction process.) Each bottle is typically stamped with a pressing date and an expiration date to guarantee freshness. Once opened, this oil should ideally be used within a month. If never opened and kept frozen, it may last for six months or longer. It should be kept refrigerated, even when unopened.

In the 1950s Dr. Max Gerson successfully used fresh flax oil to dissolve tumors, his patients using about two tablespoons per day.[12] According to Udo Erasmus, flax oil has the following benefits:

- Its omega-3s lower high blood cholesterol and triglyceride levels by as much as 25% and 65% respectively. Its use decreases the probability of a clot blocking an artery and lowers high blood pressure. Omega-3s dissolve tumors, as shown by the work of Gerson, Budwig, and others.

- It will aid in the treatment and prevention of diabetes, arthritis, asthma, PMS, allergies, and inflammatory tissue conditions.

- It is also of great benefit with skin conditions, lack of vitality, stress, and virtually all degenerative conditions.[13]

OIL AND PROTEIN TOGETHER

Good protein and good fat require each other if either is to be used properly. This is perhaps why they are so typically found together in most whole foods. It is recommended that the essential fatty acids be consumed along with a good source of protein, for the essential fatty acids become water soluble when combined with the sulfur-containing amino acids, methionine and cysteine. Dr. Johanna Budwig notes that "it is specifically at the unsaturated bonds in these fatty acids chains that protein is easily incorporated. This fatty acid becomes water-soluble as a result of combining with protein."[14] These water soluble fatty acids are then highly useful within the body, due in particular to their ability to readily reach the cellular level. All animal proteins are good sources of methionine and cysteine, while most protein from plant sources has relatively little of these two sulfur-containing amino acids. Garlic and onions, however, are good sources of methionine and cysteine.

Udo Erasmus uses the analogy of a "life battery" to express this fundamental relationship between proteins and oils:

> Biochemically, the poles of our life battery are the good oils and good proteins—oils rich in EFAs, and sulphur-rich proteins: oils containing many slightly negatively charged cis-double bonds and proteins containing many slightly positive charged sulphydryl groups. On our life battery, good oils are the negative pole and good proteins the positive pole. Between these two poles, our life currents, produced by the metabolism of carbohydrates and other molecules, flow when the circuit of essential nutrients is complete.
>
> In biological terms, one could call good oils the female pole, because eggs and female bodies contain more of these oils, and good proteins the male pole, because sperm and male bodies contain more sulphur and more of these proteins. But both males and females need both poles for health. Present-day diets are usually protein-rich but lacking in good oils. The result of an unbalanced life battery is lowered capacity to withstand stress, easier breakdown of health, and degeneration.[15]

VITAMINS

Vitamins are a normal constituent of most foods, and were we to consume a diet primarily composed of high quality foods, our vitamin needs would probably be met fairly readily. Yet let us recall the findings of Weston Price.

He compared the typical Western diet of the 1930s, which was probably better than the typical contemporary diet, with the traditional diets of peoples around the world who were successful in maintaining healthy bodies from one generation to the next. These traditional diets contained on average *four* times as much of the water-soluble vitamins and *ten* times as much of the fat-soluble vitamins as the typical Western diet. Given this result, it is apparent that if we are to meet our vitamin needs through diet alone, we will need to greatly improve the quality of our food supply as discussed earlier.

There are at least fifteen known vitamins. These are substances which are necessary for a variety of bodily processes. Some vitamins are required only in minute amounts, while others are required in much greater amounts. Fat-soluble vitamins such as A, D, E and K are more readily stored in the body. As a result, daily ingestion of the fat-soluble vitamins is not absolutely essential so long as we receive enough of them over time. The water-soluble vitamins such as the B-complex, C, and P are not stored in the body to the same extent. As a result, daily ingestion of the water-soluble vitamins is recommended. Symptoms of B deficiency can be apparent within a few days, while symptoms of C deficiency can be apparent within a few weeks.

Vitamin A is essential in many ways: for the eyes and vision, healthy skin, normal tissue growth and repair, liver function, the immune system, as an antioxidant, for protein digestion and utilization, bone formation, blood formation, reproductive function, fighting infections, mineral utilization, and numerous other functions. Rich sources of vitamin A include good quality butter and eggs, organ meats, and seafoods. Vitamin A is only found in animal products. Beta carotene or provitamin A is found in yellow, orange, red, or dark green vegetable and fruits. While many claim that the human body is capable of converting beta carotene to vitamin A sufficiently well to meet its needs, much research suggests that this is not the case. It is not possible to convert sufficient beta carotene to vitamin A if our thyroid is underactive or if there is insufficient fat in our diet. Weston Price found that to reverse dental disease in his patients it was necessary to have a rich source of vitamin A in addition to several other factors. He relied on high quality butter for this purpose.

The *B vitamins* play a broad range of roles. They are needed for the nervous system; the cardiovascular system; proper digestion; the skin; combating stress, anxiety and depression; memory; red blood cell formation; growth and maturation; liver function; and more. Whole and unrefined grains are probably the best source of most B vitamins. They are also found in eggs, organ meats, seafood, and various fruits and vegetables. Under optimum circumstances, our intestinal bacteria will also produce B vitamins. Vitamin B_6 (necessary for the function of numerous enzymes) is primarily found in animal products. And vitamin B_{12} (necessary for growth, red blood cell formation, and maintaining nerve fibers) is found primarily (or exclusively according to some researchers) in animal products.

Vitamin C is essential for the formation and maintenance of all body tissues, especially bones, cartilage, teeth, gums, collagen, and the walls of blood vessels. It is also a potent antioxidant and is necessary for wound healing, adrenal function, and lactation. Sources of vitamin C include citrus fruits as well as other fresh fruits and vegetables, and some animal organs. Rosehips are an especially rich source. Vitamin C is destroyed by heat, so these foods must be consumed raw in order to retain their vitamin C content.

Vitamin D is necessary for calcium absorption as well as its deposit into our bones. Vitamin D also plays a role in the metabolism of phosphorous; hence, it is vital for the health of our bones. A portion of vitamin D, known as vitamin D_3 is actually manufactured by the body in a process involving sunlight as well as cholesterol. But the remaining portions of vitamin D must come from our foods. Weston Price found that to reverse dental disease in his patients it was necessary to have a rich source of vitamin D. He relied on a high quality butter for this purpose. He noted in particular, however, that vitamin D_3 alone was not sufficient to reverse dental degeneration, but that other aspects of vitamin D were also necessary. Vitamin D is only found in animal products. Good sources include quality eggs and butter, seafood, and organ meats.

Vitamin E is also an antioxidant, and essential for wound healing, tissue repair, sexual function, circulation and cardiovascular health, kidney function, muscle activity, and normal growth. The more unsaturated fatty acids we consume, the greater our requirement for vitamin E. Without sufficient vitamin E, the amount of unsaturated fatty acids at the cellular level decreases. This leads to a variety of problems with the mitochondria, lysosomes and the cell membrane. Sources of vitamin E include nuts, seeds, grains and legumes as well as oils made from them; quality butter; organ meats; and dark green leafy vegetables.

Vitamin K is necessary in order for blood to clot properly. It is ordinarily manufactured by bacteria in the large intestine. If these are absent for any reason, then a dietary source will be needed. Vitamin K is found in egg yolks, liver, whole and unrefined grains, and in cruciferous and dark green leafy vegetables.

Vitamin P is also known as bioflavonoids. These act synergistically with vitamin C. Bioflavonoids may be found in citrus peels, buckwheat, grapes, and peppers.

As noted above, it may be difficult to obtain sufficient quantities of all necessary vitamins from the available food supply. For this reason, many people take vitamin supplements. However, despite claims to the contrary, natural vitamins from whole food sources are not the same as synthetic vitamins made in a laboratory. Natural vitamin supplements are generally more expensive and of lower potency than their synthetic counterparts. And given that most people are unaware that there is a difference, synthetic vitamins tend to dominate the marketplace. But there is much evidence to suggest that synthetic vitamins do not perform the functions of natural vitamins. In addition, there is much to suggest that synthetic vitamins are actually detrimental to our health. For these reasons, it is strongly recommended that only natural vitamin supplements be used.

Synthetic versus Natural Supplements

SYNTHETIC VITAMIN C IS CLEARLY NOT THE SAME AS THE NATURAL VITamin C. As discussed in Chapter Nine, synthetic vitamin C actually destroys our friendly intestinal flora. However, natural vitamin C will not harm these friendly microbes. In the production of his various products, Alan Meyer has noted that various friendly bacteria require certain B vitamins as necessary growth factors: without these B vitamins, they will not grow. When asked about the use of synthetic B vitamins for this purpose, Alan stated that while the synthetic B vitamins will not kill the friendly bacteria, they will not allow them to grow either. Certainly our microbes can tell a difference between synthetic vitamins and the real thing.

Francis Pottenger's works show that cats can also tell the difference. Pottenger was a medical doctor, and he conducted some remarkable experiments with cats on various diets. These experiments involved over 900 cats and a period of over ten years. Pottenger observed the impact of various diets on the health of these cats over many generations. He discovered that on a diet of raw milk, raw meat (meaning organ, bone and muscle), and cod liver oil, these cats were able to maintain optimum health generation after generation. He called such a diet a *healthy* diet. Other cats were fed what he called a *deficient* diet. This was identical to the healthy diet except that either the meat was cooked or the milk was altered in some manner such as using pasteurized milk, condensed milk, or fortified milk in place of whole raw milk.[16] On the deficient diet, cats quickly degenerated in all regards. This degeneration was progressive from one generation to the next. The experiment could only last for about three generations, for by then the cats were no longer capable of producing viable offspring. With regard to the deficient diets involving milk, one utilized milk from cows fed dry feed without greenery. This milk was fortified with synthetic vitamin D. Yet the cats on this diet developed rickets. Since rickets results from a deficiency of vitamin D, this would clearly suggest that synthetic vitamin D is not the same as natural vitamin D.

Light, Oxygen, and Electrons

BESIDES MINERALS, AMINO ACIDS, FATTY ACIDS, AND VITAMINS, WE MIGHT mention a few other "nutrients" that are often not included in lists of essential nutrients. These include water, oxygen, sunlight, and electrons. Water and light have been discussed in Chapter Five. Oxygen and electrons will be discussed in this chapter, with some additional reference to light insofar as it relates to essential fatty acids, oxygen, and electrons.

SUNLIGHT AND ESSENTIAL FATTY ACIDS

Exposure to natural sunlight is required for optimal health, but exposure to lighting with a spectrum dissimilar to that of natural sunlight can have a negative impact upon our health. Therefore, we should enjoy moderate exposure to natural sunlight on a daily basis and use full spectrum lighting in place of conventional lighting wherever possible .[17]

Many people are concerned and confused about the advisability of exposing the skin to the sun to any great extent. Certainly burning the skin in the sun is not a good health practice. According to Dr. Johanna Budwig, pioneer in the study of essential fatty acids, the detrimental effects of the sun upon many people today is largely attributable to the lack of rich essential fatty acids in the diet and the abundance of toxic altered fat substances. She notes that "the electrons of the highly unsaturated fats of seed-oils, being on the same wavelength as sunlight, are able to attract solar energy, to store it, and according to need, to release it as pure energy, making it available for life functions."[18]

Due to the proximity of their double bonds the essential fatty acids have the ability to generate a cloud of electrons on the same wavelength as the sun's rays. When we consume an abundance of essential fatty acids we are able to benefit greatly from the sun's rays. Dr. Budwig elaborates upon the interplay between the essential fatty acids, electrons, the sun, and photons. "We can store solar energy, and living tissue is capable of withdrawing energy from this reservoir of electrons, according to need. When this reservoir is empty, the person becomes irritable, tired and the limbs become heavy. But we can replenish these reservoirs again by ingesting electron-rich seed oils. These are tuned to the reception of solar energy."[19]

All life as we know it is dependent upon the sun's rays because each member of the food chain is dependent, at least indirectly, upon the process of photosynthesis. For it is through this process that plants convert the sun's rays into the nutrients we may all utilize. Yet in addition to our indirect dependence via the plant kingdom, we may also be dependent upon the sun more directly. Dr. Budwig explains the mechanism whereby we may receive and store this solar energy.

> The electrons from our foods act as a resonance system for solar energy. Electrons derived from foods are real nutrients. They attract the photons of sunlight with their electromagnetic field. These photons—active, energetic, in constant motion, without

which even the physicists say there would be no life—these photons which are on the same wavelength as the electrons of seed oils, that are in resonance with solar energy, operate as the life element. This interaction between the solar energy of photons and the electrons in seed oils governs all life functions.[20]

Udo Erasmus also discusses the ability of the essential fatty acids to store sunlight and pass it on to us. As we move further from the equator to areas with less and less sunlight, the amount of these highly unsaturated fatty acids and their various derivatives will increase in the plants and animals found in that area. And as we move towards the equator and to greater amounts of sunlight, the amount of these fatty acids will decrease in the plants and animals found in these regions. The same type of plant will typically have a greater amount of these fatty acids when grown further from the equator. Thus, nature seems to naturally provide more of these fatty acids wherever there is less sun.[21] This would certainly offer some indirect corroboration of Budwig's theories on the matter.

OXYGEN

Properly oxygenated tissues are essential to our health, and the oxidation of foods is quite fundamental to our metabolism. Much information on this subject can be found, for example, in *Oxygen Therapies* by Ed McCabe. Yet there is also much information currently available on the perils of free radicals and the vital role of various antioxidants. And so the average person is probably confused. If we are to truly understand this, we must consider both sides. Udo Erasmus offers an interesting analogy in *Fats that Heal, Fats that Kill*. Substances such as glucose, fatty acids and oxygen are referred to as pro-oxidants. These are what starts and maintains "the fire of life within us." Erasmus compares free radicals to sparks, and suggests that antioxidants are needed to control sparks and prevent the fire from getting out of control. Some authorities suggest not only using antioxidants, but decreasing our consumption of certain pro-oxidants such as essential fatty acids in order to prevent free radical damage by slowing down the fire. Erasmus reveals the nonsense of this advice by noting that "it is true that we can prevent sparks by decreasing the fire. In fact, the only way that sparks can be completely prevented is by extinguishing the fire which, in our analogy, means death."[22]

As Erasmus notes, we have a tendency to focus upon one side of an issue to the neglect of the other. Oxygen and the fuels that it burns are important. Antioxidants are equally important. If we stray to one extreme and ignore the other, we either smother the fire or have a blaze raging out of control. For our health, we need a fire that is simultaneously vigorous and under control.

INCREASING OXYGENATION

Most efforts to increase oxygenation tend to focus upon taking in more oxygen. Yet the ability of the body to utilize oxygen may also be improved greatly with the ingestion of essential fatty acids and chlorophyll.[23] Chlorophyll helps to build up the hemoglobin, thus greatly increasing the blood's ability to carry oxygen. The chlorophyll molecule is quite similar in structure to hemoglobin, a principle difference being that chlorophyll has magnesium whereas hemoglobin has iron. Whatever the mechanism involved, it is clear that ingestion of chlorophyll can rapidly increase our hemoglobin. Flax oil will assist in oxygenating the body because the essential fatty acids have a significant ability to attract oxygen. The essential fatty acids, due to the proximity of their double bonds (the areas in which they are unsaturated), generate electrons, which in turn attract oxygen. As noted by Dr. Budwig "as soon as two unsaturated, double bonds occur close together in a fatty acid chain, the energy is increased, and an electron cloud is generated in the highly unsaturated fats . . . a real electrical charge which can be quickly discharged in the body, which can be activated, recharging the living tissues, especially the brain and nerves."[24] Also, "electrons have a very strong affinity for oxygen—they love oxygen. That is why they crowd to the surface. They attract oxygen and stimulate our respiration, our whole being."[25]

Oxygenation of the tissues can certainly be improved through the use of nutrients such as chlorophyll and the essential fatty acids in flax oil. In addition, it is imperative that we avoid all substances that are oxygen inhibitors, such as sodium fluoride and food preservatives, if our body is to be thoroughly oxygenated.

The importance of oxygenating the tissues is widely recognized as an important part of the natural treatment for cancer because cancer exists in a largely anaerobic environment. Maurice Finkel notes in his *Fresh Hope With New Cancer Treatments*:

> Koch, Warburg, and others have firmly established the fact that oxygen deficiency and certain toxic substances block the oxidation process, and that in this condition energy is then produced by fermentation instead of oxidation. This is the pathological basis for malignant, viral, bacterial, and allergic diseases.
>
> The pathogenicity, virulence and parasitism of micro-organisms is due to the same blocking of oxidation in these organisms. When normal oxidation is established in these organisms they lose their pathogenicity, virulence, and parasitism.[26]

Finkel also notes in discussing the work of Dr. Issels that "... any substance that reduces aerobic oxidative potential for any cell tends to convert that cell into one that will rely more and more on anaerobic respiration. Should that be a cell with the potential for becoming a cancer cell, then such cells will thrive anaerobically. They become cancer cells and grow wild."[27]

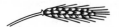

Chapter Eleven

Avoiding Detrimental Food Choices

For every thousand hacking at the leaves of evil, there is one striking at the root.

Henry David Thoreau

W E NOW HAVE SOME IDEA OF WHAT NUTRIENTS WE MUST HAVE in order to regain and maintain health. While an identical and ideal diet for everyone does not exist, and foods that one person digests well may cause problems for another, a few simple recommendations apply to most of us. Besides seeing that we take in essential nutrients, it is recommended that the following foods and practices be avoided entirely if possible. At the very least, their use should be greatly reduced. With very few exceptions, these foods and practices are detrimental to all of us, though the degree of damage may vary from one person to the next. But ultimately, if our aim is to maintain or regain our health, we should avoid the following.

Refined, Skeletonized, or Processed Foods

W HEN WESTON PRICE CONDUCTED HIS RESEARCH IN THE 1930S, HE was able to compare the health of various isolated peoples on their traditional diets with that of people on a "civilized" diet. In addition, he was often able to observe the disastrous effect upon these same peoples as their traditional foods were displaced by modern foods. The rapid and shocking decline in their health has been discussed extensively elsewhere. The main two items that came into the diets of these peoples, and thus were primarily responsible for their decline, were white sugar and white flour. Certainly canned foods, vegetable fats, and other items also played a role. Yet Price noted through his contact with the trading ships that inevitably ninety percent of what was sold or traded to these formerly isolated peoples was white sugar and white flour. I would suggest that the destructive impact of these two *skeletonized* foods was not simply a result of direct damage but that part of the enormous detrimental impact of such refined foods is also indirect. For when we eat these empty foods rather than foods rich in nutrients, our health suffers. The problem with highly refined foods is not just what they *are*, it is also what they *are not*. They are often quite detrimental to us in specific ways. And almost without exception, they are not capable of meeting our nutritional needs. Only with such "foodless" foods does it become common to be overfed, undernourished, and obese. If we wish to regain or maintain our health, we must leave white sugar and white flour as well as other devitalized foods behind us.

WHITE SUGAR

There is not much challenge in coming up with negative things to say about white sugar. (Brown sugar is not much different than white sugar.) Sugar is one of the most harmful items in most diets, and it will almost always be a priority to eliminate this noxious substance. Sugar is present as an additive in the vast majority of processed foods, so most people are consuming large amounts of sugar whether they realize it or not. The average American now consumes over 120 pounds of sugar per year. Sugar consumption per person has increased by a factor of three in a century, and by a factor of fifteen in two centuries. Sugar consumption can be linked to numerous problems including stroke, heart attack, high blood, diabetes, hypoglycemia, kidney disease, obesity, all manner of endocrine disorders, cancer, and nutritional imbalance in general.

Anyone who needs convincing that eliminating refined sugar from their diet is of the highest priority should read *Sugar Blues* by William Dufty and *Nutrition and Physical Degeneration* by Weston Price. One interesting indication of the severity of white sugar's impact upon the body was noted by George Meinig in *Root Canal Cover-Up*. Enamel typically covers most of the exposed portion of a tooth, while the bulk of the tooth substance is known as *dentin*. Dentin contains numerous hollow tubules known as *dentin tubules*. Fluid normally flows through these tubules carrying nutrients to the tooth structure. The enamel also has these tubules to some extent. Meinig notes that "it is this fluid which flows through all parts of teeth and is responsible for sustaining their life."[1] It turns out that the ingestion of sugar has an interesting effect upon this fluid flow, for it actually reverses it! Meinig continues.

> By now many scientists have documented this interesting phenomenon and have demonstrated that the fluid flow in the dentin tubules from the pulp outward is actually reversed when a person eats sugar. In more recent years, Dr. Ralph R. Steinman, Professor Emeritus from the Loma Linda University Dental School, found in studies of rats that the flow reversed when he injected glucose (sugar) under the skin of their abdomens.
>
> He also introduced sugar directly into their stomachs through the use of a stomach tube and had the same result. This showed that, contrary to popular belief, sugar doesn't have to touch teeth at all for its presence to result in a severe amount of tooth decay. These investigations clearly demonstrate that the reversal of fluid flow in the dentin tubules could be created by detrimental nutritional changes which, in turn, would be responsible for severe systemic changes to the bodies of humans and animals.[2]

As Meinig notes above, sugar's deleterious effect upon teeth cannot be attributed to mere contact with the teeth. Rather, it must be related to its impact upon our entire nutritional balance. The late dentist Melvin Page spent many decades researching the relationship between body chemistry, nutrition, dental health, and overall health, and his work confirms this.[3] Weston Price and other previous researchers had noted a relationship between calcium and phosphorous levels in the blood and dental as well as overall health. Melvin Page demonstrated that it was not simply the levels of calcium and phosphorous, but quite specifically their ratio to one another. He showed that a ratio in the near vicinity of ten parts calcium to four parts phosphorous was necessary if dental and overall health were to be maintained. In addition, he found that there were entirely opposite types of dental and other health problems associated with departure from this ratio in either direction. High calcium and low phosphorous had one set of consequences, while low calcium and high phosphorous had another. People whose ratio remained close enough to the ideal ratio would enjoy immunity to dental problems as well as a relative immunity to degenerative illness. And when a person's ratio could be changed so that it stayed within this ideal range, dental problems would be arrested and reversed and overall bodily degeneration would also reverse.[4]

Melvin Page's primary means of correcting the ratio of calcium and phosphorous was through correct nutrition. In particular, white sugar and white flour needed to be removed from the diet.[5] He noted in particular that "sugar disturbs calcium-phosphorous balance more than any other single factor."[6] The ingestion of sugar throws this ratio out of balance, increasing calcium and decreasing phosphorous. Also, "these two things, white sugar and white flour, are the most common and the most harmful items in our diet."[7] As to precisely how sugar disrupts our body chemistry, Page noted the following:

> A brief explanation of the relationship of sugar to our bodily processes may make clear the reason for this harmful effect. Sixty-eight percent of the food we eat is broken down through bodily chemical processes into sugar. Sugar, water, the amino and fatty acids, and mineral salts in solution are capable of permeating the intestinal wall and directly entering the blood stream. If we take refined sugar into our systems it does not need to be changed greatly in order to permeate the intestinal wall. It enters the blood stream in a flood. And as in a flood, someone must come to the rescue to prevent disaster. If there is more than one teaspoon of sugar in the entire blood stream or less than one-half teaspoon, we court disaster. But we are most remarkably built and the liver and the pancreas form a rescue team and turn this sugar into glycogen and store it for future use. Now that may be very

well in an emergency, but think of the abuse which most of us inflict on our systems daily. It is astonishing that any of us are well. [Given that] the intake of sugar increases the calcium assimilation and that resistance to degeneration and bacteria are dependent upon the maintenance of a proper ratio between calcium and phosphorous, you can not but be impressed by the necessity to use this drug with care. As mentioned earlier, nine chocolates can throw the calcium-phosphorous levels out of balance within two and one-half hours and keep them below the margin of safety for immunity to dental decay at least thirty-two hours.[8]

Along with white sugar, all other refined sweeteners including corn syrup, dextrose and glucose should be avoided entirely. And natural sweeteners such as maple syrup and honey should only be consumed in extreme moderation, as they too can have severe consequences on the body chemistry when used in excess.

WHITE FLOUR

White flour, like white sugar, has little to recommend it. Rats and bugs will generally avoid it in favor of whole grain flour. Whole grains are full of nutrients, which is not surprising, given that a new plant may grow from each grain. However, by the time it has been refined into white flour, very few of these nutrients are still present. Even most of the fiber is gone. White flour is perhaps the epitome of the term "empty calories." Some consider white flour to be detrimental in a direct fashion. Others suggest that it is harmless in itself, but that it causes much indirect harm by replacing other foods that would nourish us. This basically amounts to a debate as to whether white flour is harmful or merely useless. In either case, to be healthy we should avoid it, and also its cousin, white rice.

MARGARINE OR PARTIALLY HYDROGENATED OILS

Margarine and other partially hydrogenated oils would also be serious contenders for the dubious distinction of being the greatest cause of disease, degeneration and suffering of any foods we eat. Margarine originally came about as an inexpensive substitute for butter and is typically made from various inexpensive vegetable oils. These oils, which contain high levels of unsaturated fatty acids, are quite liquid at room temperature and thus unsuitable as a butter substitute. However, through a process known as hydrogenation, these oils can easily be hardened to precisely the extent desired.[9] Unsaturated fatty acids have one or more double bonds, at which point there will be space for several hydrogen atoms. If there is one such double bond, the fatty acids is known as *monounsaturated*. If there is more than one double bond, then the fatty acid is known as *polyunsaturated*. At each double bond, several configurations are possible. A trans-fatty acid will be straight at the double bond. A cis-fatty acid will be bent at the double bond. Our body requires its essential fatty acids and other unsaturated fatty acids in the cis-form. (Saturated fatty acids are neither in the cis-fatty acid nor the trans-fatty acid form, for there are no double bonds present. This is one reason saturated fatty acids are more stable.) Unsaturated fats will begin to be transformed from the healthy cis-fatty acid form into the potentially dangerous trans-fatty acid form at about 320 degrees Fahrenheit or 160 degrees Celsius. A trans-fatty acid can be a serious problem for the human body, for it is similar enough to the desired cis-fatty acid that it is often capable of taking up its space. Unfortunately, it is not capable of doing the job of the cis-fatty acid. Some have compared the trans-fatty acid to a key that will fit in a lock but will not operate the lock, and further, it will not readily be removed from the lock. Such a key is worse than no key at all, and we can look at trans-fatty acids the same way.

The process of hydrogenation hardens some of the unsaturated fatty acids by forcing hydrogen into the area where there is room for it. These fatty acids are basically turned into saturated fatty acids. If the process of hydrogenation were allowed to run its course, the entire oil would become saturated with hydrogen. This would result in a finished product that would be so hard as to be useless for most commercial purposes. So instead, oils are only partially hydrogenated, to a certain point of hardness. The process of hydrogenation takes place at considerably higher temperatures than necessary to form trans-fatty acids. Hence, a major problem with margarine or any partially hydrogenated oil is that it contains trans-fatty acids. But all sorts of other altered fatty molecules are also produced. Some or all of these may be as detrimental as trans-fatty acids or perhaps even worse, nobody really knows. For this reason, some refer to margarine and partially hydrogenated oils as *funny fats*. Udo Erasmus explains:

> Trans-fatty acids encourage fatty deposits in the arteries, liver, and other organs, and trans-fatty acids also make platelets more sticky, increasing the likelihood of a clot in a small blood vessel, leading to strokes, heart attacks, or circulatory occlusions in other organs ... trans-fatty acids change the permeability of membranes. This means that some molecules, which ordinarily would be kept out of the cell, can now get in, and that some molecules which would ordinarily remain in the cell can now get out. The protective barrier around the cell, which is vital to keeping the cell alive and healthy, is impaired by trans-fatty acids.... We have to look no further than altered molecules and their capacity to impair, derail, or interrupt the natural flow of energy from molecule to molecule within the body, to explain the degenerative diseases on the molecular level. Trans-fatty acids constitute the major class of these altered molecules.... Finally, the trans-fatty acids disrupt the vital functions of the essential fatty acids...by interfering with the enzyme systems which transform the fatty acids into other important molecules....[10]

Dr. Budwig also notes another important reason to avoid the hydrogenated oils: "chemical manipulation of the unsaturated oils destroys the electrical field, removes their ability to incorporate protein, thereby destroying their capacity to remain water soluble in the body fluids. These fats are no longer operative on the surface and capillary level, i.e. they can no longer penetrate the tiny blood capillaries.... The solidified fats which have lost their solubility and the ability to combine with protein, no longer have the ability to penetrate the tiny capillaries. They thicken the blood and cause circulatory problems."[11]

Consuming these inactive fats, particularly when our diet is deficient in the active essential fatty acids, also harms us because the essential fatty acids generate an abundance of electrons, which is vital to our health. The altered inactive fats lack this ability, as noted by Dr. Budwig. "In the maintenance of the structural integrity of the living cell, the bipolarity—the electrical differential between fat and protein—is fundamental. If there is a breakdown in the bipolarity between the highly unsaturated fats and the sulphur-rich proteins as a result of first solidifying the fats, removing their electrical charge and effectively removing the opposing pole necessary to maintain the electrical potential, then the battery is empty. It is exactly the same as in a car battery. When one pole is disconnected, the current no longer flows."[12]

As mentioned earlier, margarine and other partially hydrogenated oils may finish a close third behind white sugar and white flour in the damage they have done to mankind. Some would argue with this and place them at the top of the list. But how we rank them is not as important as understanding that they are all three nutritional disasters. However, margarine is undoubtedly different from the others in one important way. I think it is the most successful nutritional "scam" or "con" ever perpetrated on the public. Allow me to explain. Few people eat white sugar or white flour out of a belief that they are more healthy for them. Yet people have replaced butter with margarine in response to a sustained and effective deluge of advertising and misinformation that has ended up convincing everyone that margarine is actually good for them, nutritionally superior to butter. And this campaign of misinformation was largely successful for many decades. Only in very recent times are newspapers beginning to report that margarine may not be so good after all.

HEATED OILS

That trans-fatty acids are formed from unsaturated acids beginning at 320 degrees Fahrenheit or 160 degrees Celsius tells us that frying or even baking with unsaturated fatty acids will produce these detrimental substances as well as other altered fat molecules. Thus, it is probably best to avoid cooked fats and oils entirely. If we are going to cook with fats at all, there are several simple recommendations. The first is to use fats that are primarily saturated, such as butter, rather than oils. Oils should not be used for cooking purposes. (A pretty good rule of thumb is that the better a given oil would be for us in an unheated and otherwise optimum state, the worse it would be for cooking. The best raw oils make the worst cooked oils.) The second is to use lower cooking temperatures whenever possible, especially when fats or oils are involved. Frying, especially deep fat frying, is best avoided entirely. When baking, set the oven to about 300 degrees Fahrenheit or about 150 degrees Celsius for a longer time. Many recipes using oil can also be adapted easily enough to avoid the problems associated with heating the oils. In many instances, the oils can be added at the table instead of during the cooking. In other instances, food can be sauteed in water or butter instead of oil. Poaching and steaming are good cooking methods as they limit the temperature involved to 212 degrees Fahrenheit or 100 degrees Celsius as well as lessening oxygen exposure during cooking.

When we consume heated oils, artificially hardened oils, and various other altered or detrimental fats, we are harmed in many ways. One of these is the health of our cardiovascular system. We have been told that margarine is good for our heart because it has "no cholesterol," is "polyunsaturated," and contains "essential fatty acids." All of these are true claims. Yet none of them indicates that margarine is good for the heart. As will be discussed in the next section, cholesterol may have little to do with cardiovascular problems. And while margarine does contain fatty acids that are polyunsaturated and essential, they are not only no longer in a form to benefit the body, they are extremely detrimental. Budwig notes a few of the many ways these types of fats can harm the heart.

> The functioning of the heart is particularly affected by faulty fat metabolism—actually in three ways. The digested and assimilated fats are transported by the lymphatic system. Before the venous blood—the oxygen-poor blood that returns from the body—flows into the right ventricle of the heart, a dose of lymph enters into the blood stream with each heart beat—lymph containing fats absorbed directly from the intestines. The blood that fills the left ventricle comes from the lungs where it has just picked up oxygen. The difference in electrical potential between the fat-laden venous blood in the right chamber, and the oxygen-rich blood in the left chamber of the heart is directly involved in generating the heart-action impulses. This is anatomically evident, and can be studied in detail. If the new electrical impulses are not generated by this reloading with fats, and if this fat consists of

inactive and paralyzing fats, then the heart says "NO"—it rejects these fats, which then deposit in the coronary vessels and in all muscle tissue. At the same time—and this is scientifically established—the heart is deprived of a substance that plays an essential role in the oxygenation and regeneration of the heart muscle. This substance ... was identified in America as "Cytochrome Oxidase," and is identical to the substance that Warburg called "the yellow respiration enzyme." Thus, when the heart isolates these solid fats, indicating that the incoming fats are unsuitable, the beneficial fats required for proper heartfunctioning are also missing. In precisely this situation, these highly unsaturated fats are also deficient in the bloodstream. The absorption of oxygen by the blood in the lungs is impaired, and so the heart has to pump three to four times as much blood through the body in order to adequately supply the tissues with oxygen. The third component is the fact that only the natural fats can be easily pulsed through the tiniest capillaries without excessive resistance. The solidified, inactive, heavy fats cause further obstructions in the blood.[13]

Homogenized Dairy Products

We have all heard the cholesterol myth enough times. Dietary cholesterol causes cholesterol deposits in the arteries, which lead to heart attacks and other problems. And cholesterol is, of course, only found in animal fats. The only problem with the myth is that it is completely unsupported by evidence or common sense. A few salient facts in this regard are noted by Mary Enig and Sally Fallon in "Separating Myth from Truth in Nutrition." To paraphrase a few of these facts:

- As heart disease has increased, animal fat consumption has decreased while vegetable fat consumption has increased.

- Artery clogs are primarily composed of unsaturated rather than saturated fats.

- People with serum cholesterol levels below 180 mg/dl are more likely to die of all causes than those with levels above this.

- Both cancer and heart disease increase with consumption of large amounts of vegetable oils.

- Those who eat margarine have double the rate of heart disease of those who eat butter.

- Vegetarians have as much arteriosclerosis as those who eat meat.[14]

Cholesterol is normally produced within the body and is a necessary substance with many functions. Whether we eat it or whether we make it ourselves, it will be present and it should be present. Where it becomes a danger is when it settles out as deposits on the arterial walls. Arteriosclerosis may be defined as "the abnormal thickening and calcification of the arterial wall ... with the additional accumulation of fatty material in the artery wall."[15] What is little understood concerning the development of arteriosclerosis is the deposits of cholesterol and plaque in the arterial walls are not a cause but rather an effect. The deposits form in response to lesions in the arterial walls. That is, these deposits are a protective reaction by the body to an injury in much the same manner as a scab would form were the skin cut. Therefore, if we would reverse or prevent arteriosclerosis, it is not enough to clear out the cholesterol. We must also remove the cause by determining what exactly is damaging the arterial wall in the first place. A book that should be read by all on this subject is *The XO Factor* by Kurt Oster, M.D. and Donald Ross, Ph.D.[16] According to their research over several decades, a main culprit of damage to the artery walls is the consumption of homogenized cow's milk, for this introduces an exogenous source of the enzyme xanthine oxidase (XO) that is highly available biologically.[17] The xanthine oxidase in raw cow's milk is not in a form that is capable of passing through the intestinal wall into the circulatory system; it is part of a larger fat molecule. But once the milk is homogenized, the molecular structure is so greatly altered that the XO can now enter into the circulatory system. Once there, it causes much damage to the arterial walls. It breaks down a substance known as *plasmalogen,* which is vital to the structural integrity of the wall. It appears that this exogenous XO is a major source of arterial lesions, and the body's response to the lesion is to deposit cholesterol and plaque within the wall. Clearly, then, the consumption of all homogenized dairy products must be halted immediately if the disease is to be reversed.[18] Other harmful effects can be minimized if we avoid pasteurized dairy products or at least ferment them. Good quality dairy products seem to work quite well for some people, and not so well for others. If we include dairy products, they should be raw or unpasteurized. It would be even better for them to be fermented and unpasteurized. (If they have been pasteurized, they can still be fermented, which will greatly improve their value to us.) When a raw dairy product is pasteurized, its food enzymes are destroyed and other nutrients may be harmed as well. Fermentation, whether of raw or pasteurized milk, will improve its nutrient value, increase its enzyme content, and make it more easily digested. Certainly many cultures around the world have utilized raw fermented dairy products from a variety of mammals, including cows, for thousands of years.

Sprayed Foods or Foods Grown with Chemicals

We should certainly eat organically produced food whenever possible. The detrimental effects of pesticides, herbicides, fertilizers, fumigants, antibiotics, and other agricultural chemicals are extensively documented. Eating organic foods is not always possible and is often more expensive. If we are unable to eat all organic foods, we can at the least minimize our exposure to chemicals, for instance by washing produce thoroughly.

Canned Foods

Most canned foods are of questionable nutritional value. It should tell us something that canned meat and fish are less expensive than fresh. If this meat or fish could have been sold fresh, it would have been, for the profit would have been much greater. When it is not of sufficient quality, it can always be put into cans. Much of the nutritional value of canned fruits or vegetables has also been lost along the way. Canned foods (along with white sugar, white flour and vegetable fats) were another of the major foods that displaced the traditional foods in the cultures that Weston Price researched.[19]

Pork

Pork, ham, and bacon are best avoided entirely. Some suggest that this is because pigs have relatively poor elimination of toxins, and that these toxins will tend to remain in the fat of the animal. Much of this fat is imbedded in the muscles, so we take in these toxins when we consume pork, ham, and bacon and so forth. Sally Fallon notes the following in *Nourishing Traditions:* "Investigations into the effects of pork consumption on blood chemistry have revealed serious changes for several hours after pork is consumed. The pork used was organic, free of trichinosis, so the changes that occurred in the blood were due to some other factor. In the laboratory, pork is one of the best mediums for feeding the growth of cancer cells. The prohibitions against pork found in the Bible and the Koran thus may derive from something other than a concern for parasite contamination."[20]

SHELLFISH?

Shellfish present an interesting quandary. On the minus side, there are serious and legitimate concerns about parasites as well as pollutants. Shellfish live on the bottom of coastal areas, and the waters there may be highly polluted, as the worst industrial pollutants are heavy and are thus likely to concentrate in shallow waters. Certainly many religious traditions do make a point to avoid certain types of bottom feeders or scavengers.

Yet on the plus side, shellfish are rich in a broad variety of nutrients. Weston Price states several times that the most physically impressive people he observed anywhere in his travels were the Maori in New Zealand, which is quite a statement given the number of places he studied in his travels. The Maori ate large amounts of shellfish in addition to other seafood, and it certainly seemed to work for them.

Some may choose to include shellfish in their diet, some may not. If they are included, we should be certain they are fresh and make every effort to obtain them from the cleanest waters possible.

Other Things to Avoid

CAFFEINE

Caffeine and related substances are found not just in coffee but in black tea, colas and many other soft drinks, and chocolate. Caffeine is detrimental to the body in numerous ways. The energy boost we get from caffeine does not come for free; we are simply borrowing against our future. As with any stimulant, the long term effect is that the initial problem of exhaustion only gets worse. Caffeine can mask the problem, but only for so long. Caffeine can also create havoc in the endocrine system, especially the adrenal glands. In addition, the routine consumption of caffeine-containing beverages instead of water is a major contributing factor to chronic dehydration with all its related problems. Thus, while it is best avoided entirely, if we do drink a caffeinated beverage, we must at the very least be sure to consume extra water so as to dehydrate as little as possible.

DISTILLED ALCOHOL

Alcohol is a poison and toxic to the body. If that were all, it would be simple to recommend avoiding it entirely; however, alcoholic beverages such as wine and beer are produced through fermentation (in other words, made by microbes) and may be of some benefit. Their concentration of alcohol will rarely be above about thirteen percent as a result of how they are produced. Distilled spirits, on the other hand, have far higher concentrations of alcohol, some as high as seventy-five percent. Such distilled spirits as whiskey, bourbon, vodka, gin, and rum, are best avoided entirely. Bearing in mind that our friendly microbes can be killed by alcohol concentrations of fifteen percent or higher, it is clearly possible to wipe out our gut flora to some extent if these spirits are consumed undiluted.

As for consuming wine and beer, on the minus side, the alcohol is still a poison. And certainly much of our wine and beer is full of chemicals, pasteurized, or of less than ideal quality. Also, we can abuse wine and/or beer just as we can any other alcohol. Drunkenness, frequent and excessive, is destructive to our health physically, emotionally, mentally and spiritually. On the plus side, there is much evidence to suggest that moderate consumption of wine and beer is beneficial to the health. Wine and beer have been consumed in moderation by people of many cultures for thousands of years. Wine and beer can also be considered as predigested foods. They may contain many nutrients, enzymes, microbes, etc. Certainly some of the studies done in France with red wine consumption suggest that this wine contains certain highly beneficial substances. If wine and beer are to be consumed, they should be unpasteurized, free of chemicals, and most importantly, taken in moderation.

Microwaved Foods

Heating foods in a microwave oven bears little relation to conventional cooking. Any cooking will result in alterations of the food; however, heat in conventional cooking comes from the outside in. In the case of microwaving, the heat is a result of friction, and this friction comes from the molecular bonds being torn apart due to activity of the microwaves. This produces all manner of toxic and carcinogenic substances that do not exist in nature, and is reason enough to avoid microwaved foods. In addition, water is greatly altered by microwaving. As we noted in Chapter Five, water can pick up information or energy, and this energy can be passed on to us when we consume that water. This means that we ultimately receive the energy of the microwave on some level by ingesting the microwaved food. It is also known that microwaving destroys a greater amount of nutrients than conventional cooking. Bearing in mind that microbes require proper nutrition to survive just like we do, I once asked Alan Meyer about the effect of microwaved foods on beneficial microbes. He responded that while the microwaved foods would not kill them, they could not live on them either as they did not have sufficient nutrient value.

In Tulsa, Oklahoma in the 1980s there was an interesting court case. Several patients in a hospital there died from blood transfusions. Blood for a transfusion is normally brought to body temperature in equipment designed for that purpose. But as established in this court case, a nurse used a microwave oven to warm the blood for the transfusion. It was shown in the court case that the transfusion of this microwaved blood was the cause of death. This is especially staggering when we consider the vast number of infants whose bottles are warmed in a microwave.[21]

Irradiated and Genetically Modified Foods

The human race has already served as unwitting guinea pigs in a big experiment to test the effects of such items as white sugar, white flour, margarine, processed foods, chemically grown foods, microwaved foods, and others. We have found that eating these foods is disastrous for our health. It would appear that we are currently being manipulated to serve as guinea pigs once again, for both irradiated foods, and, more recently, for genetically modified foods. There has been an impressive amount of consumer backlash, especially with regard to genetically modified foods. Perhaps if the public outcry is sufficient, these experiments will be discontinued. If not, a few decades from now, people will be able to write books about exactly how these new perils affect us, that is, of course, if there are enough of us left around to read these books.

FOOD PRESERVATIVES

Food preservatives are added to foods to prevent spoilage. In most cases, these food preservatives are chemicals that prevent or hinder the oxidation of these foods. Such chemicals, of course, will continue to work once they are ingested and will interfere with respiration within the body. To put it simply, they are respiration poisons.

ARTIFICIAL COLORINGS

The negative effects of white sugar upon the moods and behavior of children are quite pronounced. This is especially apparent to parents whose children consume white sugar only occasionally. Yet the negative side effects of white sugar pale in comparison to the effects of artificial colorings. While brightly colored foods may be more appealing to some, I would suggest that artificial colorings are yet another nightmare. Fortunately, they are one that we can avoid for the most part.

ARTIFICIAL SWEETENERS

As bad as white sugar might be, it is possible that in the case of artificial sweeteners we may have come up with something even worse, which is impressive in a bizarre way. The most commonly available today is aspartame, sometimes known as nutrasweet. It is linked to a huge variety of symptoms as well as a number of deaths. When ingested, one of the results of its breakdown is the formation of methyl alcohol, or wood alcohol, which is highly toxic. We should avoid artificial sweeteners.

ALUMINUM COOKWARE

Aluminum has been linked to Alzheimer's disease and various other problems. We can remove a prime source of exposure to aluminum by avoid-

FIGURE 10: DETRIMENTAL FOOD CHOICES

skeletonized or processed foods

white sugar

white flour

margarine or partially
  hydrogenated oils

heated oils

homogenized dairy products

pasteurized dairy products

sprayed foods or foods grown
  with chemicals

canned foods

pork

caffeine

distilled alcohol

microwaved foods

irradiated foods

genetically modified foods

food preservatives

artificial colorings

artificial sweeteners

aluminum cookware

ing aluminum cookware. Stainless steel, cast iron, and glassware are all better alternatives.

Chapter Twelve

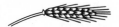

Principles of Eating Wisely and Well

Someone who believes that he has made a new discovery, but as a scientist cannot express it in terms that others can comprehend, has not discovered anything new at all.
Max Planck

Think *and* Feel about Foods

GIVEN THE TREMENDOUS VARIATION BETWEEN PEOPLE NO "ONE SIZE fits all" diet will work for everyone. The previous chapter presented a straightforward and simple set of rules about what not to do. In this chapter, a set of rules about what to do will be presented. Within the wide parameter defined by these two sets of rules, an optimum diet for each of us can be found. While logic and reason may often play significant roles in arriving at this diet, intuition and feeling will play equally important roles for most of us: a balance must be achieved between what we *think* about our foods and how we *feel* about our foods. Thought and feeling will not always agree, at least not at first. But if we enjoy the process and see it as an adventure, the combination of thinking and feeling will eventually work far better than exclusive reliance on either in helping us to regain and maintain our health.

Some people will eat certain foods that they think are good for them despite consistent and clear feelings of aversion to them. Or people will avoid certain foods that they think are bad for them despite consistent cravings for these foods. (I am not talking about passing aversions or cravings.) This reliance upon thinking to the exclusion of feeling is bound to result in trouble. Of course, if we were to totally rely upon our feelings and ignore all reason, many of us would consume prodigious quantities of chocolate and other goodies, much to our detriment. Instinct alone is probably not the safest of guides either.

Natural Instincts

MANY ANIMALS RELY UPON INSTINCTS FOR FOOD SELECTION. UNDER natural circumstances, these instincts tend to serve them well; however, sometimes instincts lead creatures astray. Certain flies will go for sweetness. If provided with saccharine water as well as a variety of nutritious foods, they will go for the saccharine water and ignore the other foods until they starve to death. Melvin Page notes an interesting example of this as well: "A scientific experiment with the sea-anemone, a water organism, provides an amusing illustration of the folly of being misled by labels. Sea-anemone live on meat, but it is the creatine in the meat which attracts them. That is their one sense of taste. However, if the meat from which the creatine has been extracted is placed in the water, the sea-anemone will ignore it, but if blotting paper soaked in creatine is placed within reach, they eat it with relish. They eat the label and leave the substance. Silly, isn't it? But how about us?"[1]

Page poses the question how about us? The formerly isolated peoples that were studied by Weston Price in the 1930s provide an answer. So long as only natural foods were available to these people, they flourished. But in general, once imported foods have become available, the same sad pattern has been observed all too consistently. The physical deterioration of these once healthy peoples has inevitably followed the introduction of processed foods. Despite the continued availability of the local foods that had nourished them for countless generations, these traditional foods were forsaken for the "civilized" foods. It appears that humans will also eat the label and leave the substance.

We humans have instincts much like most other animals. It is all too evident that our natural instincts often fail when faced with perverted foods. Yet perhaps under more ideal circumstances these same natural instincts might serve us very well. We also have a high level of reason, which can be our misfortune or our good fortune depending upon how we exercise this faculty. Through using this power of reasoning to the neglect of anything else we have managed to create our modern nutritional predicament. Yet we can still use our thinking to restrict our choices in keeping with the basic parameters set forth in this chapter and the preceding chapter. And within these parameters, our feelings will doubtless be a safer guide than they might be otherwise.

Eat Whole and Natural Foods

FRUITS, VEGETABLES, NUTS, SEEDS, GRAINS, LEGUMES, DAIRY PRODUCTS, seafood, eggs and meats in various combinations have formed the basis of human nutrition for millennia or perhaps longer. Traditional methods of preparing these foods worked because they minimized nutrient loss and in many cases improved the nutritional value of these foods. Twentieth century science abounds with examples in which the benefits of various traditional practices have been confirmed. Remember that these practices were followed because they worked, and they worked long before science could explain them. However, modern methods of processing these whole foods have a track record that is mostly disastrous. We have strayed from these traditional methods in the interest of efficiency, economics, commercial interests, shelf-life and many other factors. But the most significant food factor of all—the nutritional value of the finished product—has somehow been neglected.

Eat Organic and/or Biodynamically-Produced Foods

WHOLE FOODS CAN VARY TREMENDOUSLY IN QUALITY DEPENDING upon a number of factors such as soil quality (including mineral levels and microbe activity) and the presence or absence of various agricultural chemicals. As we learn to follow our feelings about food, we will realize that we have been able to taste the difference all along. Organically produced foods are a good start, but even in the absence of chemicals, the soil itself may be of poor quality. Various methods of soil improvement can be used with great result. One method of farming which produces high quality food is biodynamic farming, and there are others. Basically, we must make sure the whole foods we are consuming are of the highest quality possible.

Use Fermented Foods

FERMENTED FOODS HAVE A LONG AND IMPRESSIVE TRACK RECORD around the globe. Fermentation increases the enzyme content of food. Fermentation also greatly increases the nutrient value of food. Fermented foods are a good source of friendly microbes. Fermented foods are more readily assimilated, for they have been predigested to some extent. The lactic acid acts as a natural preservative, which means these foods will keep for long periods. And on top of all that, when we do it ourselves, fermented foods are very inexpensive.

Eat Fresh Foods

CERTAIN FOODS WILL KEEP QUITE READILY, INCLUDING NUTS, SEEDS, grains, and legumes. Fermented and dried foods will also keep. For such foods being fresh and in season is probably not important. So long as the nuts, seeds, grains and legumes are still capable of germination, they are fine to eat when properly prepared. So long as the fermented and dried foods have not spoiled, they too are fine. But nutritional value of most other foods will be much greater when they are fresh. For foods that spoil, there is a continuum. They will have a peak stage of nutrition, and long before they have deteriorated to where we would consider them spoiled, they will have strayed from their peak state. For example, we might leave some grapes in the fruit bowl for a week and eat some each day. Suppose on the seventh day we decide not to eat them anymore as we judge them spoiled. We still ate them on the sixth day, although their nutritional value by then was far from what it was the first day.

Eat Mostly Local Foods in Season

SOME SUGGEST THAT THERE IS A REASON SOME FOODS ARE ONLY AVAILable at certain periods of the year. Perhaps such foods are not as good for us at different times of the year. Perhaps some foods are needed at certain times and not at other times. We do not have to go back too many generations to a time when foods being in season was not an issue, for when people only had foods available from their own vicinity, eating these foods was the only option. However, the mass transportation of foods, especially produce, has changed all that. Now we can eat many of the same types of fruits and vegetables all year long, and few will question this practice.

There is a certain wisdom to the idea that our local area will produce the foods we need and at the season that we need them. So for the most part I agree with the idea of eating local foods in season whenever possible. As noted with respect to fatty acids, for example, the unsaturated and essential fatty acid contents of plant and animal foods tends to vary with latitude. Closer to the equator where sunlight is more abundant, these are reduced, while further from the equator where sunlight is scarce, these will increase markedly. But there are other sides to this, and I would suggest refraining from being overly rigid about it. To follow such a principle completely may not be a good idea, if we can learn anything from history.

The healthy people that Weston Price studied consumed primarily foods that were local. But he noted exceptions to this rule. Salt was imported from elsewhere by many societies, and often when it was neither easy nor inexpensive. Price noted in particular that the isolated tribes in the high Andes of Peru consumed fish eggs and kelp from the Pacific Ocean. To obtain them involves a lengthy journey down from the heights and across the desert. Price noted:

> It was, accordingly, a matter of great interest to discover that these Indians used regularly dried fish eggs from the sea. Commerce in these dried foods is carried on today as it no doubt has been for centuries. When I inquired of them why they used this material they explained that it was necessary to maintain the fertility of

their women. I was informed also that every exchange depot and market carried these dried fish eggs so that they were always available. Another sea product of very great importance, and one which was universally available was dried kelp. Upon inquiry I learned that the Indians used it so that they would not get "big necks" like the whites. The kelp provided a rich source of iodine as well as of copper, which is very important to them in the utilization of iron for building an exceptionally efficient quality of blood for carrying oxygen liberally at those high altitudes.[2]

It would seem then that including some foods that are not local may be necessary in many instances, so it would be foolish not to include them as needed.

We must also consider our genetics. Perhaps the local area would supply all the appropriate and necessary foods for those whose ancestors had been living in that area or at least in a similar climate for thousands of years. Yet people whose genetics are vastly different from this might do quite poorly on the local fare. Their ideal diet may need to be some sort of compromise between their genetics and their new environment. Perhaps there are significant reasons besides comfort and familiarity that various ethnic groups will often go to great effort to cling to the foods of their ancestors. In Auckland, New Zealand, where I have lived the past five years, there are substantial populations from many of the tropical and subtropical Pacific Islands. Many of the native foods from these islands will not grow in New Zealand. It is a very common sight in the Auckland airport to see people returning to New Zealand from a visit to their native island lugging large sacks full of coconuts or taro. Maybe these foods provide more than a sense of comfort and familiarity: maybe they provide nutrients not available in local foods.

Eat Raw Foods

THE NUTRITIONAL SUPERIORITY OF MANY RAW FOODS OVER THEIR cooked counterparts has been discussed in Chapters Nine and Ten. It is sufficient to reiterate here that all of the successful diets studied by Weston

Price contained some raw foods.[3] As explained in Chapter Ten, the essential amino acids lysine and tryptophan are denatured at about 110 degrees Fahrenheit or about 43 degrees Celsius. This makes them of little use to us. Raw protein on a regular basis is therefore essential. Weston Price noted that all of the healthy peoples that he studied included some raw animal protein in their diets.

The body appears to respond to the ingestion of most cooked food with a distinct immune response, possibly indicative of the body viewing these foods as foreign. These same foods, when consumed in an appropriate raw form, will not typically trigger any immune response. Additional experiments have been done with combinations of raw and cooked foods at the same meal. So long as half or more of the meal consisted of raw foods and the raw foods were consumed before the cooked foods, no immune response would occur.

For this reason, raw foods should be consumed prior to the cooked foods at a given meal. While raw foods may not be a big part of every meal, they should be eaten before the cooked foods when both are consumed at a given meal.

However, the diet should contain a significant percentage of raw foods on a consistent basis. Some may find this difficult in cold weather, especially if they define raw foods as fruits and vegetables. Yet please note that the culture that has come closest to consuming an exclusively raw diet is the Eskimos, who eat primarily various raw animal products. Again, many people's diet may not reach the ideal figure of half raw foods, but everyone should include a percentage of raw food on a consistent basis.

Use Good Quality Salt

THE COMMON RECOMMENDATION TO AVOID SALT IS A PRIME EXAMPLE of throwing out the baby with the bath water, and it was one that I followed myself and made to others for about ten years. The refined salt that is commonly consumed is indeed a health hazard. This type of salt has had almost all of its trace elements removed, reducing it primarily to sodium chloride. It also contains harmful additives whose main purposes are to keep it free flowing and to give it a nice white color. For table salt to flow readily from the salt shaker, it must be dry. Natural salt will retain and/or pick up a certain amount of moisture; thus it tends to cake. So refined salt is conditioned in such a manner that it will not readily combine with fluids. One result of this tendency to not combine with fluids is that it does not tend to do us much good anyway. In addition, the refinement of salt involves sufficiently high temperatures that the few remaining minerals in the finished product may no longer be of any value to us. Refined table salt is of little benefit and may be detrimental.

Yet salt itself is another matter. With the possible exception of the Eskimos, all traditional societies have used natural unrefined salt. As Weston Price noted, many of these peoples went to considerable efforts to obtain a supply of salt. Edward Howell suggests that given salt's powerful effect upon enzymes and hence our digestion, only those on an all raw diet won't need any salt. And as noted by Batmanghelidj in his research on water, the body requires salt as well as water in order for it to be properly hydrated.

The best quality natural salt is light grey and somewhat moist in comparison to refined table salt. (Do not be misled by the term "sea salt." All salt is technically from the sea, so even highly refined table salt can truthfully use this term. If the salt we are using is white, it will be highly refined.) Whereas refined salt will be virtually ninety-nine percent sodium chloride, a quality natural salt will contain over approximately eighteen percent trace elements. These trace elements are necessary for health, and they will be in a form that the body can use when the salt is properly produced. Basically, sea water is allowed to dry in the sun using basic techniques that have been used for centuries. Probably the best readily available source of this salt is the Celtic Salt which comes from the salt marshes of the coast of Brittany in France.

Deactivate Phytic Acid and Enzyme Inhibitors

AS DISCUSSED EARLIER, ALL NUTS, SEEDS, GRAINS, AND LEGUMES IN A living but inactive state will contain substances known as enzyme inhibitors. Such enzyme inhibitors will interfere with the digestion of these foods if they are consumed in this state. However, if they are soaked sufficiently to neutralize the enzyme inhibitors, they may then be consumed safely and with great benefit. Enzyme inhibitors will also be destroyed by cooking. So roasted nuts, for example, will no longer contain enzyme inhibitors. Of course, they will no longer have enzymes either, and some of their proteins will be denatured, and trans-fatty acids will have been produced if the temperature was sufficiently high.

There is a substance known as *phytic acid* which is found in the bran of all grains. If the phytic acid is not properly neutralized, then the ingestion of whole grains will hinder our absorption of calcium, phosphorous, iron and zinc by binding with them. Thus, eating whole grains in which the phytic acid is not neutralized can cause serious deficiencies of these vital minerals. Fortunately, it is simple to neutralize the phytic acid: soaking grains overnight will do the trick. So will fermenting or sprouting grains. And the traditional sour leavening process used in real sourdough breads will also neutralize the phytic acid.[4] As noted by Weston Price, traditional cultures have always prepared their grains using one or more of these simple methods.[5]

Eat Leafy Greens

LEAFY GREENS ARE A RICH SOURCE OF MANY NUTRIENTS. MANY ARE BEST consumed raw, although there are a few such as spinach which should generally be steamed first due to the oxalic acid content. Greens are rich in chlorophyll. Whether due to the similarity of chlorophyll to hemoglobin or for other reasons, it has consistently been observed that daily ingestion of chlorophyll works wonders to build up the blood in people with anemia. For this and many more reasons, consume leafy greens (including raw greens) on a consistent basis.

Combine EFAs and Sulfur Proteins

AS DISCUSSED EXTENSIVELY IN CHAPTER TEN, THE GOOD OILS NEED THE good proteins and vice-versa. In the same way a battery needs both a positive and a negative pole, life requires both proteins and fats together.

Make Soups from Bones and Organs

MANY TRADITIONAL CULTURES HAVE USED ANIMAL BONES AS WELL AS other parts of the animal to make highly nutritious soups. The gelatin from the bones may play vital roles in maintaining our health. Animal organs will tend to have a much higher concentration of nutrients than the muscle meats people typically consume nowadays. Clearly all predators go straight for certain vital organs after the kill is made, rather than concentrating on the muscle meats as we do. Grandma's chicken soup does indeed have healing properties. Or Grandpa's fish head soup.

Use Healthy Methods of Food Preservation

FERMENTING FOODS AND DRYING FOODS AT LOW TEMPERATURES ARE both effective methods of preserving foods for later use. Both methods do a good job of preserving many of the nutrients, and with fermented foods there is an increase in many nutrients.

Eat Foods That Have a Good Historical Track Record

SOMETIMES IT IS BETTER TO FORGET ALL THE HYPE AND CONSIDER whether a given food has much of a track record historically. If a given food has been consumed for generations by various healthy peoples around the world, and if it is grown or produced as well as prepared in a similar fashion today, then it is probably still a good food choice. On the other hand, if a food has only been consumed for a few generations, we might be advised to view claims about its benefits with a healthy degree of skepticism. Fats and oils provide a fine example of this principle. As noted by the Price-Pottenger Nutrition Foundation, "these nutrient-rich traditional fats have nourished healthy populations for thousands of years: butter; beef and lamb tallow; lard; chicken, goose and duck fat; coconut, palm and sesame oils; cold pressed olive oil; cold pressed flax oil; and marine oils."[6] Furthermore, "these newfangled fats can cause cancer, heart disease, immune system dysfunction, sterility, learning disabilities, growth problems, and osteoporosis: all hydrogenated oils; soy, corn and safflower oils; cotton-seed oil; canola oil; and all fats heated to very high temperatures in processing and frying."[7]

Use Only the Best Types of Cookware

As NOTED IN THE PREVIOUS CHAPTER, ALUMINUM COOKWARE SHOULD be avoided. Some suggest that teflon cookware should also be avoided. The best types of cookware will typically be stainless steel, cast iron, and glassware. Some ceramic and enamel cookware are fine, but there are instances where as a result of poor quality such cookware may not be acceptable.

Use Only the Best Methods of Cooking

WHILE ALL COOKING WILL DESTROY ENZYMES AND OTHER NUTRIENTS to some degree, some methods of cooking are better than others. Lower temperatures as well as lesser exposure to oxygen during the cooking will tend to minimize nutrient loss. For baking, try and keep the temperature as low as effectively possible. Three hundred degrees Fahrenheit, for example, would be greatly preferable to three hundred fifty degrees Fahrenheit. Steaming is a good means of preparing many foods as it keeps the temperature low, minimizes oxygen exposure, and also prevents nutrient loss into the water. Frying should be avoided, and cooking with a microwave oven is very harmful.

FIGURE 11: EATING WISELY AND WELL

Eat whole and natural foods.

Eat organic and/or biodynamically produced foods.

Use fermented foods.

Eat fresh foods.

Eat mainly local foods in season.

Eat raw foods.

Eat raw protein.

Eat raw food first if possible.

Have a high ratio of raw to cooked foods.

Use good quality salt.

Deactivate phytic acid and enzyme inhibitors.

Eat leafy greens.

Combine EFAs and sulfur proteins.

Make soups from bones and organs.

Eat foods that have a good historical track record.

Use healthy methods of food preservation.

Use only the best types of cookware.

Use only the best methods of cooking.

Chapter Thirteen

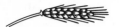

The Use of Supplements

The doctor of the future will give no medicine but will interest his patients in the care of the human frame, in diet, and in the cause and prevention of disease.

Thomas A. Edison

Diet versus Supplements

HEALTH AND HEALING ARE DEPENDENT UPON WHAT WE'VE TERMED *nutrient saturation,* defined as a state wherein all the essential nutrients including minerals, enzymes, essential amino acids, essential fatty acids, and vitamins are available to the cells of the body in sufficient amounts. Clearly this state of nutrient saturation is possible using diet alone: Weston Price's research offers convincing evidence of that. Yet there are certain inherent difficulties in doing so. These include the mineral deficiencies of our soil, the quality of the available food supply, and people's tendency to consume a less than ideal diet.

As for remedying the deficiencies of a poor diet, even the most extensive program of supplements can only do so much. Nutritional supplements are not designed as a substitute for proper diet. As their name suggests, they are for *supplementing* a diet in order to improve the nutritional status of the individual. However, many people, convinced of the merits of their supplements, use them to justify or excuse a deficient diet.

There is no substitute for a good diet, naturally rich in essential nutrients. Should such a diet be faithfully adhered to, the need for additional nutritional supplements would be considerably less than the amount needed when following a conventional diet. However, even the best of diets can probably be improved substantially with the use of high quality natural supplements. A more thorough state of nutrient saturation may be achieved in this manner.

There is no reason that dietary approaches and supplemental approaches to establishing a state of nutrient saturation need be thought of as contradictory or competing approaches. They may be more properly seen as complementary approaches. Quality nutritional supplements can augment the nutrients available in a proper diet, and also certain supplements can greatly increase our utilization of the nutrients already present in the diet. However, supplements are not intended to replace a good diet or to serve as an excuse to continue in poor dietary patterns. Supplements are intended to work in conjunction with a good diet.

All supplements are by no means equal in quality. There are high quality natural supplements, reasonably priced, and also high quality supplements, which due to their price are simply not cost effective. Then there are numerous supplements of mediocre quality. And finally, some supplements on the market are detrimental to health and should be avoided entirely.

The Most Essential Supplements

NUMEROUS TYPES OF SUPPLEMENTS ARE AVAILABLE, FOR SPECIFIC PURposes or roles in the human body.[1] A certain herb, for example, might be intended to benefit a specific organ or gland. Or a specific isolated nutrient might be required for one specific function in the body. Other supplements are designed for a more general purpose, to benefit the body in numerous ways. I have observed over the years that when the general needs of the body are taken care of first, a majority of the specific problems will disappear without any need to address them individually. However, when specific problems are addressed without attending to the general needs of the body, success is often not forthcoming until the general needs are addressed as well. For these reasons, I suggest that the initial focus of supplementation be upon the general needs of the body as opposed to the specific.

ENZYMES

All bodily processes depend upon an adequate supply of enzymes, and to maintain our "enzyme bank account," we must make deposits and not just withdrawals. An enzyme deficiency is a precursor to many health problems, while robust enzyme activity is necessary for the maintenance and preservation of health. All other nutrients are dependent upon the presence of enzymes for their proper function and utilization within the human body. As Dr. Howell so succinctly puts it, "The length of life is inversely proportional to the rate of enzyme expenditure."[2]

While the consumption of raw and fermented foods is greatly beneficial, people should consume a high quality food enzyme supplement that will contain protease, lipase, amylase and cellulase. Protease will assist in protein digestion; lipase will assist in fat digestion; amylase will assist in carbohydrate digestion; and cellulase can help break down plant fibers. Quality food enzyme supplements are typically available in capsule and powdered form. The amount taken can vary somewhat as potencies will vary between manufacturers. In general, one or two capsules per meal is sufficient for most people given the potencies typically available as of this writing. Given the tremendous role enzymes play in the body, a food enzyme supplement should probably be the first priority for most people.

MINERALS

The many roles of minerals in the human body are well documented, and the relative lack of minerals in most available foods due to soil mineral deficiencies and other factors suggests that most everyone will benefit from a quality mineral supplement. For best results, this mineral supplement should be naturally chelated as well as colloidal. It should also contain a broad spectrum of minerals, including necessary trace elements. High quality mineral supplements of this nature are available in liquid form as well as in freeze dried capsules. For health maintenance purposes, one to three capsules per day or one to three ounces (thirty to ninety milliliters) of the liquid is generally sufficient. Higher amounts are often needed in dealing with various health challenges. A mineral supplement is probably the second highest priority after food enzymes for most people.[3]

Amino Acids, Including Raw Protein

If quality protein sources are included on a daily basis (including good sources of raw protein), then it is certainly possible to obtain adequate amounts of amino acids from the diet, depending upon our ability to digest and assimilate protein. This ability is deficient in many people for various reasons. An inadequate output of stomach acid is one. An overall enzyme deficiency is another. Poor thyroid function also interferes with protein utilization, as does a deficiency of vitamin B_6. For these reasons and others, many people may benefit from natural supplements rich in amino acids in a form that is easily assimilated. (Synthetic amino acids, like synthetic vitamins, are not the same as the real thing, and should be avoided.) Two or three tablespoons of bee pollen daily is often added to the diet for this purpose. An excellent protein supplement has been developed by Alan Meyer in which various grains and greens have been predigested by beneficial microbes and then dried at low temperature until powdered.[4] A great advantage of these powders is not simply their high nutrient content but the fact that the nutrients are readily available to the body. Through the activity of the microbes and their enzymes, proteins have already been broken down into amino acids, fats into fatty acids, and carbohydrates into simple sugars. One or more tablespoons per day of these powders can be used as an additional source of raw protein.

Essential Fatty Acids

The need for essential fatty acids can certainly be met from the diet with the appropriate inclusion of various foods. Yet this may not be so easy. According to Udo Erasmus, by 1980 the typical consumption of omega-3 had decreased to a sixth of what it was in 1910. During this same period, consumption of omega-6 doubled.[5] Taken together, these two factors result in an increase of the crucial ratio of omega-6 to omega-3 by a factor of twelve! Two tablespoons of flax oil daily will assist greatly in restoring this ratio to its proper bounds, given flax oil's high percentage of omega-3. However, if the ratio goes too far in the opposite direction of too much omega-3 to omega-6, problems can result. Therefore, the diet must also contain sufficient omega-6, which is readily available from a variety of sources. Oil blends (that contain flax oil as well as other oils) are available which contain a more ideal balance of the two essential fatty acids, and these can be used instead of flax oil.

Friendly Microbes

If we consumed a diet rich in fermented foods and if our habits didn't place our friendly microbes under continual attack, then the need for a supplement of friendly microbes might not exist. Yet our diets are typically lacking in fermented foods, and our microbes are under continual assault from antibiotics and other medications, as well as various pollutants. Please bear in mind that a substantial portion the world's annual production of antibiotics is applied directly to our food supply. Of the 50 million pounds of antibiotics currently produced in the United States on an annual basis, "human treatment accounts for roughly half the antibiotics consumed every year."[6] The remainder are sprayed on crops and fed to livestock on a massive level. So whether or not we have ever taken prescription antibiotics, most of us ingest antibiotics on a continual basis.

There are numerous *probiotics,* or sources of friendly microbes, available. (*Antibiotic* basically means "against life." In contrast, *probiotic* means "for life.") These probiotics are not all equally effective. If we recall the earlier section on friendly microbes (Chapter Nine), good bacteria will not have an offensive smell to our nose. Assuming we have minimized or discontinued most factors that would destroy friendly bacteria, it is pretty simple to ascertain whether or not a probiotic is actually benefiting us. If it is, the offensive smell of the feces and flatulence should be greatly reduced and possibly disappear. If the smells remains strong, then most likely the probiotic is doing little to benefit us.

Some probiotics containing acidophilus and other beneficial bacteria in a capsule form work fairly well. However, the most effective probiotic I have come across is manufactured by Alan Meyer in Brisbane, Australia.[7] It is in a liquid form, and it contains at least twelve different beneficial strains of lactobacillus as well as two highly beneficial types of friendly yeast. It is worth noting that in a healthy human digestive tract, there should be a variety of beneficial microbes all the way from the mouth to the anus. This particular probiotic is formulated to supply this variety. Many other probiotics supply only a few bacteria, rather than the whole crew. In this liquid form, one or more ounces (thirty milliliters or more) can be taken daily as a maintenance dose, while more is often used for particular applications.

ADDITIONAL PROTEASE

Many people have difficulties digesting protein. As mentioned in Chapter Nine, papayas, kiwi fruit, figs and pineapple all contain natural proteases which will aid us in protein digestion when consumed with our meals. Various concentrated protease supplements are also available in capsule, tablet, and powdered form for this same purpose. The mature green papaya supplements manufactured according to Dr. Kurt Koesel's original formulations are an especially good source of extra protease.[8] Suggested dosage will vary depending upon the product. In addition to its ability to assist in protein digestion, protease also has a significant ability to enhance immune function, and that the immune system is inadequate to a varying degree in the majority of people is another major reason to utilize extra protease.[9]

Other Supplements and Aids

BESIDES THESE ESSENTIAL SUPPLEMENTS, NUMEROUS OTHERS CAN BE used with good effect. What follows is no exhaustive list, but simply a few of the highly effective supplements known to me through experience. There are undoubtedly many others.

Schweitzer formula. A small packet of crystals is heated and dissolved in pure water to make up one gallon (approximately four liters) of Schweitzer fluid. Drinking one or more teaspoons per day can boost the immune system, as evidenced by live blood cell analysis. It may also help to eliminate any abnormal tissue, a valuable asset when dealing with any tumor. While the exact mechanism by which this is done is not known, it has been observed that ingestion of Schweitzer fluid will create a condition of hyperthermia in any abnormal tissue, which may act like a localized fever to help eliminate the condition.[10] Schweitzer fluid is also extremely healing when applied to the skin. It is especially effective with burns and scar tissue, upon which it can be applied topically one or more times per day.

Lymphatic enzymes. These have been designed to assist in cleaning out the lymphatic system, which is frequently congested. The lymphatic enzymes are a concentrated source of protease and amylase, which means they will digest protein, breaking it down into amino acids, and carbohydrates, breaking them down into simple sugars. (As a result of this release of sugars, diabetics are advised to use lymphatic enzymes with extreme caution.) One to four capsules or up to one level teaspoon, one to three times per day may be taken. This is best done on an empty stomach with a large glass of water.

Lecithin, lipase, and flax oil. In the event of clogged arteries in which deposits of cholesterol have accumulated, it is important not only to change the diet so that no further accumulation occurs but also to take steps to remove existing deposits. An effective, safe, and noninvasive manner of doing this is to use lecithin, lipase, and flax oil, which work most powerfully when used together. Lipase digests fats, including cholesterol, but is only able to work on the surface of the cholesterol. Lecithin emulsifies the cholesterol, breaking it down into smaller particles so that the lipase can more readily digest it.[11] Flax oil will also assist greatly in removing deposits of cholesterol by helping to liquefy the cholesterol. Some recent research suggests that cholesterol by itself has a melting point of about 300 degrees Fahrenheit; thus, it is quite solid at body temperature. When lecithin is present, the melting point drops to 180 degrees Fahrenheit; thus, it will still be solid at body temperature. However, when the essential fatty acid omega-6 (linoleic acid) is also present along with the lecithin, the melting point of cholesterol drops all the way to 32 degrees Fahrenheit. Thus, it would appear that in the presence of sufficient quantities of both lecithin and omega-6, cholesterol will be liquid at body temperature and the danger of cholesterol deposits greatly reduced, if not removed entirely. One or more capsules each of lecithin and lipase per meal may be taken, along with flax oil.

Sensitive leaf tea. Sensitive leaf tea is an excellent herbal tonic for the central nervous system. The Latin name for it is *Mimosa pudica*. One cup or more per day may be taken.

Betaine hydrochloride. Taken between fifteen to forty-five minutes after the meal, this will lower the pH in the stomach to activate the enzyme pepsin to continue protein digestion in the lower stomach. If taken too late it is ineffective. If taken too soon it will interfere with primary digestion by lowering the pH below the range in which the food enzymes function optimally. When taken at the correct time it will greatly assist protein digestion for those with insufficient output of hydrochloric acid. One capsule approximately a half hour after each meal is best.

Compressed leaf alfalfa. Taken for its mechanical scrubbing ability, this is an excellent means of keeping the large and small intestines clean and functioning efficiently. These tablets function like miniature scrub brushes to keep the system free from debris. Five to ten tablets per meal may be taken.

Cascara sagrada. An herbal laxative, *cascara sagrada* stimulates peristalsis temporarily by irritating the intestines, resulting in increased elimination through the colon. However, it should not be used habitually as it is addictive and eventually overstimulates the intestines, with the result of actually weakening peristalsis in the long run. Its proper use is as a temporary measure to evacuate the bowel. All true laxatives function in this manner, that is, as irritants to the system; thus, all true laxatives will weaken the peristalsis sooner or later if taken habitually. *Cascara sagrada* has the advantage over harsh chemical laxatives in that it is a substance that the body eliminates fairly promptly, and it does not appear to have any bad effect upon the body when used infrequently as a temporary expedient. The same can be said for senna, another common herbal laxative.

Kelp and/or dulse. Both kelp and dulse are rich sources of organic iodine, necessary for proper thyroid function. A deficiency of iodine is known to result in goiter, once common in certain areas of the USA where the soil is lacking in iodine. One or more tablets per meal may be taken or it may simply be used as a condiment on food.

Licorice root. An excellent herb to support the adrenal glands. One to two capsules per meal may be taken.

Cedar berries. This herb will assist the pancreas to function better. Pancreatic function is poor in many people. In addition to insulin production, the pancreas secretes chymotrypsin. This substance helps digest abnormal tissue. One or two capsules per meal may be taken.

Ginseng, gotu kola, and damiana. All excellent herbs for supporting the reproductive organs. Ginseng is more typically for men, while damiana is more for women. Gotu kola is good for everyone. One or two capsules per meal of one of these herbs may be taken.

Niacin. A niacin flush, ideally once per day, is an excellent means of boosting the circulation in the entire body, especially in the skin and extremities. Start with a small dosage to see how much is required to obtain a flush. With a quick release niacin, many people will flush with 50 mg or less. With a time release niacin, higher dosages are typically needed for a flush. Niacin is a vasodilator; thus, it dilates the capillaries and sends extra blood to the extremities. A niacin flush is especially beneficial to the skin. During the flush is also an excellent time to spray the skin with Schweitzer fluid. During a niacin flush, the individual may reexperience old sunburns and other skin traumas. It is common to see the outlines of old bathing suits as the old sunburns reappear.

Skin Zyme. Skin Zyme is made from mature green papaya and is rich in papain. It has a wonderful ability to heal the skin through the breaking down of abnormal tissue and is excellent in particular for moles and age spots as well as wrinkles.[12]

Chaparral, black walnut, garlic, wormwood, and cloves. These are all effective at driving parasites out of the body by means of suppression, as with chemical vermifuges. While ultimately it is best to bring the body to a condition of health so that parasites are not capable of existing in it, these herbal suppressants may need to be employed by people whose quality of health is not yet so high (probably most of us). While many effective combinations of these herbs work, most herbs that can be used to kill parasites are somewhat toxic to humans. Such herbs should clearly be used intermittently if at all.

Dandelion root or yellow dock. These are each effective herbs to support the liver. One or two capsules of either per meal can be taken.

Juniper berries. These are an excellent herb for the kidneys as well as the bladder. One or two capsules per meal may be taken.

Mullein and lobelia. These are two excellent herbs for the lungs, especially when used together. Mullein helps to gather debris from the lungs, while lobelia assists in expelling it. One or two capsules per meal of each may be taken.

Stabilized oxygen drops. These are an excellent means of oxygenating the tissues of the body. As is shown by the work of Dr. Otto Warburg (twice awarded the Nobel Prize) and also Dr. William Koch, cancer and other abnormal tissues thrive in oxygen-poor environments but do not proliferate well in tissue that is properly oxygenated.[13] Dosage varies depending upon the brand involved.

Cayenne pepper. This is an excellent herb for the heart and circulation. One or two capsules per meal may be taken.

Oxy-Mag. This is an effective means of oxygenating the tissues of the body. It is helpful to take a quarter teaspoon or more up to three times per day as per the directions. Larger amounts often trigger intense intestinal cleansing.[14]

Eyebright formulation (without capsicum). This remedy is an effective means of helping with a variety of eye problems. Two capsules may be taken in a half cup (120 ml) hot water. Make strong tea, strain, cool, add to eye cup along with ten drops chelated colloidal minerals. Wash each eye three times per day for five minutes. (The eyebright herb may also be taken internally. One or two capsules per meal may be taken.) The eyewash will often trigger fairly intense discharge or drainage from the eyes, including pus and other materials. While this may appear unsightly, it is an excellent means of cleaning out the eyes.

Natural vitamin supplements. Chapter Ten discusses these. Avoid synthetic vitamins.

Wheatgrass juice. Wheatgrass juice consumed immediately upon extraction is abundant in many valuable nutrients including chlorophyll and neuropeptides. The latter aid the transmission of nerve impulses across the synapses. When grown at home wheatgrass juice is an inexpensive means of obtaining a broad range of nutrients, especially when grown in soil that is full of minerals. For those with the small amount of time and space needed to grow their own wheatgrass, there are few less expensive means of obtaining such a broad array of quality nutrients. Excellent results have been obtained by individuals on high amounts such as a pint (500 ml) or more per day of fresh wheatgrass juice. Most people will do well if they take about one ounce (30 ml) per day.

Spirulina. Spirulina is a good source of many nutrients, including B vitamins. To the best of my knowledge, nobody has truly succeeded in producing a dried spirulina at temperatures low enough to preserve all the amino acids. Nevertheless, it has many valuable nutrients.

Aloe vera juice. This is an excellent means of maintaining a colon free from constipation. One ounce (30 ml) or more per day may be taken.

Colloidal calcium. Calcium is one of the single most important elements for the body. In a colloidal form, it is readily assimilated. One may take one or more tsp per day. Please note: consuming too much calcium and too little magnesium can lead to serious imbalance and a host of health problems associated with hardening or calcification of the tissues. The body needs abundant magnesium in order to be able to utilize calcium properly.

Beneficial Health Practices

IN ADDITION TO TAKING SUPPLEMENTS TO ENHANCE OUR HEALTH AND nutritional status, our daily routine may be supplemented by various healthy practices.

Consuming drinks at moderate temperature. Extreme temperatures are damaging to the stomach lining and should be avoided. Warm drinks should be cool enough to dip the finger into comfortably, while cool drinks should not be straight out of refrigerator or with ice but should be allowed to warm up to where they are cool, not cold. Warm and cool are each fine. Hot and cold are to be avoided for the sake of the stomach lining. Many people are numb to such an extent that they do not find it uncomfortable to drink fluids that are so hot as to be most unpleasant if poured on their skin.

Colonic irrigation. Colonic irrigations are an excellent means of clearing old impacted debris from the colon. Care should be taken that the water used is pure, that all equipment is properly sterilized, and that the water is introduced at low pressure, e.g. with a gravity feed system, so as not to injure the colon. An initial series of colonic irrigations several times per week is often helpful, while in the long run it may be done with good results at intervals of one or more months. Enemas as well as self-administered colemas or high enemas are also quite beneficial for colon health, and hence for the health of the entire body. While a clean bowel is certainly not the only factor involved in good health, it is nonetheless an important factor that should not be ignored. Many health problems elsewhere in the body will respond positively to colonic therapy. Colonics are primarily for those in poor health. Once the bowels are functioning properly, colonics should only be used occasionally if at all.

Two ounce mineral retention enema. This may be done with liquid minerals either straight, or diluted, or with a mineral capsule rehydrated. The exact strength of the solution is not vital. The fluid is inserted into the rectum using an enema syringe, and is retained up to twenty minutes. The procedure is excellent for individuals with problems in the lower bowel, especially the sigmoid colon and rectum. Schweitzer fluid may also be used in the retention enema with good results, as strictures are generally accompanied by scar tissue which the Schweitzer will help to dissolve.

Exercise. As the motion of the muscles is a primary mover of the lymph throughout the lymphatic system, simple forms of exercise such as walking and swimming will be of great benefit to the lymphatic system and hence the entire body.

Exercise on mini-trampoline or rebounder. Start with thirty seconds three times per day and work up to five minutes three or more times per day. This is a highly efficient form of exercise for the lymphatic system, excellent for the entire body and suitable for most everyone. It literally benefits every cell in the body. For those who lack agility or balance, this may be done to good effect while leaning against a wall, in a doorway, or in some other way supported so as to avoid injury. It is not necessary to jump high or vigorously to achieve benefit from this excellent form of exercise.

Dry skin brush. The skin is an important organ of elimination. Dry skin brushing with a natural bristle brush helps to keep it clean and functioning well. Brushing should be done over the entire body except the face and neck, and it should be done in the direction of the heart so as to work with the return flow of blood as well as the lymph. Follow brushing with a lukewarm shower without soap, followed by a cool splash. Extreme water temperatures should be avoided in bathing as in drinking as they damage the skin. By finishing with a cool splash, the pores are left in a closed position. Soap should be used as little as possible for several reasons. Anything used on the skin is absorbed into the body to some extent; thus, if a substance is not fit for ingestion it should not be used on the skin either. Also, soap removes the natural oils on the skin, which must be there and in contact with natural sunlight in order to form vitamin D_3, which is necessary for calcium metabolism.

Chapter Fourteen

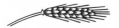

Degenerative Diseases

The strength or weakness of a society depends more on the level of its spiritual life than on its level of industrialization. Neither a market economy nor even general abundance constitutes the crowning achievement of human life. If a nation's spiritual energies have been exhausted, it will not be saved from collapse by the most perfect government or by any industrial development. A tree with a rotten core cannot stand.

Alexander Solzhenitsyn

But what about human liberty? Is there no spiritual freedom in regard to behavior and reaction to any given surroundings? Man can preserve a vestige of spiritual freedom, of independence of mind, even in such terrible conditions of psychic and physical stress. We who lived in concentration camps can remember the men who walked through the huts comforting others, giving away their last piece of bread. They may have been few in number, but they offer sufficient proof that everything can be taken from a man but one thing: the last of the human freedoms—to choose one's attitude in any given set of circumstances, to choose one's own way.

Viktor Frankl

WHEN A DEGENERATIVE DISEASE SUCH AS ARTHRITIS OR CANCER is present, it must be recognized that the condition of the physical body is the end result of a host of factors, both physical and otherwise. The successful course of treatment must take as many of these factors into account as possible. In addition, a degenerative condition has most likely been many years in its development, even though there may have been few apparent symptoms during much of this time. Thus, complete recovery from such a condition is unlikely to occur without a sustained effort over a period of time, which will be dependent on numerous factors. Paavo Airola notes, for example, that "arthritis is not a local disease of a particular joint but a systemic disorder, a disease which affects the whole body. It could have taken years and years of abuse to bring about the systemic disturbance in bodily functions which eventually leads to a breakdown of the health and the functions of the joints."[1] Maurice Finkel concurs, stating that "what most physicians will not recognize about cancer is that the entire body is affected with the disease. The tumor is simply the outward sign."[2]

Modern Medicine

THE RELIANCE OF MODERN MEDICINE ON SURGERY, CHEMOTHERAPY, drugs, and radiation for the treatment of degenerative and other disease conditions with little or no recognition of any of the underlying factors which have caused the disease flies in the face of all reason. If the cause of a condition is unknown and ignored, determining an effective course of treatment is virtually impossible. This is akin to focusing our efforts on killing the mosquitoes in the living room without paying attention to the fact that there are no screens on the windows and a swamp outside. We may kill the mosquitoes, but they will keep coming back until we address the underlying causes behind their presence. We might extend this analogy further by pointing out that such methods might be equated with trying to drive the mosquitoes from the living room with poison or fire, forgetting that in the process the living room will be rendered uninhabitable.

These four methods are all gross violations of the fundamental dictum "Do no harm." In many situations modern medicine is the most appropriate treatment. Yet when dealing with degenerative diseases, destructive methods such as these are largely counterproductive and will only further slow the process of rebuilding the body, if they do not make it virtually impossible. Both chemotherapy and radiation are extremely destructive to the immune system, as well as to the overall health of the body, and even the anesthesia from an operation is very detrimental. While it is outside of the scope of this book to consider just why modern science has put all its efforts into surgery, drugs, chemotherapy, and radiation, some of the underlying economic and political factors have been discussed elsewhere. One of the most exhaustively documented and extensive of such books is *Murder By Injection: The Story of the Medical Conspiracy Against America* by Eustace Mullins. The tone of this book is certainly not designed for the timid reader, and doubtless it will offend many. But given the voluminous documentation of verifiable facts, it is difficult to find fault with the author's coverage of this subject.

Numerous Factors in Degenerative Disease

WHILE NOBODY CAN SAY WITH CERTAINTY WHY ANY OF US DEVELOPS a particular degenerative disease condition, numerous factors may contribute to its development. Some of these factors are largely beyond our control; however, many others are well within our ability to change. While it is important to be aware of the former group, since these factors have influenced the genesis of the disease and might influence the course of treatment, we should focus on the factors we can change and let these form the heart of successful treatment for a degenerative disease. If the conditions that originally contributed to the genesis of the disease remain unaltered, a permanent recovery from the degenerative condition is highly unlikely: the best that can be hoped for is a suppression of symptomology. However, reversing as many of the causes as possible should not only be a major part of the treatment for an existing degenerative condition, but also an effective program for prevention.

Individual Constitution and Past Health History

OUR CONSTITUTIONAL MAKEUP IS A MAJOR FACTOR THAT IS BASICALLY beyond our control. Some of us possess a robust and vigorous constitution with few if any weaknesses, while others have considerably less inherent vitality. For many of us the inherent vitality of the various tissues of our body also varies. Some may have particular inherited weaknesses in the major organs and glands. Other factors over which we have no control include illnesses, injuries, traumas, and operations which have occurred in the past.[3] All these factors, and perhaps others, must be taken into account if the condition is to be reversed.

When any part of the body is sick, the entire body is involved, and this is especially true when a degenerative condition is involved. The inherently weaker tissues of the body, as determined by genetic makeup and previous traumas and illnesses, will have a more pronounced tendency to be the site of disease in the future. That is, when the seeds of degeneration are sown and the conditions are right, they will ripen first in the weakest areas of the body, and which these are is partially predetermined.

Toxic Environment and Toxic Attitude

THE FACTORS THAT ARE MORE OR LESS WITHIN OUR CONTROL MUST BE extensively considered, and these include the quality of our food, air, water and overall environment. In addition, our emotional resistances such as suppressed states of anger, fear, grief, and so forth, will have a pronounced effect on our physical wellness. Negative attitudes can thus be a major factor in the genesis of degenerative conditions as well as a major obstacle to recovery from such conditions.

OVERALL ENVIRONMENT

The quality of the air we breathe, the water we drink, prepare our food with, and bathe in, and, of course, the food we eat, will all be of great significance for our health. Many environmental factors should concern us, as we are routinely exposed to numerous toxic substances and other environmental hazards. The avoidance of pesticides, chemical fertilizers, food additives, and the many other contaminants in much of our food supply would free much of the body's vital energy from the task of dealing with these toxins and make regeneration of the body far less difficult than it would be were the ingestion of such substances to continue. These toxic substances place an enormous strain on the body's elimination systems. The eventual result is that sooner or later the elimination systems begin to fall behind in their task. Toxins begin to accumulate in the tissues of the greatest relative weakness, where they wreak metabolic havoc. While it may be impossible to entirely avoid such exposure, nonetheless, much can be done to minimize it. Air quality is another concern, both at home and at work, as well as elsewhere. In some cases it can be greatly improved using either air filters or houseplants or both. In other cases the environment which includes poor air quality must simply be avoided, which may require a change of occupation and/or a change of address. The typical modern building with its airtight insulation and toxic gases in the indoor air as a result of household products, building materials, and other factors can be a major contributing factor to health problems, a fact which is only recently beginning to draw the amount of attention it deserves. A move from the polluted air of the city to the cleaner air of the country may be necessary, particularly when dealing with respiratory conditions.

Finkel notes that given the numerous carcinogenic substances that abound in this day and age, cancer is a threat for virtually everyone unless precautions are taken: "If one can keep the supply of food materials, as well as our sources of air and water, as free of toxins as possible, then we might all escape this scourge."[4]

ATTITUDE

Successful treatment must not only involve major changes for the better in our air, food, water, and overall environment, but also in our attitude. One of the major hurdles to overcome is correctly noted by Finkel when he states that most people want to continue with the old habits that gave rise to the tumor originally. While in many cases successful treatment will require other measures, certainly it must involve change in toxic attitudes and habits. Dr. Alec Forbes states that "one can evade the question cancer asks, but the cancer itself cannot be evaded. It is my experience that those who struggle against chronic illnesses and change their attitudes, lifestyle, and diet, recover more often than those who do not and drift passively along under treatment from their practitioners. This applies particularly to cancer."[5]

Cultivating a positive attitude, one of continual enthusiasm for all of the experiences of life, will be a vital part of the treatment. In my experience there is no other factor of as great importance as a positive attitude. While many people with serious physical problems will undergo similarly rigorous treatments, the people who become better are those who attain and maintain good attitudes during the long succession of healing crises that they must pass through on the road to renewed health. I have seen severely ill people succeed against all odds when their enthusiasm is maintained. I have also seen people accomplish far less in the face of much less severe conditions, despite a rigorous program of physical treatment, largely because of a poor attitude. Many people would rather die than change their lifestyle and attitude. And yet, whether they understand it or not, this is precisely the choice with which they are confronted. The nature of our reactive patterns is such that many of us will struggle in our quest for change and emancipation from their bondage. The chains of death that bind each of us are quite sturdy. While outside sources can help us change our attitude for the better, ultimately the change must come from within us. Airola notes the same in reference to arthritis: "The importance of proper attitude on the part of patients is emphasized in all clinics. After years of pain and suffering, persons afflicted with arthritis are often irritable, tense, bitter, and resentful. These negative emotions can do much to make efforts to regain health difficult, even impossible."[6]

Other Toxins We Can Avoid

SODIUM FLUORIDE

A significant contributing problem to much chronic and degenerative illness is sodium fluoride. A very comprehensive book on the subject of sodium fluoride is *Fluoride the Aging Factor* by Dr. John Yiamouyiannis. This toxin is added to municipal drinking water in many places and is also present in most brands of toothpaste. It allegedly helps prevent tooth decay, although many who have examined the raw data of the studies used to support such a claim suggest that it is utterly false.[7] The many known detrimental effects of fluoride even at doses much lower than are found in drinking water should prevent us from deliberately ingesting it, in our water or our toothpaste. Among the most significant of the detrimental effects is its impact on the immune system, demonstrable at doses as low as 0.1 ppm. (Drinking water typically contains one to two parts per million, or ten to twenty times this amount.) According to Finkel, "Fluoride then becomes a very important factor in the conversion of normal cells into cancer cells because it effectively blocks aerobic respiration through its inactivation of magnesium. The intake of fluoride on a daily basis year in and year out *must* have a heavy influence upon the onset of cancer."[8] It should be obvious that any substance which destroys our immune system *must* be eliminated from our body. In my experience it is difficult to achieve any improvement in the condition of an individual who continues to use fluoridated water, and all dental products which contain even the slightest amount of sodium fluoride should be avoided. This includes the vast majority of commercially available toothpastes.

Fluoride is also an enzyme inhibitor. Many of its detrimental effects can be directly attributed to its disruption of numerous enzyme systems within the body. I once interviewed Dr. John Lee, a medical doctor from just north of San Francisco, on a radio show. He told me an interesting story. As a medical doctor, he was on a local committee whose job it was to make a recommendation regarding fluoridation. He entered into the job with an extremely strong bias in favor of the use of fluoride. After all, in medical school he had been indoctrinated in the view that fluoride helps prevent tooth decay. As he told me, his only initial question was not whether or not to fluoridate, but how much to use. But being a thorough man, he carefully began to examine the scientific literature. Much to his surprise, he soon discovered that in his own words "the Emperor has no clothes!" He could find no evidence for fluoride's effectiveness or safety, and quite a bit of evidence to the contrary. He then devised his own study. With the help of patients from his medical practice who volunteered, he set up a careful double blind study. All patients in the study would obtain all their drinking water from the local pharmacist. Neither Dr. Lee nor the patients would know whether they were receiving fluoridated water or nonfluoridated water at any given time during the study. The pharmacist would keep record of what type of water each patient was receiving at various intervals during the study. Both Dr. Lee and the patients would keep careful track as to whether they seemed to be improving or deteriorating with respect to their various health complaints. Only after the study was completed would Dr. Lee be able to correlate patient progress with the type of water they received. The results were dramatic and clear. Regardless of their complaint, patients got worse when drinking fluoridated water. When drinking nonfluoridated water, their conditions improved. When I asked Dr. Lee why he thought this was so, he said that since fluoride was an enzyme inhibitor, it interferes with practically all bodily processes.[9]

Numerous water filtration devices are available today. Some shower filters will remove the chlorine as well as many of the other contaminants. However, to my knowledge there is no on demand filter capable of removing fluoride. The best quality reverse osmosis filters will apparently not remove sodium fluoride completely. There is evidence that the Grander units may cause the fluoride to be suspended so that we do not absorb it. I suggest that to be on the safe side (if it is truly not possible to have a water supply without fluoride), that we use reverse osmosis and then a Grander unit for best results in removing fluoride.[10] Those who live in fluoridated areas can involve themselves in the issue of water fluoridation and attempt to get it removed from their water. It may not be an easy battle.

ELECTROMAGNETIC POLLUTION

Other environmental factors involved in much degenerative disease include proximity to nuclear plants, industry, and so on. One factor drawing increasing attention is the electromagnetic pollution emitted by power lines, VDTs, and numerous other sources, including common household appliances such as microwaves, televisions, refrigerators, fluorescent lights and so forth. Some of this information is covered in the books *Cross Currents* by Dr. Robert Becker and *Currents of Death* by Paul Brodeur. The detrimental effects of electromagnetic pollution on the individual have been shown in many experiments. The bottom line is that our exposure to such hazards must be minimized. At this juncture in history it is unlikely that it can be eliminated entirely. Care should be taken that the spaces in which we sleep, work, and live are as free as possible from electromagnetic fields. These fields fall off greatly with distance; thus, an electrical appliance one foot from our head while sleeping may be an extreme hazard, while the same appliance five or six feet away may not be significant. A broad range of gadgets currently available purport to protect us from electromagnetic pollution. In many cases, neither the theory behind a certain gadget nor whether it actually does what its proponents claim has been objectively proven. This does not mean that it does not work, but merely that we often simply do not know. Objective evidence suggests strongly that a few such gadgets do benefit the user in a tangible way, but I am not an authority, and I will not offer any specific recommendations. The best approach is to reduce our exposure to electromagnetic fields as much as possible.

Tobacco

At the risk of stating the obvious, tobacco in cigarettes, cigars, pipes, and chewing tobacco is detrimental to health, and its continued use will make it extremely difficult to regain or maintain health. While people with especially vigorous constitutions will manage to live to a ripe old age despite these habits, it should be clear that this is despite the tobacco and not because of its use.

Recreational Drugs

Recreational drugs, including marijuana, cocaine, LSD, ecstasy, heroin, amphetamines, and so on are incredibly detrimental to health on all levels. Do not be deceived by the suggestions that marijuana is harmless. It has a half-life in the vicinity of about four days, and lingers in the body tissues for weeks or longer. This means that people who smoke it on a frequent basis are "stoned" continually, whether they realize it or not. Marijuana can be used as a painkiller for the simple reason that it numbs or deadens a person physically. It has a similar effect emotionally. It has been my consistent observation over the past fifteen years that a history of marijuana is an obstacle that must be overcome if healing is to take place. And continued use of marijuana is choosing to continually throw obstacles in our own path.

Mercury and Dental Amalgams

Another factor of great significance is the mercury found in silver amalgam dental fillings. While many in the dental profession continue to deny the hazards of mercury, extensive research proves that the mercury in silver amalgam dental fillings poses a significant health risk. Much information on this subject can be found in the excellent books *Silver Dental Fillings: The Toxic Time Bomb* by Sam Ziff and *It's All in Your Head* by Dr. Hal Huggins and also in the booklet *A Patient's Guide to Mercury-Amalgam Toxicity* by Dr. Roy Kupsinel. Many believe that the presence of dissimilar metals in the mouth, which creates electrical current, also poses a health risk, as it tends to short circuit energy meridians to various organs and glands. Thus, even gold fillings may be a health risk, albeit a considerably lesser one than that posed by amalgams.

Mercury from dental amalgams is highly destructive to the immune system, thymus, thyroid, and pituitary glands. It also appears to adversely affect the nervous system. Some individuals diagnosed with Multiple Sclerosis have made impressive recoveries upon removal of all dental amalgams. Even its proponents freely acknowledge that mercury is highly toxic. Its use in dentistry has been defended based upon the erroneous belief that it does not escape from dental fillings and is therefore harmless to the body. Yet repeated tests have shown that hazardous levels of mercury vapor are actually released from dental fillings simply from the compressive forces involved in chewing. Autopsy studies show a strong correlation between the number of amalgam fillings and the amount of mercury present in various tissues. Also, though when an amalgam filling is initially placed, it is in the vicinity of fifty percent mercury, when amalgams from extracted teeth have been tested years later after extraction, they have been found to contain a much lower percentage of mercury. These facts are clear evidence that mercury does not remain safely within the fillings. Mercury released into the mouth may also react with bacteria present there to produce methyl mercury, a substance many times more toxic than mercury itself.

I strongly recommended that all amalgam fillings be removed at the earliest possible point by a dentist who understands the proper manner in which this must be done, as outlined by Dr. Huggins. Amalgam fillings should be replaced with a suitably nontoxic type of filling. As certain individuals will react with some of the replacement materials, specific materials should be tested in advance for individual compatibility. In choosing an appropriate replacement material, nontoxicity and durability would both be significant considerations. Numerous options are available, with new ones regularly appearing, and the best material for one person may not be the best for everyone. Rather than suggest any specific material, I simply recommend that a state of the art dentist be consulted.

ROOT CANALS

Another significant contributing factor to chronic and degenerative illness, which is only recently starting to become more widely known, is root canals or root canal filled teeth. What is particularly tragic about the situation is that Dr. Weston Price conducted an exhaustive study on the subject of root canals which demonstrated beyond any doubt that this practice was extremely hazardous to health. This study was done over a period of twenty-five years. Sixty of the leading scientists in the United States worked under Dr. Price's supervision. And the entire research program was directly under the auspices of the Research Institute of the American Dental Association. And this took place over seventy years ago!

Somehow or another, the results of Price's research were buried for years. As a result, much human suffering which could easily have been averted has been allowed to happen. Two excellent books on the subject are *Root Canal Cover-Up* by George Meinig[11] and *The Price of Root Canals* by Hal Huggins.[12] Both Huggins and Meinig are dentists.

A root canal is a process in which the pulp of a tooth is removed and this area filled, and the bony part of the tooth is left in the mouth. Most dentists have been trained that a tooth can be "saved" in this manner. What Weston Price's research demonstrated, however, is that these root canal filled teeth remain a permanent source of infection in all cases. Price demonstrated that it was simply not possible to sterilize such a tooth completely, and even today, nobody has yet succeeded in sterilizing such a tooth. There are miles of microscopic tubules through the dentin and even the enamel. In a root filled tooth, these become the permanent home to numerous pathogenic bacteria. To put it simply, what is left in the mouth is a dead tooth.

Worse than that, it is a dead tooth that is a constant source of potential trouble elsewhere in the body due to these bacteria.

> One of the most important revelations of Dr. Price's research concerned how the bacteria in teeth act much like cancer cells that metastasize to other parts of the body. These bacteria in teeth similarly metastasize and as they migrate through one's system they infect the heart, kidneys, joints, nervous system, brain, eyes— can endanger a pregnant woman, and in fact may infect any organ, gland, or body tissue. In other words, root canal filled teeth always remain infected. Even worse ... these infections are responsible for a high percentage of the degenerative disease illnesses which are so epidemic in our country today.[13]

Weston Price performed some interesting experiments to demonstrate the perils of these dead teeth. He demonstrated repeatedly that when healthy teeth were surgically implanted under the skin of a rabbit, this did no apparent harm to the rabbit. (These were teeth that had been extracted for various reasons but were alive and well when extracted.) Similarly, when sterilized coins were implanted under the rabbit's skin, the rabbits were not harmed. He then took a root canal filled tooth that had been extracted from a patient with severe arthritis. The rabbit developed severe arthritis within only two days, and died from the infection within ten days. However, the patient recovered from the arthritis after the extraction. Price repeated this procedure numerous times with root canal filled teeth extracted from various ill patients, and also with cultures from these same teeth. Almost inevitably, the rabbit developed the same or a similar disease as the patient. The majority of these rabbits died within three to twelve days. And many of these chronically ill patients made complete recoveries after all their dead teeth were properly extracted.

Obviously most people are quite reluctant to "lose" a tooth, and therefore, many will choose a root canal to "save" the tooth. Many who read this will be reluctant to even consider removing any dead teeth they already have. My response to the idea that we do not want to lose a tooth is that if it requires a root canal or has already had one, we have already lost this tooth. It is dead, and if we leave this dead tooth in our mouth, we are asking for trouble sooner or later. Some will suggest that if the tooth in question is not a problem, it can safely be left alone. Melvin Page, also a dentist, offers an interesting perspective on that idea:

> A dead tooth may be so well surrounded by an armed force of the body's permanent police that the hostile bacteria are walled in and are harmless for the time being. Nevertheless they are potentially dangerous. Let the body forces be needed elsewhere in an emergency and the walled off bacteria are quick to strike. Only a few have to get through the wall to start a serious invasion for their rate of multiplication is so great that in a few hours they become an army of great number and vigor. To the patient's query, "May I not leave the dead tooth as long as it is useful and not harmful?" We answer that when the tooth is found to be harmful, it may be too late to do anything for you. The body is continually surrounded by infection. We stay alive because our power to fight this infection is greater than the power of the infection to fight us. We should not put our defensive systems under a continuous handicap. In an emergency that handicap might mean the difference between life and death.[14]

It should be noted that when a dead tooth has been left in the mouth for any length of time, it is quite likely that there will be infection and decay in some of the surrounding jaw bone. This may not be apparent upon x-ray. There will often be holes in the bones that are referred to as *cavitations*. When a dead tooth is extracted, it will be necessary to thoroughly examine the bone in the area, and in many cases a certain amount of the decayed bone must be removed by grinding it away until healthy bone is exposed. In the case of any tooth extraction, care must be taken to remove the ligaments from the socket and to do all that is necessary to prevent future problems in the bone. An extraction must be done right.

In the event of missing teeth, there are several factors to consider. Given the importance of proper mastication of our food, our health may be compromised if we cannot chew our food sufficiently. In addition, when gaps are left between our teeth, over time the teeth will often tend to *drift*. As a result, our bite is thrown off, which can lead to a vast number of problems in the TMJ, skull, spine, and elsewhere in the body. Also, each tooth has a reflex effect upon specific glands and organs. These glands and organs benefit in a reflex fashion from the mechanical pressure of chewing on that portion of the jaw. Certainly the best situation would be to have all of our own teeth in good condition. But if we are already missing teeth, the best option that I am aware of is removable partial dentures. There are materials for this purpose that are fairly biocompatible for most people. They are also nonmetallic, so there is no problem with electrical currents in the mouth and consequent corrosion. Unlike bridgework, partial dentures do not require any drilling of the adjoining teeth and consequent damage to them. As these removable partial dentures fit directly upon the jawbone, pressure will be exerted upon the jaw bone much as if there were a tooth there, with the reflex benefit that goes with this stimulation to the corresponding glands or organs.

VACCINATIONS

The subject of vaccinations is a controversial one, beyond the scope of this book to treat in great depth. Yet a few brief comments might be made. To begin with, despite the claims of its proponents that vaccination is responsible for the eradication of numerous infectious illnesses, statistical evidence paints quite a different picture. My final semester at Harvard, I took a course in demographics. Vaccinations was a subject to which I had given little thought at that time, and like most other people I simply accepted without proof that vaccinations conferred immunity upon us and were responsible for the virtual elimination of many diseases. I was quite surprised one day when my professor mentioned that from a statistical point of view the premise that vaccinations had ever eradicated a single disease was absurd. For most of the major illnesses which were allegedly eliminated by vaccination had largely been brought under control many decades prior to the advent of vaccinations. In fact, the use of vaccinations had typically caused dramatic increases in the prevalence of these diseases among those vaccinated. This professor attributed the control of most infectious diseases primarily to better hygiene and sanitation. So we must consider whether or not vaccinations truly work. There are numerous books available on the subject, and one is *The Poisoned Needle* by Eleanora McBean.

In many areas there are also private organizations which help to educate people as to the perils of vaccinations.

A more important consideration for many, especially parents, is the safety of vaccinations. I have met quite a number of children who are "vaccination casualties." These children were perfectly healthy until they received a vaccination. Within hours or days, they suffered a severe adverse reaction to the vaccination, typically causing massive brain damage and leaving them crippled and incapable of taking care of themselves for the rest of their lives in some cases. The anguish of their parents is unimaginable. Cases of what is referred to as sudden infant death syndrome or crib death are also far more common shortly after vaccinations, and the number of children maimed or killed by them is far more than the official government statistics will ever admit. In the United States, for example, severe adverse reactions to vaccination are supposed to be reported to a particular federal agency, which is how the official numbers are generated. Yet a survey of medical doctors in several mid Atlantic states revealed that nine out of ten doctors were unaware of this agency or the requirement to report adverse reactions. So right from the start, ninety percent of the cases would not make the statistics. And given the ramifications of acknowledging that a vaccination you have given has caused any damage, it is pretty optimistic to assume that even those medical doctors who are aware of this agency would report such incidents. (Apparently the vaccination rate among children of medical doctors is *less* than that among the general population.) In Western Australia I met a family with a vaccination casualty. The doctor and the government had fully acknowledged to these parents that the vaccination had been the cause of the crippling of their son. They were also assured that this was only the second such incident in Australia ever. This family appeared on a television show and told their story. In a short time, they were contacted by over 350 other Australian families with the same sad story to tell.

Faulty Nutrition

It can be reasonably stated that virtually all degenerative disease has its roots in faulty nutrition. Furthermore, the successful treatment will almost inevitably involve an extensive level of nutritional therapy in the form of sweeping dietary changes. Both Airola and Finkel state emphatically that nutrition is the single most important factor in both the genesis and the successful treatment of arthritis and cancer. Airola notes that "faulty nutrition is singularly the most important causative factor in the development of arthritis. An unbalanced diet of devitalized, overprocessed, and over-refined foods combined with toxic and foodless items ... together with other negative environmental factors, brings about a general deterioration of health, biochemical imbalance, and systemic disturbances. Therefore, the first step in an effective program of treatment for arthritis must be a complete change of nutritional patterns."[15]

Finkel notes as well that according to Dr. Bircher-Benner "faulty nutrition is the basis of cancer."[16] And if we recall the research of Weston Price, degenerative illness was extremely rare in the populations he studied so long as they remained on their traditional diets. Melvin Page has demonstrated that if proper body chemistry can be achieved and maintained, then not only dental but overall physical degeneration can be halted and even reversed to a great degree.[17]

POOR ELIMINATION

The health of the body is dependent upon the health of its cells. Cells will in most cases thrive as long as they are supplied with proper nutrients and as long as their wastes are removed in a timely fashion. When either of these fundamental processes is interrupted or impaired, the health of the cells begins to suffer. This results in an undernourished body suffocating in its own waste products. It is essential that the proper nutrients are supplied as well as assimilated and that all bodily wastes are eliminated at both cellular and whole body levels. Many authorities mention chronic constipation as an underlying cause or precursor to either arthritis or cancer.

There is a long period of deterioration that occurs before a tumor or other obvious abnormality develops. Finkel notes in reference to Dr. C. Moerman that "he does not believe that cancer develops out of sound tissue, but out of sick tissue. First the tissues become sick, and then come the tumors."[18]

When wastes are not eliminated fully they begin to accumulate in the tissues of greatest weakness as determined by a host of factors. These tissues have diminished nerve supply and circulation, and they grow progressively weaker as a result of toxic accumulations. Gradually lymphatic congestion sets in. And as the electrical potential of the tissues continues to decline as this dwindling cycle continues, the tissues grow ever more susceptible to the proliferation of unhealthy bacteria, viruses and parasites. These organisms will not exist in truly healthy tissue. Eventually a point is reached where the process of degeneration has reached such proportions that a "disease" is said to exist. The tumor is not the disease but merely a natural reaction of the body to some very fundamental metabolic dilemmas. A more advanced state of degeneration is indicated when the tumor begins to spread into the surrounding tissues. The integrity of these tissues can no longer be maintained. When dealing with such an extreme condition, during the healing process the first priority will be to restore integrity to the surrounding tissues. This is in accordance with Hering's Law wherein healing will occur in reverse order to the original development of the disease condition. On this point Finkel comments that "the ultimate hope for cancer victims lies in normalizing body chemistry so that it will no longer support the tumors present. When this happens, the tumors break down and dissolve. Any treatment that ignores this fact is doomed to failure. Any treatment that further aggravates and disturbs the metabolism will ultimately reduce the body's resistance and stimulate the development of tumors."[19]

Colonic irrigations, enemas, and other methods are employed in most programs as a means of restoring and maintaining full ability to eliminate. Virtually all successful natural treatments for degenerative disease stress the necessity of extensive detoxification. Finkel notes for example that "the first step is to detoxify, plain water enemas must be given at least twice a day. Any cancer treatment that does not keep the colon clear will have a greatly reduced success. The poisons in the colon must not be allowed to be re-absorbed. The use of the enema may continue for many months until the patient is thoroughly detoxified."[20]

Keeping all channels of elimination open is always important; when working with any degenerative condition it will be absolutely imperative. This will include not just the colon but the respiratory system, skin, urinary system, and lymphatic system, as well. Therefore, such means as breathing exercises, dry skin brushing, massage, the rebounder, niacin, appropriate herbs, and many others, may be employed to insure that the channels of elimination are kept in smooth operation.

Conclusion

FACTORS WHICH ARE INVOLVED IN THE DEVELOPMENT OF DEGENERATIVE conditions, such as our constitutional makeup, as well as previous traumas, illnesses and operations, are largely beyond our control but must nonetheless be considered. Such factors which have contributed to the genesis of a degenerative condition will in most cases make recovery more difficult and will influence the course of treatment. Other factors which are to some degree within our control are the quality of food, air, and water, our attitude, and other environmental factors. Any such factors which have contributed to the development of a degenerative condition must be altered if the condition is to be reversed. If the cure is to be lasting, individuals can never go back to their old ways. In general the conditions which will promote recovery from the condition will be identical to those which will prevent its development in the first place. And these will be opposite to those which will lead to the development of degenerative conditions in the body.

Poor nutritional habits are almost inevitably involved in any degenerative condition; thus, a major component of most successful treatment programs will be nutritional in nature. A degenerative condition almost always develops over many years. Hence, recovery will also take time. When the body is given proper food, air, water, and overall environment, when a positive attitude is attained and maintained, and when other appropriate and harmless methods are suitably employed, virtually any condition can be overcome. We need patience, as a degenerative condition which has been years in developing may take months, if not years, of disciplined effort to completely overcome. The "cure" will ultimately involve far more than a change of physical habits. For the underlying patterns of resisted thought, word and emotion must eventually be met and transmuted if success is to be obtained.

Part Three describes a modality of healing called Body Electronics. The principles underlying the discipline and practice of Body Electronics are in agreement with the principles of health and healing outlined previously in this book. Yet while it is important to consider the underlying principles of a given modality, and to examine critically whether these principles do indeed coincide with the overall principles of health and healing, this alone is insufficient reason to adopt the given modality. For while a particular modality may claim or appear to be working according to a particular set of principles, and while these principles may be sound, things are not always as they seem. For this reason it is desirable to have some set of tangible criteria by which to judge the efficacy of a particular course of treatment or modality.

If healing is to occur we will anticipate the appearance of a healing crisis or a series of healing crises with the accompanying symptoms. However, even then it is possible to be deceived. For example, a healing crisis may result in severe intestinal cleansing, including diarrhea, nausea, gas, and other generally unpleasant symptoms. These exact symptoms may also appear as the result of a negative environmental or dietary influence. In either case the symptoms will be much the same. If we observe carefully the progression of symptoms, we may be able to see if they are progressing in accordance with Hering's Law of Cure: that is, from the head down, from the inside out, and in reverse order of how they occurred originally. If a modality is really working in accordance with the basic principles of health and healing, then positive and constructive changes will take place in the tissues of the body. As the various crises come and go, each new state of balance attained will result in a higher level of health and well-being than before the crisis.

There is certainly an appropriate time, place and purpose for all things under the sun, including such treatments as will suppress the life force. Surgery and drugs are two such examples. However the proper place of such treatments is not within the natural healing arts. A modality may alleviate symptoms to an extraordinary degree and yet produce no significant changes in overall health or vitality. In such a case we must realize that the modality in question is simply balancing the body without actually contributing to its regeneration. Such modalities do indeed have their proper place in the healing arts, for there is often a need to simply relieve symptoms, if only for a time. If this can be done without harm to the body, it may be considered a blessing. However, many treatments which reduce symptoms are powerful suppressants which reduce the life force of the body and retard true healing. If the relief of symptoms through balancing the body is the goal, as opposed to the regeneration of the body by passing through a series of healing crises, then it is far better that this balancing be achieved with little or no harm to the body. Thus, an observation of what positive or negative changes in health and vitality occur as a result of a particular modality is a reasonable means of determining the effects of the given modality.

In the case of Body Electronics, tremendous healing crises are routinely triggered through its application in conjunction with a state of nutrient saturation. The nutritional program alone brings about significant positive changes, and when this is augmented with Body Electronics, far more significant changes for the better have been routinely observed. This establishes that Body Electronics is helping to bring about the regeneration of the body. Many serious medical conditions have been completely reversed through Body Electronics. The routine occurrence of healing crises and positive changes in health unquestionably establish Body Electronics as a successful modality for promoting the regeneration of the body.

PART THREE

Body Electronics Fundamentals

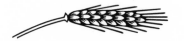

A healing crisis will occur only when an individual is ready both physiologically and psychologically. The basic foundation for all healing crisis is nutritional preparedness. A healing crisis (cure) will begin from within out, in reverse order chronologically as to how the symptoms have appeared, tempered by the intensity of the trauma. The individual will have the opportunity to reexperience each trauma, both physiological and psychological, beginning with the trauma of least severity. It must be recognized that traumas involving emotions, which include all traumas, will be released in order beginning with unconsciousness, then apathy, grief, fear, anger, pain, and eventually enthusiasm (love), in conjunction with the appropriate word patterns for each emotion and thought patterns (sensory memory) which are accessible at each level. Unconditional love and unconditional forgiveness are the keys to apply to transmute any resistance at any level once these resistances are brought to view through the application of the laws of love, light and perfection.

John Whitman Ray

THE NEED FOR PHYSICAL AND PSYCHOLOGICAL READINESS CANNOT BE overemphasized if the healing process is to be successful. Much of the physical readiness is the state of nutrient saturation which has been covered in Part Two. The psychological preparedness consists of several factors including an understanding of the concept of the healing crisis, a willingness to reexperience the suppressed physical and emotional traumas locked into the tissues of our body, and the willingness to be fully and enthusiastically responsible for our own situation at all times. When we are prepared both physically and psychologically, then it is time to begin Body Electronics.

Chapter Fifteen

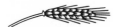

The Basic Theory of Body Electronics

Men stumble over the truth from time to time, but most pick
themselves up and hurry off as if nothing had happened.
Sir Winston Churchill

T HE PROCESS OF RETURNING TO A STATE OF HEALTH IS MADE POSSI-
ble on a physical level by establishing good nutritional habits and
other beneficial practices (covered in the Part Two). However, as
explained in Part One the condition of our bodies is dependent upon consciously or unconsciously held patterns of thought, word, and emotion.
Inner essence (cause) and outer manifestation (effect) are inseparable yet
distinct.

The process of healing may be greatly facilitated by outside intervention, by a healing modality which addresses the body in ways that have an
impact on emotional and mental levels, that address patterns of resistance.
Body Electronics is a healing modality which works very much in accordance with the principles outlined so far in this book.

Healing Includes Dissolving Crystals

W E EACH EXIST WITHIN THE CONFINES OF A PHYSICAL BODY. EACH
body has its particular genetic inheritance, whether this entails an
excellent constitution and vigorous health or a host of inherited health

problems. Within the crystalline structure of our body will be encoded suppressed patterns of thought, word and emotion which will include traumas and other events of our lifetime, as well as patterns reflecting the Hereditary Level, the Soul Level, and the Entity Level. The condition of the physical body will be greatly influenced by physical factors such as diet and lifestyle. The underlying reactive patterns that we possess will also exert a tremendous influence on our health. Our experiences, our perceptions of these experiences, and our physical health will all be influenced by the information locked into our crystals. This information will be at various frequencies, and as like attracts like, certain experiences of a similar vibration will be drawn to us as to a beacon. On the outer level health varies from person to person. On the inner level we each exist within parameters and limitations determined by our own crystals.

Nutrient Saturation Begins the Process

THE PROCESS OF HEALING MUST BEGIN AT THE PHYSICAL LEVEL, WHERE we work to dissolve the crystals. In Body Electronics this is commenced quite effectively through establishing a state of nutrient saturation in the body through diet and supplements. That this condition of nutrient saturation is necessary for the successful application of Body Electronics was discovered by Dr. Ray well over thirty years ago as a result of his own experimentation with numerous individuals,[1] and this has been repeatedly demonstrated by numerous other individuals since that time. The healing crises necessary for the regeneration of the body, which are triggered by the correct application of Body Electronics, are dependent upon the presence of all necessary nutrients.[2] One of the factors which indicates that Body Electronics is working properly is that the pointholder experiences tremendous heat in the points during the session. A lack of heat, a lesser amount of heat, or a minimal duration of heat in the points are all frequently experienced when the person being held has not been sufficiently prepared nutritionally. In such cases after more extensive nutritional preparation, another pointholding session will result in much heat and impressive results. In numerous instances where the points have begun to cool down prematurely, indicating that there are insufficient nutrients to continue the process, it has been observed that the points rapidly heat back up when certain supplements, notably chelated colloidal minerals, are administered.[3]

Body Electronics and Crystals

SUPPRESSED PATTERNS OF THOUGHT, WORD AND EMOTION ARE STORED in the body in *crystals,* which may also be considered as "organic computer chips" or *melanin-protein complexes.* (See Chapter Twenty-Two.) Basically they are storehouses of information, in the form of thought, word and emotion, which are held in a continual state of creation by our resistance to life. True healing cannot take place without this information being accessed and transmuted with unconditional love and unconditional forgiveness. The catch is that as long as this information remains locked in the crystals, it is effectively at the level of unconsciousness, characterized by a lack of awareness, existing at the bottom of the scale of emotions. (See Figure 3, Chapter Two.) As long as this lack of awareness persists, transmutation of these patterns, and thus healing, is not possible, for as Dr. Ray has expressed it, we certainly cannot transmute that which we cannot even remember. We must begin the process of true healing by dissolving the crystals.

As the crystals dissolve, the information in them is released sequentially. With respect to the scale of emotions, this means that we move from unconsciousness up to apathy, grief, fear, anger, pain, and eventually enthusiasm. Traumas are also released in order of increasing severity. Traumas of lesser severity will be released before those of greater intensity. This is where the state of nutrient saturation enters into the picture, for in addition to providing the physical materials necessary for healing, nutrient saturation helps to initiate the dissolving of the crystals and the consequent release of the information contained therein. It is a common experience upon beginning on this program of nutrient saturation to reexperience various emotions, memories, and associated word patterns prior to receiving any Body Electronics. Old memories which have not been recalled for years may surface. Intense emotions such as grief, fear, or anger may surface for no apparent reason as we begin to reexperience the information locked into our crystals.

Accelerating the Process with Body Electronics

THE PROCESS OF DISSOLVING THE CRYSTALS IS ACCELERATED CONSIDER-
ably through the appropriate use of Dr. Ray's unique method of sustained acupressure known as Body Electronics. As the crystals dissolve, the
information which has been locked into them begins to come up so it can
be experienced. We move through the emotional body in reverse order from
unconsciousness up to enthusiasm. Each of the emotions is transmuted by
experiencing it with enthusiasm. The process of transmuting that particular emotion involves encompassing the emotion with enthusiasm. In other
words, enthusiasm is experienced to the encompassment of the lesser emotion and not to the exclusion. To pretend that the resisted emotion is not
present is to continue the process of suppression. Rather, the resisted emotion is acknowledged and then transmuted by enthusiastically experiencing it. If we feel anger, for example, we simply acknowledge that we do,
accepting ourselves for feeling that way, rather than trying to ignore the
anger. Various thought patterns are experienced along with the associated
emotional patterns as well as the word patterns or verbal expressions. The
thought patterns are the sensory patterns of time, place, form and event.

Dissolving Crystals to Bring a Change of Consciousness

AS WE RISE UP THE SCALE OF EMOTIONS AND SPECIFIC MEMORY GRADU-
ally returns, at last the pain level is reached. At this level the full memory returns and is accompanied by the burning pain of the kundalini fire in
which the regeneration of the physical body occurs. During the kundalini
experience, we literally feel as if we are burning up from the inside out. Emotional body resistance is burned out by this experience. As we then rise to
the level of enthusiasm, the mental body may be accessed. Resistance originates in judgment, which originally occurs on the mental body level when
we identify with one side of a given duality to the exclusion of the other. At
the mental body level we now have the opportunity to once more view both
sides of the duality. When the duality is encompassed with unconditional
love, wherein each side can be simultaneously viewed from a position of

equanimity and impartiality, the resistance and judgment are transmuted. At this point we are simultaneously aware of both sides of the duality and have neither resistance nor attachment to either. This is *change of consciousness*. When a change of consciousness occurs, the associated crystals which have been dissolved during the process do not reappear later. If crystals simply dissolve or are broken up without any ensuing change of consciousness, they will eventually form again. However, the situation is not all or nothing. Rather, the extent to which consciousness remains unchanged is the extent to which crystals will form again.

Such a change of consciousness is indeed true healing, for not only has the physical body been transformed in the process but also the emotional body and mental body. Healing has occurred on all three levels. In the absence of resistance and crystallization in a given area, from that point on we will experience health and a lack of limitation on all three levels. Each area of resistance and judgment may gradually be mastered in this manner. The dramatic improvements in physical health that occur during this process are merely the tip of the iceberg. The far more magnificent process of transmutation occurs at the higher levels of the emotional and mental bodies. The visible changes on the outer level are permanent and lasting because they are the result of a change on the inner level. The physical symptoms which were the reflection of various resisted patterns of thought, word and emotion will not return because the underlying cause for them no longer exists. It is that simple.

In Body Electronics work with nutrition and the pointholding are only the beginning of the process. The ultimate goal of all such activity is not simply to remove physical symptoms, but to change consciousness by transmuting the underlying reactive patterns. This can and has been done by many people, and whenever a dramatic and permanent physical change has occurred it has been the direct result of such a change of consciousness.

Chapter Sixteen

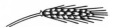

The Practice of Body Electronics

For my part, whatever anguish of spirit it may cost, I am willing to know the whole truth, to know the worst; and to prepare for it.

Patrick Henry

The Basics

IN BODY ELECTRONICS, PRESSURE IS APPLIED TO VARIOUS POINTS LOCATED throughout the body in such a manner as to bring out the pain and suppressed trauma which are locked into the crystalline structure. The pressure applied to these points helps to dissolve the crystals, thus releasing the suppressed patterns of thought, word and emotion which are the inner essence underlying all outer manifestations, including physical symptoms. However, Body Electronics is far more than the pressure applied. The dissolving of the crystals is in many ways simply the beginning of the process, as the reactive content of the crystals is then available for us to *observe, receive, recreate, and release* through the discipline of proper obedience to the laws governing the physical, emotional and mental bodies.

POINTS USED

Numerous points may be used in Body Electronics. Many are specific points which will be found on everyone; others may be points that are unique to the individual, for example, the site of some specific trauma such as a fracture. Some of the points commonly used in Body Electronics are unique to Body Electronics. The vast majority are points that are also used in such modalities as acupressure, acupuncture, shiatsu, or reflexology. Body Electronics differs from other modalities more in how points are held than in which points are actually held. Typically a point that is used effectively in any of these other modalities will also work effectively in Body Electronics.

Points may be held directly on the skin or through light clothing, although the former is generally preferred. When a specific point is selected, there are generally charts which indicate the basic location of the point, anatomically precise descriptions of where the point is to be found, or both. In some cases, the point will simply be chosen because there is tenderness in the area. In any case, once the general area is located, the pointholder can move around ever so slightly with subtle variations in both location and angle of pressure. In this manner the precise point will be found, which will be the point of greatest tenderness. Many individuals can immediately locate the precise point through some combination of experience, extreme sensitivity in their fingers, intuition, and perhaps the ability to perceive energy patterns visually or otherwise. These are certainly useful abilities to possess, and they may help us to be more effective pointholders. Most pointholders will find that they have wonderfully sensitive fingertips once they get their intellect and their self-doubt out of the way. Also, it is important to bear in mind that the individuals whose points are being held are ultimately the best judge of whether we have hit the precise point or not. They can generally give us precise feedback. There really does not need to be any great mystery about how to find points.

In many cases several points might be in close proximity to each other, and thus we have some doubt as to whether we are actually on the right point. Virtually any point that is sore is ultimately worth holding. Hence, even if the point is not the intended point, it is still the right point. In many cases we will simply hold sore points without knowing just what they are. In the words of Dr. F.M. Houston, "If you find in your explorations a sore spot and do not know its name or number as listed, treat it anyway. It is calling for help."[1] This is expressed by Dr. John Ray in the phrase, *find the pain and push.*

With a few notable exceptions this basic principle of find the pain and push is a good one, as any sore spot does need some attention. The exceptions involve being aware of any possible damage that might be caused by the pressure applied. Excessive pressure should be avoided in the abdomen, for example, and great care should, of course, be taken in such areas as the throat and eyes. Also, extra caution should be the rule in holding points whenever we are working on any individual who has inadequate nerve supply or numbness, as these individuals may not be able to feel if trauma is occurring as a result of the pressure being applied. Severe osteoporosis also indicates need for caution, as pressure that would be quite safe on an average person could result in damage to a bony area. In most areas of the body it is extremely unlikely that the amount of pressure applied with a finger or thumb would be enough to cause any tissue damage. However, points should *not* be held in the vicinity of a tumor until the individual is extremely well prepared nutritionally and then only under the guidance of someone who is well qualified. If there is any doubt, it is better to not hold points in such an area. A good rule of thumb in Body Electronics is *when in doubt, don't.*

How to Hold the Points

There are several things to bear in mind regarding the manner in which a point is held during Body Electronics. They are generally held for fairly lengthy periods of time. The duration of a session is not known at the outset. A complete pointholding session is rarely less than ninety minutes with two to three hours being typical and four to five hours not unusual. In many cases sessions have gone much longer. (I have held points as long as eight hours at a time and have heard of sessions as long as eighteen hours. However, the vast majority of sessions will be less than four hours.) It is important to maintain contact with the point at all times. If possible, we should not switch fingers, and if we must, it should be done as unobtrusively as possible by sliding the new finger onto the point as the old finger is slid off in such a manner as to never break contact with the point. If contact is broken, up to thirty minutes may be needed for the point to regain the level of intensity that it had. Thus, Body Electronics may be quite demanding for those holding points. Most find it quite difficult the first few times they do it. But most people who hold points quickly find that they are capable of maintaining more pressure for a longer time than they would have believed possible.

The points will generally be held with the index finger, thumb, or middle finger. An elbow may be used, but only in situations and areas of the body where this amount of pressure is considered safe. When using an elbow, it is extremely important that the other hand be used to hold the elbow steady, as slipping can be quite traumatic to the pointholdee. (The pointholdee is the person whose points are held. The pointholders are those holding these points.) A steady firm pressure is much more effective than sporadic bursts of increased pressure.

A cardinal rule of Body Electronics is never give the person more pain than they are capable of lovingly and willingly enduring. The intention of Body Electronics is to bring out or elicit the pain that is already locked into the tissues of the body. There is a distinction between pain that is being brought out by the pointholding as opposed to pain that is being caused by the pressure applied. When we apply more pressure than can be lovingly and willingly endured, we are definitely in the latter realm. The basic idea is to bring out as much pain as possible within the limits of what can be lovingly and willingly endured. There is no therapeutic value in going beyond this level, as this simply adds more trauma to that which is already there.

Who Holds the Points

While points may be held on one's self, due to the nature of the Body Electronics process it is generally more effective to have other people hold our points so that we can concentrate upon other things. The aim is to reexperience suppressed trauma and various memories as our points are held. With other people holding our points, we can concentrate on the various patterns of thought, word, and emotion as they arise up out of unconsciousness. Another advantage is that in most cases, more pressure can be applied by another person. It also allows us to lie in a comfortable position during the process rather than contorting the body to reach a point.

Points can be held by one or more people on an individual at a given time such that many points may be held simultaneously. It is fairly typical for there to be two to three pointholders on one person. I have seen as many as twelve pointholders at a time on a given person. (After a certain point, it is almost impossible to add any more pointholders as it is too difficult to have that many people clustered around the pointholding table.) In most cases each pointholder will hold two points simultaneously, one with each hand. As a Body Electronics session can last for several hours or more, and as it is typical to have several pointholders at a time, Body Electronics is not especially suited to a practitioner/patient situation, although this is possible and does occur. More typically, pointholding takes place in a cooperative group situation in which one or more in the pointholding group have attended seminars in Body Electronics and is sufficiently knowledgeable to teach the others the basic principles of Body Electronics. Indeed, most seminars in Body Electronics are designed to teach people how to hold points so that they in turn can teach others.

Body Electronics is highly experiential and cannot be learned intellectually. Please do not attempt to practice Body Electronics without proper instruction and initial supervision by someone with adequate training in Body Electronics, ideally including the successful completion of a Body Electronics Instructors Seminar. Body Electronics cannot be fully learned from videos, books or other indirect methods. These methods are intended for use in conjunction with proper instruction and supervision. They are not intended to replace proper live instruction. There is no substitute for experience. People who have attempted to practice Body Electronics without proper training or understanding have often spent considerable time and money with little benefit. More importantly, they have needlessly placed themselves and others at risk of certain potential contraindications for the application of Body Electronics. Without proper training, they would have neither the ability to recognize these contraindications nor the experience and understanding necessary to handle them should they in fact arise.

SENSATIONS AND EXPERIENCES OF THE POINTHOLDEE

Both the pointholder and the person having points held should have some idea of what types of sensations they may experience during the process.

The pointholdee will normally experience pain in the points initially. The degree of pain felt throughout the session may vary considerably, ranging from extreme pain to total numbness. The pointholdee, or person "on the table," will normally reexperience the various suppressed patterns of thought, word and emotion locked into their body. The traumas of least severity will normally be reexperienced prior to those of greater severity. In many cases a particular trauma will be reexperienced over time in various layers of successively greater intensity. The various emotions will typically be reexperienced from the bottom up. Thus, unconsciousness will come first, followed by apathy, grief, fear, anger, pain, and eventually enthusiasm. The role of memory is also crucial. The full memory of the trauma must eventually be reexperienced in order for the trauma to be completely released, as we cannot release that which we cannot even remember. This will not occur until the pain locked into the tissues is no longer resisted but is lovingly and willingly encompassed.

At the level of unconsciousness, we will often experience numbness in the body, including the reexperience of anesthesia, drugs, alcohol, or any other experience that numbs the body. At the pain level the full memory is reexperienced. At this stage we will often experience the burning searing pain of the kundalini either throughout the entire body or in some cases confined to a particular area. This experience is described by many who have experienced it as hotter than a fire but coming from the inside out. If we are unsure whether this has occurred, then it probably has not, for the sensation is so intense as to leave little doubt. At this point of kundalini many of the more stunning physical changes and transformations have occurred through Body Electronics. All manner of other physical symptoms may be experienced on the table at some point during the experience.

An additional experience which often occurs bears mention. Many individuals will experience either extreme heat or extreme cold during Body Electronics. During the former, we will feel like we are in the midst of an intense fever and may be dripping with sweat. During the latter, we will feel quite cold and may shiver. On many occasions I have felt the skin of the individual and found it to be extremely cold and clammy. On many occasions I have witnessed the heat or cold that has been so intense that it can be felt several feet or more from the individual. These experiences of intense heat or cold are quite commonplace in Body Electronics.

A probable explanation for such experiences can be inferred from the work of Dr. Louis Kervran, author of *Biological Transmutations*. Dr. Kervran discusses the transmutation of the elements as it occurs in living tissue, which he was able to demonstrate conclusively. In other words, controlled atomic reactions can occur under the right conditions in living organisms. Simpler elements being transformed into more complex elements will require an input of energy as electrons will necessarily be moved into more external orbits or higher states of energy. Such reactions are known as *endothermal reactions*. The energy required is seemingly drawn from the surrounding environment and is experienced as a lack of heat, or in other words, as cold. When more complex elements are transformed into simpler elements, energy will be released as electrons move to lower states of energy; this will be experienced as a surplus of energy, or as heat. Such reactions are known as *exothermal reactions*. Thus, these experiences of intense cold and heat may be endothermal and exothermal reactions respectively.[2] These phenomena of intense heat and cold have been experienced by too many people to be disregarded, and for those of us who have experienced them in our own bodies they are undeniably real. A more extensive explanation of biological transmutations will be found in Chapter Twenty-One.

SENSATIONS AND EXPERIENCES OF THE POINTHOLDER

Various phenomena may be experienced by the pointholder depending on the degree to which the person on the table is prepared nutritionally. In most cases the pointholder will experience a considerable degree of heat in the fingertip. In some cases this heat is moderate, while in others it is absolutely excruciating, like a blowtorch applied to the finger. Mild blisters on the fingers are fairly common. On a few occasions I have even observed brown or black marks similar to those which occur when a paper match sticks to the finger as it is being lit. These blisters and other marks are often gone by the next day. (When elbows are used for pointholding, the heat can also be felt, although in some cases it is not.) The heat experienced by the pointholder may not be experienced by the person on the table simultaneously. Also interesting is that although the sensations of heat on the point are undeniable and the resulting blisters are real, the surface temperature is still inexplicably normal. In addition to heat, throbbing or pulsing sensations are routinely reported which are distinct from the circulatory pulse of the heart and not necessarily at the same frequency or in synchronization. These pulses typically tend to approach seventy-two beats per minute.[3] Another common sensation is numbness in the finger. This numbness may extend well up the arm, even reaching to the shoulder in some cases. The pointholder may also experience what feels like an intense sensation of electricity coming out of the point. This may vary from a mild current to an excruciating sensation as if the finger is stuck in a light socket. Considerable fortitude is required to continue holding points under such conditions. I have seen pointholders with tears in their eyes on more than a few occasions, although such extreme electricity is not routine. These sensations of heat, throbbing, numbness, and electricity may occur separately or simultaneously, and they may disappear and reappear throughout the session.

How Long to Hold the Points

The duration of a session is not generally known at the outset. Several factors determine when the session is complete. Basically, we look for the cessation of all heat, throbbing, numbness, and electricity before pulling off a particular point. The point should generally feel complete to the pointholdee as well. Some tenderness may remain, but the bulk of the activity should have finished. Usually no harm is done by pulling off a point too soon, but the point is simply left incomplete. There are exceptions to this, however, where if a point is not complete, the pointholdee may be left in the middle of a healing crisis for an extended period. In those cases where time does not permit the completion of all points, it is recommended that all incomplete points be finished at the earliest possible opportunity.[4]

An interesting phenomena involves pulling off when the finger is still numb. When this is done, the finger often stays numb for days or weeks. If we plug back into the point later and wait until the numbness is gone, it can be finished, and the numbness can be resolved. It is ideal to continue the pointholding session until all heat, throbbing, numbness, and electricity have ceased. However, practical time constraints may make this impossible. An opportunity to stop may not present itself for many hours. Thus,

---

people should not plug in if they will not be able to stay until the very end. It should also be noted that even after all activity has ceased on a point, it may resume activity again if we stay plugged into the point.

Another interesting and common phenomena is that of the finger seeming to literally penetrate into the point, not in the sense of piercing the skin, but rather as if the finger and the other body were occupying the same space. In some cases, up to a half inch of the finger will disappear and there will be a distinct sensation that the finger is literally embedded in the other person. In such cases, when the point is unplugged at the end of the session, we may often feel as if we actually have to pull to remove the finger from the point.

A Basic Sequence of Points

THERE IS A GENERAL ORDER OF PRIORITIES FOR HOLDING POINTS. WITHIN this general order, specific choices are made based upon the readiness of the individual as well as this person's needs. Specific needs and weaknesses are determined by a variety of means, chief among these being an Iris-Sclera Integrated Diagnosis. (See Chapter Twenty.)

NERVE SUPPLY AND CIRCULATION

The first priority is to reestablish or improve nerve supply, as it is nearly impossible for the body to heal otherwise. *If we cannot feel, we cannot heal.* Circulation appears to proceed from nerve supply. To test for the degree of nerve supply, we use a simple pinch test. If adequate nerve supply exists throughout the body, a moderate pinch using the thumbnail and the nail of index or middle finger will be experienced as a distinct and sharp sensation just about anywhere on the skin. If only pressure is experienced with no sharp sensation, this indicates a lesser degree of nerve supply. As this is quite subjective, a comparative pinch test is used wherein the subject is pinched at various points along an arm or leg so they may compare the degree of sensitivity. Even in people with extremely poor nerve supply, a sharp sensation should be experienced if we pinch the underside of the arm near the armpit or on the inside of the thigh near the groin. In most people, an equivalent pinch may be experienced as quite sharp in the armpit or groin area and yet as simple pressure with no sharpness on the finger or toe. If we work distally along the limb out towards the extremities, we will see quite readily that sensitivity in most people drops off quite noticeably. If the pinch is not experienced as a sharp sensation clear out to the tips of the toes and fingers, this indicates some degree of inadequate nerve supply. Most people experience at least a minor degree of numbness. Inadequate nerve supply would therefore seem to be an almost universal condition.

Specific points known as the *STO points* (Figure 12), located at the back of the neck in close proximity to the base of the skull, have proved to be extremely effective in restoring nerve supply. (The STO points take their name from the three landmarks used to locate them: the *sternocleidomastoid,* the *trapezius,* and the *occiput.* The first two of these are muscles while the third is a bone.) Having the STO points properly held will often bring obvious improvement in a single session. In other situations, these points may need to be held several times. (There are instances where other factors will hinder success with STO points, and it may be more effective to work in additional areas in order to restore nerve supply.) Along with nerve supply, having the STO points held seems to do much to improve circulation, which is of great benefit in attaining and maintaining a vibrant state of health. It is very common for people with chronically cold extremities to report this disappearing after having the STO points held one or more times. I have seen countless individuals go from an ashen or pale complexion to bright rosy cheeks in just a few hours of having these points held.

While it is preferable and easier to learn the location of points via supervised instruction, in the case of the STO a brief description is offered. The STO points will be found between the sternocleidomastoid and trapezius muscles and slightly inferior to the occiput or base of the skull. Pressure is best exerted with either the middle or index finger with the pointholdee lying on their back and the pointholder sitting at their head. The direction of pressure is approximately towards the center of the brain. Thus, pressure will be medial, superior and anterior. While the fingers may be close to the skull, the pressure is not exerted on the skull itself. (For those trained in acupuncture, the STO points are close but not identical to GB-20.)

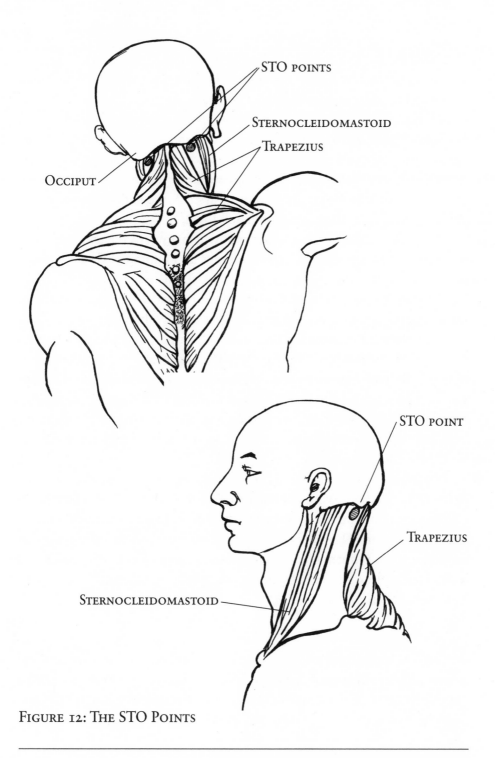

STO POINTS

STERNOCLEIDOMASTOID

TRAPEZIUS

OCCIPUT

STO POINT

TRAPEZIUS

STERNOCLEIDOMASTOID

FIGURE 12: THE STO POINTS

ENDOCRINE SYSTEM

The next priority after working with the STO points is holding points related to the endocrine system, which can be found on the feet as well as elsewhere (Figure 13). As in most cases there is more than a single pointholder, endocrine points are usually held along with the STO points in the initial sessions. The need for certain endocrine points to be held is generally determined through iridology and sclerology (Chapter Twenty). Since there is a chain of command within the endocrine system, the endocrine points are generally held from the top of the chain down.[5]

The first in order is the pineal gland, which governs the endocrine system in coordination with the hypothalamus and pituitary. These three are top priorities for most people, and are typically held in this order: pineal, hypothalamus then pituitary. Due to the neurological connection with the pituitary and its importance in governing many involuntary functions, the medulla is the next priority. The order continues with the thyroid and parathyroid, thymus, and the heart and heart firing mechanism. (The heart may properly be considered an endocrine gland in addition to its other functions, for it has been demonstrated that the heart does secrete specific hormones.) The solar plexus may be held as this will assist with nerve supply to the next priorities, the pancreas and adrenals. The spleen, liver and gonads will follow.

If many or all of these glands need attention, it is generally best to start at the top and work down, holding reflex points for each. The reflex points on the feet are used most often due to the ease of finding them and of finding pain on them. These are also areas where there is little possibility that an overzealous pointholder could do any damage. Endocrine points are also located elsewhere on the body as a given organ or gland can have numerous reflex points.

MAJOR ORGANS

After nerve supply and circulation have been taken care of with the STO points and the endocrine system is working well, attention may be required for one or more of the major organs such as the kidneys, lungs, liver, gall bladder, stomach, small or large intestines, bladder, eyes or ears. In most

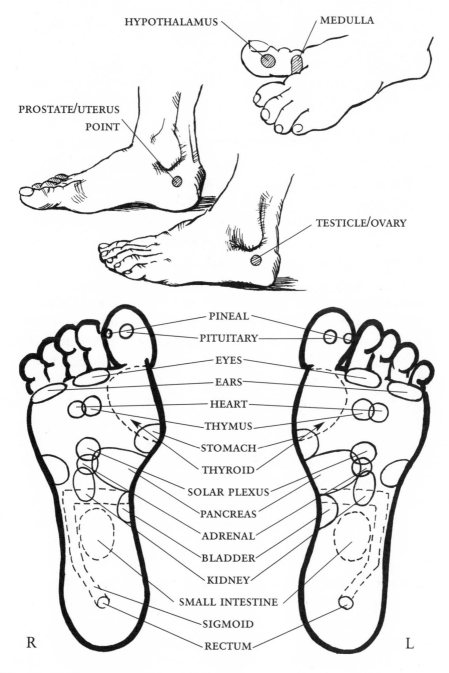

HYPOTHALAMUS   MEDULLA

PROSTATE/UTERUS
POINT

TESTICLE/OVARY

PINEAL
PITUITARY
EYES
EARS
HEART
THYMUS
STOMACH
THYROID
SOLAR PLEXUS
PANCREAS
ADRENAL
BLADDER
KIDNEY
SMALL INTESTINE
SIGMOID
RECTUM

R   L

FIGURE 13: REFLEX POINTS ON THE FEET

cases it is preferable to address general concerns such as nerve supply and endocrine function prior to working on specific problems. It is possible to work directly on a specific complaint, whether chronic or acute, but the results will be more far reaching if we take care of these basics before addressing the specifics. It is important to recognize that no problem in the body will exist or be healed independently of all else in the body.

SPINAL POINTHOLDING

The next priority is usually the spine itself. In most cases some degree of distortion and calcification are involved, adversely affecting nerve supply to various areas of the body. Spinal pointholding is best done on a massage table with a face cradle so that the person on the table can be as comfortable as possible. In most cases a person will need a number of previous Body Electronics sessions to prepare for a spinal session.

Working on the spine is fairly straightforward. We begin by locating problem areas, which is accomplished through palpation and visual observation as well as the person's own knowledge of problems in the back in terms of habitual or recent stiffness, pain, tension, or discomfort. When there are problems in particular body areas revealed through iridology or otherwise, it is also wise to double check the reflex area of the spine. (See Chapter Twenty.) Working on the spine to improve its health is important in itself and also helps improve other areas of the body. A problem in a given part of the spine results in a diminishment of nerve supply to the corresponding tissues of the body. Thus, so long as the spinal problem remains, healing the corresponding tissues will be more difficult than otherwise. (See Figure 14 for specific correspondences with each vertebra.)

While it is not always necessary to work on the spine in any particular sequence, it is typically more effective to work from the top down. We begin with the cervicals, then work down through the thoracic area, and on to the lumbar area, and eventually to the sacrum and the coccyx. Not every vertebrae needs to be held. A good method is to begin with the largest calcifications and curvatures and/or the areas of greatest significance. Pressure can be applied with a thumb, although a strong finger may be used. In some cases an elbow is used, as a thumb may not be able to supply sufficient force. The pressure is applied with the end of the forearm immediately adjacent

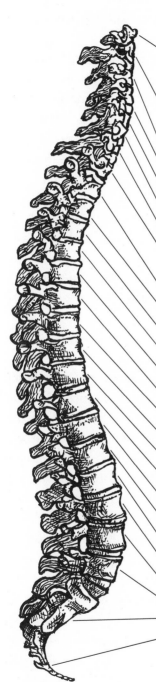

VERTEBRAE REFLEX AREAS

C1: Blood supply to the head, pituitary gland, scalp, bones of the face, brain, inner and middle ear, sympathetic nervous system

C2: Eyes, optic nerves, auditory nerves, sinuses, mastoid bones, tongue, forehead

C3: Cheeks, outer ear, face bones, teeth, trifacial nerve

C4: Nose, lips, mouth, eustachian tube

C5: Vocal cords, neck glands, pharynx

C6: Neck muscles, shoulders, tonsils

C7: Thyroid gland, bursae in the shoulders, elbows

T1: Arms from elbows down, hands, wrists, fingers, esophagus

T2: Heart including valves and coronary arteries

T3: Lungs, bronchial tubes, pleura, chest, breast

T4: Gall bladder, common duct

T5: Liver, solar plexus, blood

T6: Stomach

T7: Pancreas, duodenum

T8: Spleen, diaphragm

T9: Adrenal and supra-renal glands

T10: Kidneys

T11: Kidneys, ureters

T12: Small intestines, lymph circulation

L1: Large intestines, inguinal rings

L2: Appendix, abdomen, upper leg

L3: Sex organs, uterus, bladder, knees

L4: Prostate gland, lower back muscles, sciatic nerve

L5: Lower legs, ankles, feet

Sacrum: Hip bones, buttocks

Coccyx: Rectum, anus

FIGURE 14: SPINAL REFLEXES

to the elbow itself in a *scooping* manner. The elbow is cupped between the opposite thumb and index finger to prevent sliding.

With a curvature we usually will press against the spine medially and anteriorly at the extreme point of the curve on the side to which it is curving. With a calcification, we will press directly upon the calcification from one side or the other in a medial and anterior direction in most cases. The exact angle preferred will simply be that which will bring out the most pain. Spinal work is often more painful than that which has preceded it. Extra care should be taken never to transgress the limits of that which can be lovingly endured.

It is surprisingly easy to permanently straighten out curvatures and dissolve calcifications on an individual who is well prepared nutritionally and who has had full nerve supply and endocrine function restored, though holding spinal points before the person is ready is generally ineffective. I have felt a calcification as large as a golf ball decrease in size nearly eighty percent in twenty minutes.

STRUCTURAL SYMMETRY

A few pairs of points are very useful in restoring symmetry to the body. Since any distortion in structure will tend to be related to functional difficulties, any move towards greater bodily symmetry will tend to improve function as well. These points include what are known as the triple axis clavicle points, which help restore symmetry primarily from the diaphragm upwards. Also there are the pubic points, which help restore symmetry primarily from the diaphragm downwards. And the ischial tuberosity points will assist mainly with various problems in the pelvis and lower back.

Weston Price, Francis Pottenger and others observed that physical degeneration in succeeding generations as a result of faulty parental nutrition was accompanied not merely by a deterioration in health and vitality, but by obvious deviations from normal body symmetry, structure and proportion, including cranial and dental deformities as well as other skeletal deformities. Such deviations also included changes in overall bodily proportions, including a tendency for gender differences in bodily structure and proportions to gradually diminish. This last was noted especially by Pottenger. All of these changes were observed not simply in humans, but in cats, cows, dogs and other mammals. Weston Price used the term *intercepted heredity* to describe this type of phenomena. (See Chapter Eight.)

When animals with these deformities were fed properly themselves, they could typically produce offspring either without such deformities or at least with a less marked degree of deformity. There is no evidence that in adults these deformities were corrected, however, as a result of a return to proper nutrition.[6] This suggests that if Body and Cranial Electronics (next section) are able to correct these deviations from symmetry, then something quite extraordinary is taking place. To put it into Weston Price's language, this would suggest that the heredity that was intercepted has been retrieved and installed. Or to use an earlier analogy from this book, the particular energy overlay or transparency that contained this deviation from our full genetic potential has been overcome and released.

THE CRANIAL
Benefits

The next sequential stage of Body Electronics is what is known as *Cranial Electronics,* a revolutionary technique developed by Dr. Ray which will bring far reaching results for most. It is generally far more painful and intense than anything that comes before it. Cranial Electronics should never be attempted on anyone who is not extremely well prepared nutritionally, psychologically, and with previous Body Electronics, including spinal work. The benefits of the *cranial,* as this is called, are many: cranial sutures will come unlocked; the cranial bones will be able to move much more freely; and through reflex activity the entire body will benefit. The sutures are basically a type of joint that exists between the various cranial bones, and like any joint, they are designed to permit movement. As for the cranial bones, the degree of movement is small, but nevertheless their natural mobility must be maintained. (If we exclude the bones of the inner ear and the hyoid bone, there are twenty-two bones in the skull. Eight of these comprise the cranial group; the remaining fourteen comprise the facial group.) In addition to the cranial bones, there are many muscles in this area, and these, like all muscles, have direct reflex to certain organs and glands.

Most people have some degree of cranial distortion due to numerous causes. The work of Weston Price makes it clear that something as simple as inadequate parental nutrition is sufficient to result in cranial deformity in the offspring. In the civilized world, cranial deformity has become the norm rather than the exception. There is no more obvious and indisputable proof than the simple observation that very few adults have sufficient room for all their thirty-two adult teeth, including wisdom teeth. And even those who have all thirty-two teeth will generally have some degree of crookedness or crowding. As Price noted and as the photos in *Nutrition and Physical Degeneration* demonstrate, a properly formed human skull readily allows all teeth with room to spare.

As a result of cranial deformities and distortions, one or more of the cranial sutures will tend to calcify. As sutures lock up, the natural cranial mobility is impaired. A motion known as *primary respiratory mechanism,* or *PRM,* involves a rhythmic flexion and extension of the skull at around ten to fourteen beats per minute. The PRM is dependent upon the proper mobility of the various cranial bones along the sutures. The primary respiratory mechanism helps in the dissemination of *cerebrospinal fluid,* or *CSF,* out to the tissues of the body via the perineural and perivascular pathways. The unimpeded distribution of CSF, and hence the PRM, is a prerequisite for full health of the body.[7] Blockage of the free flow of CSF can result in lowered electrical potential in the tissues, poor circulation and nerve supply, and a general and progressive deterioration of health. One of the significant benefits of Cranial Electronics is releasing the calcifications in the various cranial sutures, which helps to restore the proper activity of the PRM and as a consequence, the unimpeded distribution of the cerebrospinal fluid.

In addition, remarkable changes in bone structure of the cranium routinely occur through the cranial. This has been extensively documented in a study conducted by the late Dr. Robert Whiteside, world famous personologist and author of numerous books including the international bestsellers *Face Language* (out of print) and *Face Language II.* In the science of personology, precise measurements are taken of various physical traits, many being specific measurements of cranial structure. These structural traits have been exhaustively correlated with specific personality traits. An individual is given a percentile score on each trait in relation to the rest of the population. When individuals are measured and rechecked over the course of many years, it is found that people normally change very little. However, when personology measurements have been done on people before and after a cranial, changes of twenty to thirty percentile points are common as a result of this extraordinary procedure. Such changes in personology measurements are independent verification of the tremendous changes in cranial structure that occur as a result of Cranial Electronics. Other evidence of significant cranial shift has been provided by individuals with full or partial upper dentures which, despite fitting perfectly prior to the cranial, no longer fit afterwards.

The Practice

The cranial as developed by Dr. Ray involves several sequential stages. Before a cranial is attempted, it is important that the spine be worked on sufficiently, including the sacrum and coccyx. The first stage of the cranial itself involves holding points on the mastoid process of the temporal bone, first on the left and then on the right. This will gradually shift the temporal bone in such a manner as to free up the sphenoid, thus laying the ground for the next stage. In the region of the cranium known as the pterion there are four bones which overlap each other (as Figure 15 shows). These four bones, the frontal, parietal, sphenoid, and temporal will tend to overlap from the inside out in alphabetical order. Thus, the temporal bone must be unlocked first in order to free those underneath. This is accomplished by holding points on the mastoid process. It might be noted in addition that each temporal bone (of which the mastoid is a portion) has on average fifteen muscle attachments. Given the reflexes between muscles and organs or glands, work on the mastoid will therefore also have enormous reflex implications throughout the rest of the body.

The cranial technique, especially the triple axis, should not be attempted on anyone not extremely well prepared nutritionally nor on someone who has not had all the necessary pointholding leading up to this. It should most definitely never be attempted by someone who has not been fully taught how to do it. The first cranial that a person gives should be done under the supervision of a person well versed in the field.

The second stage is known as the *triple axis*. This is the most intense and precise part of the cranial and requires tremendous patience on the

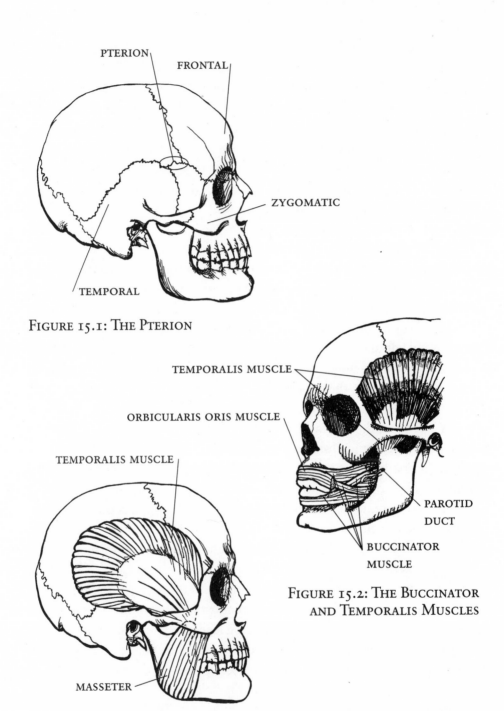

PTERION

FRONTAL

ZYGOMATIC

TEMPORAL

FIGURE 15.1: THE PTERION

TEMPORALIS MUSCLE

ORBICULARIS ORIS MUSCLE

TEMPORALIS MUSCLE

PAROTID DUCT

BUCCINATOR MUSCLE

FIGURE 15.2: THE BUCCINATOR
AND TEMPORALIS MUSCLES

MASSETER

FIGURE 15.3: THE TEMPORALIS AND MASSETER MUSCLES

part of the pointholder and much fortitude on the part of the person on the table. The triple axis is generally done first on the left, then the right, side. The left side, being the receiving side of the body, generally has less resistance and thus tends to be easier to do than the right side in most people. Once the first side has been done, bilateral reflex activity tends to make the second side easier than it would have been otherwise. When the triple axis is thoroughly completed on both sides, which may take many hours, this will shift the sphenoid, thus freeing up the parietal and frontal bones. We only have one sphenoid, as it extends through the middle of the skull. It articulates with all of the other seven bones in the cranial group in most cases, as well as many of the facial bones. In addition, the sphenoid has eleven to thirteen muscle attachments on both the left and right sides. This means that working on the sphenoid will also result in tremendous reflex effect upon the rest of the body.

Typically during the triple axis, there are striking changes in bone structure of the face, especially in the cheeks and around the eyes. A number of the muscles of mastication in particular are affected by the triple axis portion of the cranial. These include the masseter, with reflex to the pineal; the buccinator, with possible reflex to the thymus; the temporalis, with reflex to the thyroid; and the lateral and medial pterygoids, with reflex to the pituitary.

The final stage of the cranial is working on the hard palate. Special attention is paid in the event there is a condition known as *torus palatinus* where there is a ridge sagging down in the center of the roof of the mouth. This indicates that the vomer is displaced, causing the sagging of the palatine processes of the maxilla as well as the palatine bones. Such a condition, which is fairly common, is often corrected during this stage of the cranial. There are numerous reflexes from the hard palate to various parts of the skull, spine, and elsewhere in the body. Many problems in the alignment of teeth along the jaw are also frequently corrected during the cranial. People who had too little room along the jaw for all their teeth, resulting in the teeth coming in crooked have found that there was enough room after a cranial. People with extra room as evidenced by gaps between teeth have had the gaps disappear during a cranial. Prior dental trauma, including reaction to anesthetic, is often reexperienced during the cranial. It is

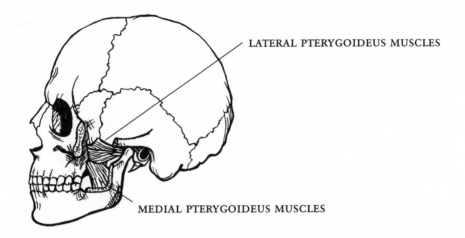

LATERAL PTERYGOIDEUS MUSCLES

MEDIAL PTERYGOIDEUS MUSCLES

FIGURE 15.4: THE PTERYGOID MUSCLES—LATERAL AND MEDIAL

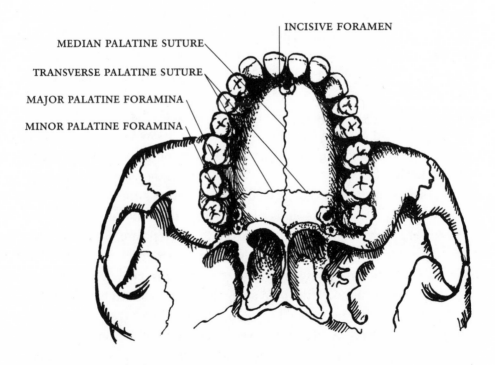

INCISIVE FORAMEN

MEDIAN PALATINE SUTURE

TRANSVERSE PALATINE SUTURE

MAJOR PALATINE FORAMINA

MINOR PALATINE FORAMINA

FIGURE 15.5: THE HARD PALATE

quite common for the lips or mouth to go quite numb as novocaine is released during healing crisis.

ADVANCED PROCEDURES OF BODY ELECTRONICS

The basic sequence of Body Electronics progresses from the STO to the endocrine and organ points, then on to the spinal and finally the cranial points. In most cases a greater level of pain is involved at each step as we move from STO and endocrine points to the spinal and then to the cranial points. There is an additional method of Body Electronics known as *advanced procedures* or *moving points* which comes after the cranial and involves the reflexes between the various muscles in the body and the various organs and glands. This technique involves pressure combined with motion and rotation on these muscles. As an advanced technique of Body Electronics, it should not be attempted on one not properly prepared up to and through the cranial, nor should it be attempted by one not properly trained in it.[8]

SELECTION OF POINTS FOR A SESSION

The selection of points to hold for a given session will depend upon many factors. The advanced stages of Body Electronics will require the preparatory steps enumerated above. In most cases, the STO and whatever endocrine points are necessary will precede any other pointholding.

Within the range of pointholding for which a given individual is prepared, there is considerable flexibility as to what points to hold on a given day. No uniquely correct set of points must be held, rather there exists a broad range of possibilities, each of which will bring about excellent results. Many logical considerations may enter the picture. For example, an individual may have problems in many of the endocrine glands as indicated through iridology. In selecting which points to hold, we might well consider the relative seriousness of the problems in the glands as well as the relative importance of these glands within the endocrine system. A severe problem in the thyroid might take precedence over a minor problem in the pineal. Were the problems more nearly equal in magnitude, then the pineal would probably take precedence over the thyroid. Somewhere in the gray area between there is more than a single appropriate response.

In addition to the use of iridology to determine which points are more critical, it is also helpful to apply pressure to the points under consideration in order to determine which is most sore. All other things being equal, it is best to hold the point that is most sore. If we plan to hold a particular point which is found bilaterally (on both the left and right, as the vast majority are), then to determine which side to hold we may use iridology as well as determining which is most sore. There are usually a great number of different points for a given organ or gland. In choosing which of these possibilities to hold, the same method is also helpful. All other things being equal, choosing points on the feet has several advantages, including the ease with which they are located.

Yet in addition to these logical considerations, the role of intuition in the selection of points should also be considered. On numerous occasions I have seen a spectacular result ensue from the selection of a point or points that did not appear initially to make any logical sense. As with nutrition, in point selection there may be an appropriate balance between logic and intuition. Reliance on either to the neglect of the other would not be advisable. Another way to explain this would be to say that once we have learned the "rules," we are in a better position to recognize the "exceptions" via our intuition.

If an initial attempt to hold points on a particular area is unsuccessful, most likely other factors have not yet been addressed. Sometimes it is necessary to get all the ducks in a row before good results will be obtained. For example, it may not be effective to work on a particular organ because the corresponding part of the spine is still a problem, or to work on the spine because the cranium is still a problem. Or a problem in the arm may not respond until the triple axis clavicle point is held to completion. There are numerous possibilities. But if results are not immediately forthcoming, it is often a good idea to consider what has not yet been done.

Situations Where Body Electronics Has Been Effective

BODY ELECTRONICS HAS BEEN EFFECTIVE WITH AN EXTREMELY BROAD range of specific conditions including broken bones, sprains, various injuries both recent and otherwise; a wide range of degenerative conditions such as cancer, heart conditions, diabetes, and arthritis; and many specific complaints such as asthma, scar tissue, chronic fatigue, spinal and back problems including scoliosis, high blood pressure, poor vision or poor hearing, various psychological conditions, and many other complaints. Body Electronics can also be extremely effective in first aid situations. In several instances when I have sustained deep gashes on my fingers which would normally require several stitches to close and would leave a scar, I have held points directly on the injury and have seen the bleeding stop and the skin completely close back up in a matter of less than five minutes, healing with virtually no visible scar. Body Electronics will routinely produce such results when the individual is nutritionally saturated and able to reexperience the trauma, including all of the associated patterns of thought, word and emotion.

Other injuries which have been routinely corrected with Body Electronics include sprains, dislocations, twists, and hyperextensions of ankles, knees and fingers. The secret of success in these instances is for the individual to be well saturated nutritionally and to reexperience the injury while the pointholder or the individual applies pressure in such a manner as to bring out the pain of the trauma. Remember: never push harder than the individual can lovingly and willingly endure. There have also been cases where Body Electronics has been used with great success in first aid situations involving injuries of much greater severity, such as simple and compound fractures. Whatever the relative severity of the injury or condition that is to be treated, it is important to understand that the basic underlying principles of Body Electronics remain the same and the manner of treatment will differ only in matter of degree.

It must also be recognized that there is a time, place and purpose for all things under the sun. This includes conventional medical techniques. The wise and discerning individual will recognize that in certain situations the threat to life is so great that the prudent course is to seek medical attention. Serious injuries resulting from accident-related trauma may require the help of a competent surgeon. Let us not be so proud as to assume that we will never need these services. Let us simply be grateful that skilled physicians exist to assist us in times of emergency. Let us also learn to care for our physical bodies and take responsibility for our thoughts, words and emotions so that our need for outside intervention may be kept to a minimum.

Contraindications for Body Electronics

BODY ELECTRONICS SHOULD BE DONE ONLY WITH GREAT CAUTION IN certain areas of the body: the basic principle of *find the pain and push* does indeed have a few exceptions. To begin with, when an individual has poor nerve supply, pointholding should be done gently or not at all in areas such as the abdomen, which is relatively unprotected. Excessive pressure to this area can be a problem, and if the individual on the table has insufficient nerve supply, they may be unaware that damage is being done. Other areas where caution should be exercised are near the throat, eyes, and varicose veins. As for the latter, should there be a blood clot present, pressure could break it loose, with potentially dangerous consequences. It is also wise to hold points only when an individual is well saturated nutritionally, especially when the individual is experiencing any serious physical ailment.

In the event of a tumor it is best to refrain from Body Electronics in the area of the tumor because there is some risk of breaking up the tumor and causing it to spread by applying pressure to it. The best approach with a tumor is to attain and maintain a thorough state of nutrient saturation in order to first contain the tumor by restoring integrity to the surrounding tissue. Then Body Electronics can be initiated, beginning with the STO and endocrine points, as it will be imperative to fully restore nerve supply and endocrine function if the condition is to be completely reversed. Because of the potential seriousness of situations involving tumors, it is better to err on the side of caution. In many cases, tumors may exist without the individual being aware of their presence. These tumors will sometimes be apparent to a competent iridologist. For this reason it is strongly urged that everyone involved in Body Electronics be trained in iridology. (See

Chapter Twenty.) At the very least, one member of each pointholding group should be an iridologist. However, no method, including iridology, will be one hundred percent effective in detecting tumors. They are a distinct possibility with almost anyone. It is best to exercise caution.

If a tumor is present or suspected, a thorough nutrient saturation program is absolutely essential if healing is to take place. It may even be dangerous to engage in Body Electronics without a nutrient saturation program if a tumor is present.[9] The six basic supplements (see Chapter Thirteen) are all necessary in such circumstances. Both extra protease and Schweitzer fluid are strongly recommended for their ability to enhance immune function. Tumors or other abnormal tissue may be far more prevalent than most people suspect. If so, then all people who involve themselves in Body Electronics should be on a thorough program that involves a good diet as well as these basic six supplements as a suitable margin of safety.

A few other potential contraindications for Body Electronics are worth enumerating, all situations where Body Electronics should only be done with extreme caution, if at all, and only after prayerful consideration. When in doubt, don't.

The application of more pressure on a point than can be lovingly and willingly endured will typically result in more trauma as opposed to being effective in helping the individual work through existing trauma. Thus, when the pointholdee asks for less pressure, it is best to back off. (There are rare exceptions to even this, but these are best left to those with the necessary experience to recognize them. They are not common.)

In the event of osteoporosis, heavy pressure should not be applied, as in extreme instances heavy pressure could result in a fracture. In any individual who is quite numb, a greater than normal degree of caution must always be applied, as such individuals may be unable to tell when damage is being done. For example, paraplegics and quadriplegics would belong in this category. It is generally best not to hold points or have points held when pregnant. This is a time when the expectant mother should be concentrating on other things and not going through healing crisis and heavy cleansing, as this is not good for the baby.

There are a number of situations in the abdomen where damage could be done if pressure were applied inappropriately. Pressure through the abdomen on an IUD, for example, could result in a severe injury. Pressure on the uterus if a women happens to be pregnant (which she might not know yet) could also be a hazard. There is a situation known as an abdominal aneurysm where the abdominal aorta is fragile and much distended. Even moderate pressure or an accidental blow could have fatal consequences, for if the aneurysm were to rupture, the person would bleed to death quite rapidly. If diverticuli or intestinal strictures might be present, only gentle, if any, pressure should be applied to the area. Basically, be careful of the abdomen, and when in doubt, leave it alone.

Some individuals have cerebral shunts to drain excess fluid off the brain. These are often located under the skin on the side of the neck and run down into the chest. Inadvertent pressure upon the shunt could prevent the fluid from draining. While this might have no consequences for a brief period given a slow rate of flow, I would prefer not to test the envelope and would recommend simply being careful not to exert any pressure on a shunt. There are other points on the cranium other than those used in Cranial Electronics, but as a good rule of thumb, no points should be held on the head until after Cranial Electronics has been successfully completed at least once.

If a person has a history of mental or psychiatric illness especially including the use of various psychiatric medications, Body Electronics might not be advisable. In healing crisis not only physical symptoms may resurface, but also emotional traumas. And in particular, anything that has been suppressed by any sort of medication is likely to eventually reappear. There are undoubtedly situations of such a severe nature that it may be prudent *not* to attempt Body Electronics, not to open Pandora's box. For once it is opened, it may not be possible to ever close it again. Put another way, it is best not to open such a box unless we are quite willing for all its contents to come out. And bear in mind that the contents will emerge on their own schedule, not ours.

If a person has had a heart attack or a stroke, it is best to be aware that they may eventually go back through this on the table. They should be well prepared nutritionally. When there are obvious problems with the heart, heart points must be held initially in order to relieve the strain on the heart and to avert an accident. Certain signs in the iris and sclera will show that a heart attack has either occurred or is imminent. In such a case, it is vital to hold the heart points as soon as the person is prepared nutritionally. A person with a known heart condition should not have their points held until they are well prepared nutritionally. In many cases people have reexperienced heart attacks on the pointholding table during healing crisis, much to the consternation of their pointholders. It is more than a little disquieting to see someone appear to stop breathing for a few minutes prior to coming out of it. Pointholders must stay plugged in to the points if this happens. It may help to plug a few more people in to other heart points. The points may be jiggled vigorously at this juncture as well. There have never been any cases where a person has reexperienced a heart attack and not gotten through it. But due to the seriousness of such a situation, it is wise to take extra precautions just to be safe. The principle of the healing crisis suggests that the individual will have the chance to reexperience each trauma. Thus, if a person has previously had a heart attack, it is likely and desirable that they will reexperience it so that they can overcome this trauma. Thus, it is best to be prepared for such an eventuality.

And finally, there are a number of unique situations where if pointholding is attempted, some interesting possibilities may result. If we are unwilling for these results, we'd better not start, as they are possible. Some people have joints where, as a result of numerous injuries, there are large amounts of scar tissue. In some cases, the scar tissue is what is holding the joint together. If pointholding is done in such an area, this scar tissue may dissolve. As the process of regenerating the joint may take place over time, what may happen is that upon the initial disappearance of the scar tissue the joint may basically "fall apart" until such time as the healing is complete and the muscles, tendons and ligaments involved are all sound again. If we stop when the scar tissue is gone but the joint not sound, in some ways we may be left worse off than when we started. According to a reliable colleague, this has happened at least once, with a shoulder. In such a situation, we should not start unless we are determined to finish the process.

There are a few other situations involving artificial body parts and organ transplants where in theory there could be serious consequences. From the perspective of the immune system, transplanted organs and artificial body parts are foreign. Were the immune system in proper shape, it might reject this foreign material. (This is why drugs are taken to suppress the immune system in the case of organ transplants.) As the body regenerates, eventually the immune system will return to full function. While on the one hand I like to think the body would have the sense not to kill itself, we really do not know what might happen. Yet it does seem possible that the body might try to reject someone else's organ or an artificial heart valve, which might be a bit inconvenient if the body needed the item in question! (This is not something I have seen or heard of happening, but it is merely a possibility we have considered.)

Conclusion: Healing as a Spiral

BODY ELECTRONICS IS FUNDAMENTALLY A SIMPLE PROCESS. IT REQUIRES nutrient saturation as well as the willingness and ability to reexperience the various suppressed patterns of thought, word and emotion in order for the process to be effective. There is a basic sequence of priorities in Body Electronics wherein nerve supply, endocrine function, organ function, proper spinal alignment, and eventually proper cranial structure and function are restored. For the advanced stages of Body Electronics it is necessary to first undergo the initial stages.

As people progress through the various stages of pointholding, first restoring nerve supply and circulation, then improving endocrine and organ function, next correcting spinal and perhaps other skeletal distortions, and eventually restoring cranial symmetry, many are discovering that the completion of this sequence with the Cranial Electronics is not merely an end but a whole new beginning as well. For as we complete our first cranial, we find that we can make even deeper progress as we engage in more endocrine and spinal work. Just as the endocrine and spinal work have paved the way to make the first cranial possible and productive, so in turn does the first cranial make it possible to reach deeper levels with the endocrine and spinal pointholding than was possible. We may consider that, on the one hand, the spinal and cranial pointholding generally must be preceded by a certain amount of pointholding to restore nerve supply, circulation, and endocrine function. Yet, on the other hand, we might also consider that "perfect" nerve supply, circulation and endocrine function is not possible so long as spinal and cranial distortions still remain. Similarly, we may consider that a certain amount of spinal pointholding must generally precede the cranial pointholding. Yet again, the spine itself will not be "perfect" so long as the cranium is still distorted. So we return to the "basics" so that we may then move again to the "advanced" points, which will in turn be more productive at a deeper level as the "basics" have been explored anew. Thus, we see that the sequence of points is truly a spiral, and each trip around the spiral brings us to a higher and deeper level. All points are connected holographically, and from any point or points we may have the opportunity to access the reactive contents of our own unconscious mind.

Chapter Seventeen

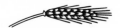

Individual Responsibility and the Pointholdee

Shine a light and people will find their own way.
Anonymous

Government should do for the people only what they cannot possibly do for themselves, and otherwise leave them alone.
Abraham Lincoln

... a wise and frugal government which shall restrain men from injuring one another, shall leave them otherwise free to regulate their own pursuits of industry and improvement, and shall not take from the mouth of labor the bread it has earned. This is the sum of good government....
Thomas Jefferson

Whomever would sacrifice any of their essential liberties for a little temporary security deserves neither liberty nor security.
Benjamin Franklin

Optimism is true moral courage.
Ernest Shackleton

"Fortitudine vincimus." (By endurance we conquer.)
Shackleton family motto

THE PHYSICAL MECHANICS OF BODY ELECTRONICS HAS BEEN COVERED in previous chapters, and much information has been given about nutrition and health on a physical level. Yet nutrition and the techniques of pointholding are still only parts of the process of Body Electronics. The true purpose of Body Electronics is to bring about a change of consciousness.

How the Body Electronics session proceeds once the person is properly prepared nutritionally, once the points have been selected, and people have appropriately plugged into these points needs clarification. In many modalities, the emphasis is placed upon what the practitioner needs to do, while the role of the patient is often ignored. However, in Body Electronics, while the pointholders play a valuable role, the primary emphasis is placed upon what must be done by the person whose points are being held. It is recognized that the ultimate responsibility for their own progression rests with each person. Let us look then at some of the principles that the pointholdee can put into practice while on the pointholding table.

Being Active and Being Receptive

CRYSTALS DISSOLVE UNDER THE COMBINED INFLUENCE OF NUTRIENT saturation and Body Electronics. The information content of the crystals is in the form of thought patterns, word patterns, and emotional patterns. The thought patterns are the sensory memory of time, place, form and event—the who, what, when, where, and how of a given experience. The word patterns are the verbal expressions, whether outwardly uttered or not. The emotional patterns are the feelings or emotions that are associated with the word and thought patterns, and these will include unconsciousness, apathy, grief, fear, anger, pain, and enthusiasm.

Those whose points are being held must learn to be simultaneously yin and yang. For it is important to be receptive to the thoughts, words, and emotions as they are released from the crystals, which is being yin. It is also important to search diligently for these very things, which is being yang.

Thus, we must at the same time let it happen as well as make it happen.

In the *Logic in Sequence* series, *Book One: The Laws of Perfection*, Dr. Ray defines four basic steps to the process: observe, receive, recreate, and release. First, we must "observe and choose to expand our ability to observe." Second, "after we observe, we make a conscious choice to be receptive pertaining to what we observe. We make a conscious choice to be 'yin,' to be receptive. This is yet incomplete for our purposes, as we are only 'Lovingly and Willingly Enduring all Things.'" Third, "after we have learned how to be yin or receptive, now we must learn how to be yang.... We selectively choose ... to recreate that energy we have experienced or received, arising out of the outer environment and inner environment. An energy of thought, feeling and spoken word has been sent into the universe and will continue to manifest itself until it is un-created. When we receive an energy of creation encoded in crystal and revealed to the inner essence, we have viewed the yin (outer manifestation) and the yang (inner creative force) simultaneously and hologramically. As we receive the yin and yang simultaneously by choice, we then choose to recreate that yin-yang energy and hold it in our mind until it no longer vibrates with the energy of transmutation." Fourth, "after the yin-yang receptivity is selectively recreated until the regenerative vibration is complete, we release with gratitude the hologramic concept we have been holding fixed in our consciousness."[1] These four steps are the essence of transmutation, and they involve activity on the part of the pointholdee. Specific practices include maintaining a state of love and forgiveness, disciplining the body, maintaining a state of enthusiasm, encompassing both sides of dualities, and looking for resistances. Let us look at each of these in turn.

Maintain a State of Love and Forgiveness

POINTHOLDEES LOVINGLY AND WILLINGLY REEXPERIENCE THE REACTIVE content of thought, feeling, and spoken word as these are gradiently released from the crystals in the body. Love and forgiveness are central to the process. As information is gradiently released from the dissolving crystals, the pointholdee should reexperience thoughts, words, and emotions with unconditional love and unconditional forgiveness for themselves and everyone else. This is not merely a passive process of lying there waiting for something to happen, but involves an active component as well. We must search diligently for the thoughts, words, and emotions. A constant attitude of enthusiasm should be maintained. Unconditional love, continual gratitude, and unconditional forgiveness should all be constant.

Yet sometimes to *feel it with love* is more than we can manage with respect to many circumstances. The next best thing might be to start by finding something we can love about the situation. If we cannot yet love the whole plate that life has served up to us, sometimes it is best to love a forkful at a time.

A given emotion is transmuted by experiencing it with love rather than by merely experiencing it, and the same can be said of a given memory which might arise during pointholding. If we go back through an experience and simply resist it all over again, we have not really mastered anything or moved through anything. It is through re-experience with love and forgiveness that we begin to release ourselves from the bondage of our own resistance.

The Importance of Specific Memory

Freedom from resistance and reaction will come as we gain access to the specific memories involved and experience them with unconditional love and forgiveness. "Ye shall know the truth and the truth shall make you free." One definition of truth is that it is "a knowledge of the way things were, the way things are, and the way things are to be." If we know the truth, we know the way things were. That is, we have clear and accurate memory, free from the bonds of our own resistance. As Dr. Ray has noted, any inability to recall the past is a sign of resistance on our part. If we have no resistance in a given area, then we can see the past clearly. We will also have a clear perception of the present, unsullied by resistance. A clear perception of the present leads to a clear perception of the future. For if we see things as they are now, we can see how things are to be, provided that we understand the applicable laws of the universe. If we know the past, we may know the present as well as the future. Conversely, if resistance stops us from knowing where we've been, then we won't know where we are or where we are going either. In the absence of resistance, all is now.

Sticking with a Memory

Sometimes it is extremely helpful in a pointholding session to stick with one specific memory for an extended period. While we may feel we have already "been there, done that" with an event that we might have looked at in many previous pointholding sessions or perhaps in other modalities as well, it is helpful to be reminded of the obvious: if we were truly done with the event in question, it would not come up. Often when people do stick with a specific event for many hours, their persistence pays off handsomely. For as one layer of resistance is encountered and transmuted, the next deeper layer of resistance is eventually laid bare so that it in turn can be accessed and transmuted. This allows people to excavate down sequentially through multiple layers of resistance to some very deeply buried core patterns of resistance. The changes people are able to experience within themselves as a result of releasing these deep resistances can be truly life changing. Deeper breakthroughs generally come about because the pointholdee is willing to keep hunting, rather than simply resting on their laurels.[2]

The Holographic Principle

Working with resistances related to specific memories is fruitful because of the holographic principle. It is the nature of a hologram that every part is connected to every other part, and every part could be said to contain the whole. Some interesting implications of this holographic principle can be applied to pointholding. Consider a given hologram involving various word patterns, emotional patterns, and thought patterns or sensory memories. Each part of this hologram provides direct access to all other parts. Every word pattern that is part of the hologram gives access to all other word patterns, all emotional patterns, and all sensory memories or thought patterns that are part of the hologram. And every emotional pattern that is part of the hologram gives access to all other emotional patterns, all word patterns, and all sensory memories or thought patterns that are part of the hologram. And every thought pattern or sensory memory (or even the tiniest fraction of a given sensory memory) gives access to all word patterns, all emotional patterns, and all sensory memories or thought patterns that are part of the hologram.

It is a fairly simple matter to use this access, for it is then a matter of repeating the part of the hologram of which one is already aware. For the repetition of any one aspect of the hologram will tend to bring up awareness of all other aspects. Hence, the repetition of a word pattern, the intensification of an emotional pattern, or going over and over any aspect of a memory or any sensory experience will eventually help bring to full awareness the entire hologram. This often requires much patience and persistence. Yet for those who do persevere, it is well worth the effort.

Discipline the Body

THE PHYSICAL BODY MUST BE DISCIPLINED SO THAT THE EMOTIONAL body might be accessed. With some exceptions, the physical body should be kept completely still. Total mastery of this discipline may require much time, effort, and experience. As long as our physical body is undisciplined, we may not be capable of fully accessing the emotional body. However, it is not merely the stillness of the body that is important, but rather that we are holding our body still. Were mere stillness the only significant factor, we could simply be strapped to the table with appropriate restraints! By compelling the physical body to obey and be still, we begin to master it. In so doing we begin to access the emotional body, which occurs from the bottom up with respect to the scale of emotions, beginning with unconsciousness first. What happens to most people when they hold perfectly still? They get numb and tired, and their limbs fall asleep. This is the unconsciousness coming out of the tissues. Most people move whenever this happens. By *not* moving, we move deeper into the unconsciousness at first, but eventually we move through it and the numbness disappears as the unconsciousness is experienced lovingly and willingly. All this is done without moving. Dr. Ray has phrased it thus: Control of the physical body must come before control of the emotional body.

But there are a few exceptions to this rule of keeping the body still. Holding the body still on the pointholding table allows the various resistances locked within to be accessed and eventually transmuted, and typically without this discipline very poor results will be forthcoming. Yet there is another side of this principle which applies in some cases. Deep traumas locked within the body may begin to surface initially as involuntary movements during pointholding, perhaps quite subtle ones at first. (However, in almost all cases, the initial physical stillness plays a huge role in bringing these involuntary motions to the surface.) There appears to be an appropriate time to actually encourage such involuntary movements. Once the trauma has been accessed sufficiently, it will probably be best to return to the discipline of physical stillness so that the resistance may be mastered on the mental level.

When to allow movement and when to keep still may be tricky to understand and put into practice. For many it may be best to simply continue to work on mastery of the discipline of stillness. But sometimes it is quite productive to shift gears briefly in order to access the trauma. A personal example might help. In one pointholding session, my arms and legs began to move involuntarily. When I allowed the movement to come out and intensify, the facilitator asked me what I felt. I quickly responded "like I'm drowning." And almost instantly, I became aware of a specific event: being thrown off a high diving board into the pond at age six during swimming class. The involuntary movements were me frantically trying to dog paddle back to the dock. Once the resistance was sufficiently identified, I was able to return to keeping still.

Maintain a State of Enthusiasm

THE EMOTIONAL BODY IS ALSO STILLED BY EXPERIENCING EACH EMOTION with enthusiasm in a controlled fashion so that the mental body might eventually be entered into. As the emotional body is accessed as a result of physical discipline, we will move up the scale of emotions from unconsciousness to apathy, to grief, to fear, to anger, to pain, and finally to enthusiasm. Each emotion is fully experienced in itself with an attitude of enthusiasm. While processing each emotion we also go through seven levels of emotion. There are levels of enthusiasm, pain, anger, fear, grief, apathy, and unconsciousness at each of these seven levels. The key to remember is that at the top of each level of emotion is always found the enthusiastic level of that very emotion. The key is to experience each emotion with enthusiasm. The enthusiasm generated by us should encompass (and not exclude) the emotion that is there. The purpose is not to gloss over any emotion, but rather to transmute it. This transmutation cannot take place without the initial admission that the emotion is there in the first place. Dr. Ray has phrased it thus: Control of the emotional body must come before control of the mental body.

Encompass Both Sides of Dualities

THE PROCESS OF HEALING INVOLVES ENCOMPASSING THE VARIOUS DUAL-ities on the mental level as they are revealed. The mental body is eventually accessed through the transmutation of the emotional body in this step by step process. On the mental body level, we are able to view the various dualities involved and to encompass each in turn. We have been identified with one end of the duality ever since the initial judgment took place in the given area. As we move back through this in reverse order, there is a point of total identification with the one side (but this time with enthusiasm, not resistance) that takes place prior to the recognition of the opposite side of the duality. Until we have overcome all resistance in the given area, we will remain unable to see the other side of the duality. The other side of the duality has been there all along; it is just that our own resistance has blinded us so that we cannot see it.

To some degree, all resistance is based upon a lie, upon less than the entire truth. Judgment, as we recall, is identifying with one side of a given duality to the exclusion of the other. The process of overcoming this judgment and the resistance that has arisen from it involves returning to the point where both sides of the given duality can be encompassed. Having a particular resistance tends to trap our attention upon the very thing we resist, and as a result, it is difficult to see anything else. The other side is often right in front of us. Sometimes in a pointholding session (or in other contexts) we are so busy looking for something that we fail to realize we have already found it. Perhaps our expectations are such that we are incapable of seeing that which is already before us. We have such strong belief systems about how things are supposed to unfold, that we are blind to what is already right before us. However, when both sides of a duality become apparent, it can be such an awakening.

These principles are well illustrated in a scene from the movie *Jumanji* with Robin Williams. Those who have seen this film may recall a scene where Robin Williams' character becomes trapped or stuck in the attic floor. His arms, legs, and most of his body dangle below, and only his head and not much else is above the floor. A bunch of giant spiders is fast approaching him and his three companions. The other adult, a woman, has her hands stuck in the floor as well, so it is up to the two children. So he shouts to the boy and tells him to go out back to the old shed and get the axe that his father used to keep inside. The boy runs frantically to the shed, intent on getting inside it so he can find the axe and get back and free the man from the floor. Much to his dismay, he finds a huge padlock on the door to the shed. He looks around in desperation, and off against the side of the shed is leaning a big axe. He grabs the axe and takes a swing or two at the padlock, still intent on getting into the shed to get the axe. All of a sudden, he turns and looks at the axe in his hands with a look of surprise and recognition. And then he runs back to save the day. Sometimes we all need to be reminded that often we are already holding the axe in our hands but just do not realize it.

To intellectually consider the opposite side of a given duality is not the same as to truly recognize it and encompass it. We can do this with a given resistance, by questioning whether it is really true or not. For the time being we assume that it is true. We work through the resistance until we are perfectly willing for it to be true. When we are perfectly willing for it to be true, it becomes totally obvious that it is not really true or at least not entirely. When we can be perfectly willing for what we resist to be true is often the moment when we can finally see the other side. A simple example of this principle will suffice. Suppose we feel that nobody loves us. We do not question the truth of it, but simply accept it as true and intensify all the resistance that goes with it. We repeat the various associated word patterns, intensify the associated emotions, go through one specific memory where we felt that way. Eventually we will reach a point where it is perfectly okay that nobody loves us, at which point we will likely see that this was never really the truth, or at least not the whole truth. Love was undoubtedly there all along, in one form or another. Perhaps not always in the form our crystals desired! But we were so busy resisting not being loved that we were unable to see that we were loved. It is generally that simple. But once again, this realization is not arrived at intellectually.

Look for Our Own Resistances

THERE ARE MANY TIMES WHERE THE PERSON ON THE TABLE BECOMES convinced that their pointholders or their facilitator is doing a poor job. This may or may not be the case, for resistance affects not just reality but perception. Our pointholders can only be as good as we let them be. Suppose we feel that one of our pointholders is not staying on the correct point but keeps sliding off. It is probably best to let them know this, and if they have moved, to help them move back to the correct point. But whether they have moved or not, it is also important for us to consider whether we have any resistance to the possibility. We may be disappointed that they have moved. We may be angry. We may feel cheated. We may feel that we cannot depend upon people. We may feel that nobody but ourselves can do it right. We may resist the situation (real or imagined!) in numerous ways.

On many occasions I have seem people who consistently feel that their pointholders are not on the right point. They feel this way session after session, no matter which pointholders are on their points. Nobody seems to be able to stay on the point. Yet I have seen most of these same pointholders have no trouble whatsoever in holding points on everybody else. So perhaps the problem is not always with the pointholder. (Certainly in some cases, it is the pointholder.) Sometimes the resistances of the person on the table have more to do with the pointholder slipping than anything else.

In the above example, what is of greatest relevance to the person on the table is not merely that their pointholder has moved off the point, but rather in what manner they resist this, if at all. If the pointholder has slid off a point, and in so doing helped reveal to us one of our own resistances, then perhaps they have done us a favor. If our pointholders or others in the room are inconsiderately conversing and we are finding it hard to concentrate, this too may reveal to us our own resistances. These people have also done us a favor. If we feel our facilitator talks too much or too little, and we resist it, this also can serve us. I am not for a moment suggesting that the person on the table tolerate conditions which do not further their healing, but we are all human. Without meaning to, at times we will help bring up resistances in each other. The person on the table can request the pointholder to get back on the point, or for the conversation to end, or whatever else. But most importantly, they can also look and see if they have any resistance. If we are able to look within ourselves and take responsibility for our own resistances, then there are countless opportunities for us to grow. None of these other people did any of these things to pop our buttons on purpose, at least in most cases. And yet they may have served us very well, if only we have the good sense to look within ourselves. Hence, the principle that we serve others in our unconsciousness at least as well as in our consciousness.

Chapter Eighteen

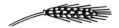

Putting It Down in Writing

It is necessary to the happiness of man that he be mentally faithful to himself.... Tis the business of little minds to shrink; but he whose heart is firm, and whose conscience approves his conduct, will pursue his principles unto death.

Thomas Paine

In the long run men hit only what they aim at. Therefore, though they should fail immediately, they had better aim at something high.

Henry David Thoreau

It is not the critic who counts, not the man who points out how the strong man stumbles or where the doer of deeds could have done them better. The credit belongs to the man who is actually in the arena, whose face is marred by dust and sweat and blood, who strives valiantly, who errs and comes short again and again because there is no effort without error and shortcomings, who knows the great devotion, who spends himself in a worthy cause, who at best knows in the end the high achievement of triumph and who at worst, if he fails while daring greatly, knows his place shall never be with those timid and cold souls who know neither victory nor defeat.

Theodore Roosevelt

T AKING INDIVIDUAL RESPONSIBILITY FOR THEIR HEALING MEANS POINT-holders not only play an active role during pointholding sessions but also work with their daily lives. One powerful technique is *the List*, which involves writing up our goals and seeking to achieve them.

The Power of the Written Word

B EFORE ANYTHING CAN BE BROUGHT INTO OUTER MANIFESTATION IN the physical universe, it must first exist on the inner. All must exist on the invisible level before manifesting in the visible. One of the most powerful means of helping to bring something from the invisible to the visible is to put it down in writing. "The pen is mightier than the sword" is indeed true on many levels. The mere act of putting something down in writing does not guarantee that it will eventually come to pass. Yet often committing things to writing helps us make concrete the healing or other changes which began on the table.

The process of regaining or maintaining physical health involves more than simply taking care of the needs of the body and overcoming our various resistances. It may also involve taking responsibility, putting order into our life, and taking definite action. Furthermore, a main purpose of improving our health and vitality may be to help us learn the lessons involving those areas of life we have not yet mastered. One of the most powerful tools to help us fulfill these purposes and more is to put things down in writing. Writing something down is at once a commitment to ourselves as well as an expression of faith in ourselves. Through this act of commitment and faith, we immediately bring ourselves closer to manifesting that which we have now committed to make manifest.

Numerous techniques may be used to harness the power of the written word. Dr. John Ray has taught an extremely simple method he refers to as *the List*. This is a deceptively simple concept, so simple that it is easy to dismiss as a waste of effort or to come up with a thousand other justifications not to do it. Yet the List will work quite well if we have the common sense to use it.

Making the List

I N PRACTICE THE LIST IS QUITE STRAIGHTFORWARD. WE MAKE A LIST which includes all our goals, desires, projects, responsibilities, uncompleted acts, areas where we have some form of amends or restitution to make, and other items that we choose to place on it. Once these items have been placed on the List, we organize them in order. The most difficult items are placed at the top and the least difficult at the bottom. We then work from the bottom up, crossing off each item on the List as it is completed. We take the time to stop and savor the completion of each act and to say, "it is good." We also revise the List on a regular basis: new items may be added, and sometimes items which have not been completed will be removed if they are no longer appropriate according to the dictates of conscience.

Moving from Success to Success

O NE OF THE MOST IMPORTANT PRINCIPLES INVOLVED IN THE LIST IS working within those areas where we can *see the end from the beginning*. When we can see the end from the beginning in a given task, we are capable of accomplishing this task. We see clearly what needs to be done to successfully complete the item on our List, and all that remains is for us to stretch forth our hand and do it. Once done, we move on to the next item. When we attempt to do something without a perceivable end, we are apt to fail because our efforts are premature. It is better to do those things that we know to do, for in doing these we expand our capacity for more complex tasks that may be still out of our reach. Thus, as we complete each item on the List we move from success to success. Those who have applied the List in their own lives can attest to the fact that by working steadily in this manner, from success to success, an incredible momentum and confidence is built, to a point where the individual is able to accomplish things that they could once only dream about. Nothing builds success like success. From time to time we may still run across the unexpected obstacle which prevents us from accomplishing an item even though we had thought we saw the end from the beginning. When this does happen, we enthusiastically accept this apparent setback as a learning experience. Such setbacks are failures only when we learn nothing from them.

Expanding Our Vision

ONE OF THE INTERESTING THINGS ABOUT THE LIST IS THAT OUR AWAREness and vision expand through diligent effort. As we work on our List, we will often find that it gets larger. We might begin with a List of fifty items. A while later, when we have accomplished twenty or thirty of these original fifty, we might find that we have added perhaps a hundred new items to our List. This is because as we begin putting order into our life by working on the simple items at the bottom of our List, we expand outward gradually such that we can be aware of more and more. We put more and more order into our life by working up our List a step at a time. As our vision expands in this fashion, we become aware of more, and our List grows.

The List is designed to help us to cultivate our vision. As we construct it, we may ask ourselves where we would like to be five, ten, or twenty years from now. We may ask what we would like to be doing, and how we would like to be living our life. We are encouraged to put these things down on our List. If we cannot see the end from the beginning, then it is wise to not waste our effort trying to do something. Nonetheless, we express faith in ourselves that we may eventually be able to do these things by putting them down on paper. Writing it down is crucial, for in so doing we begin the process of bringing it into the physical world even if the item is on our List for fifty years before we actually accomplish it.

We read through our List each day, which is an extremely important part of the process. As we do so, we come a little closer to each item on it, for in reading through our List each day, and then putting forth the effort to accomplish those items within our reach, the items higher up on our List will come a little bit more into focus until eventually we can see the end from the beginning and do them in the flesh.

Keeping It Secret

EACH PERSON MUST DETERMINE FOR THEMSELVES WHICH ITEMS TO include on their List. We determine our own responsibilities rather than simply writing down what someone else perceives our responsibilities to be. Always remember: the items on our List are our business. We keep our List secret rather than revealing it to the world. It is wise to bear in mind that "great things are done in secret." When we are busy telling people what is on our List, we are not working on it. Talking about something we plan to do before it is actually done halts our momentum and delays the completion of the task. Rather than telling people about what we might do, we let our completed actions speak for themselves. However, there may be an appropriate time and place to discuss a project with somebody else. For example, we might seek advice from an expert concerning a particular item on our List. Even then, we would be wise to reveal only that which needs to be revealed in order for them to answer our question.

In addition to our individual List, we might also construct a List with a mate or spouse, or with our family, or with a group of people. The principle of secrecy still applies here; for example, an item that is on the List of a group may be discussed by that group, but it should not be discussed beyond the group. When a List is constructed by two or more people, items are placed upon the List only by unanimous consent. When two or more people can agree to work together for a common purpose, it is a marvelous thing. Remember that a house divided against itself cannot stand, so we would be wise to confine our group Lists to only those items that all can agree upon. This does not violate the free agency of anyone, for there is no reason that a subset of a particular group may not work on their own List. The appropriate limit of our individual or collective free agency will simply be the point at which it begins to impinge upon the free agency of another.

Starting with a Personal Mission Statement

WHILE THE LIST ITSELF IS A MARVELOUS TOOL, AND WHILE IT HAS BEEN highly effective for many people as a means of putting order into their lives, in practice it typically has its limitations as well. One is that many people's use of their List tends to focus their attention upon things *to do* rather than upon their underlying states of beingness. As a result of placing certain items upon our List with the intention of completing these items and then crossing them off, there may be a distinct tendency to focus upon that activity without considering the underlying purposes and consequences, a focus upon the outer world of activity to the exclusion of the inner essence that underlies it. While this may not be an inevitable consequence of the List, it is a common experience.

A second drawback to the List is a sequential completion of items may be quite suitable for those which can eventually be brought to a state of completion, but is less suitable for items which are of a more ongoing nature. For example, we might wish to be a good parent to our children. Or we might wish to be considerate of those around us, or a more loving person. As most likely we will wish to continue to be a good parent, to be considerate and to be loving, where are such items to be included upon the List and how and when are they to be crossed off? In other words, the List by its very nature is more suitable to those things which once completed may be crossed off rather than those items which would remain indefinitely.

Another drawback to the List which many experience is that the entire List often becomes too cumbersome for daily perusal, so that in practice many people end up also constructing smaller lists of a more immediate nature. Thus, the smaller lists are used daily and the overall list is often neglected or ignored.

Some of these drawbacks can be overcome by a wonderful tool known as a personal mission statement, which is found in Stephen Covey's classic book *The Seven Habits of Highly Effective People*. The personal mission statement helps us to focus upon our fundamental values and principles, or the beingness that underlies the doingness of the List, and as such it is highly recommended as a foundation for the List itself. Once we have a personal mission statement, it makes more sense to construct a List or some similar type of time management tool. Techniques such as these can provide ways for those undergoing a healing process to take active responsibility and to apply what happens during healing sessions to their lives as they live them.

Chapter Nineteen

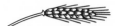

Considerations for Body Electronics Facilitators

In the long run it is far more dangerous to adhere to illusion than to face what the actual fact is.
David Bohm

The Facilitator's Role

WHILE POINTHOLDEES MUST BE ACTIVELY INVOLVED AND PERSONALLY responsible, during the pointholding session, generally one of the pointholders will assume the role of facilitator. They will talk to the person on the table from time to time, ask appropriate questions, offer encouragement, and make occasional observations and general suggestions. However, facilitators do not try to assume responsibility for the other person's progress.

One of the areas of greatest confusion for many involved in Body Electronics involves the role of the facilitator. To be of greatest help pointholders should understand their role, especially when they take on the additional task of facilitating the session.

PROPER ALLOCATION OF RESPONSIBILITY

We must always be individually responsible. The facilitator cannot ultimately be responsible for the progress of the person on the table. The facilitator's role is to help the pointholdee to come to a change of consciousness, not do it for them, and to make this as easy as possible. Please note that the word *facilitate* means literally *to make easy*.

With good intentions a pointholder may try to usurp responsibility in the misguided belief that they know what is best for a person. But "the road to hell is paved with good intentions." Body Electronics is based upon individual responsibility within a framework of cooperation and mutual assistance. The facilitator and the other pointholders are not the most important people at the session; they are nothing more than "props" who help to create an appropriate setting for the pointholdee to unfold.

The goal of the pointholdee is to simultaneously experience any thoughts, words and emotions which arise and to do so with love and forgiveness. The essence of facilitation may be summed up in two simple guidelines:

- See what the pointholdee is already doing and help them to do it better.

  This simple rule is to help the pointholdee do more of what they are already doing. If they have a thought pattern or sensory memory, we encourage them to expand upon this and uncover more of the memory. If they have a word pattern, we encourage them to intensify it, perhaps by repeating it out loud. If they have an emotion, we encourage them to intensify it and to experience it with enthusiasm. Whatever aspect of the thought, word and emotion they are already aware of, we encourage them to become more aware of that aspect: to do more of the same.

- See what the pointholdee is not doing yet and help them to do that as well.

  This simple rule is that if they already have one aspect—thought, word or emotion—we encourage them to get the other two at the same time. If the thought pattern or memory is pretty clear, we encourage them to find the emotion as well as the words that go with it. "How do you feel?" and "What are the words that go with that?" are examples of questions that might apply. If the emotion is present, we encourage them to find the words ("Can you put that emotion into words?") and the memory ("When have you felt that way before?") that go with this emotion. If the words are there, we encourage them to find the memory ("Remember a time when you felt those same

words.") and the emotions ("How do you feel as you say those words?").
We simply encourage the person to fill in the blanks.

TALKING VERSUS SILENCE

The facilitator will ask appropriate questions of the individual with the
intention of helping them to follow the steps outlined earlier. The facilitator will also have the good sense to always allow the pointholdee enough
silent time to experience the information as it is released from the crystals.
Many facilitators, particularly those under the false impression that they
are responsible for the other person, feel a strong compulsion to talk and
probe continually. This means that the pointholdee never has enough time
to actually experience anything, being too busy answering the constant
questions of the facilitator. Also, such constant questioning tends to encourage the pointholdee to generalize, rationalize, and intellectualize, and this
also makes it difficult to simply experience the information as it is released
gradiently from the crystals. Questions from the facilitator can be of great
assistance to the pointholdee, and allowing space and silence is also useful. Experience is the best teacher of when each is best. Before we ask a
question, however, we might consider whether our question will help the
person to get deeper into the experience or whether it will pull them out.

APPROPRIATE TIMING

Often facilitators will intervene at an inappropriate time, compulsively
feeling they have to do something. Other facilitators take the opposite
extreme, and are unwilling to do anything. It is wise to consider how our
own resistances will affect our actions or lack thereof as we facilitate: the
area of communication is often a major area of resistance for many of us.
Some people are programmed such that they have to talk. Others are programmed the opposite way. Both talking and not talking have their right
time: even a stopped clock is right twice a day! The key is to be willing to
do something and willing to do nothing. For then we are free to act or not
act without compulsion.

Helping the Pointholdee to Flower

A facilitator can help a person by creating a good space in which they can flower. The facilitator is like a gardener. Suppose a number of people were given the task of growing orchids using the same materials and the same basic instructions. Results would vary greatly. Some orchids might die from neglect or poor care. Some might be in poor shape but still alive. Perhaps despite their best efforts, the gardeners of these simply did not quite have the hang of it. Perhaps they tried too hard, and the orchids were watered too much. Some orchids might flourish because they received proper care and/or were cared for by people who have green thumbs. So it would seem that the gardener can be quite important and so it would be tempting to credit or blame the gardeners.

Yet we might consider that even the best gardener could not grow an orchid from a peach pit. Also, much depends on the orchid itself. Some of the gardeners might have been provided with better seeds to begin with while others were given dead seeds. It would not be possible for them to grow orchids with dead seeds, no matter what they did. So again, the orchid has to be considered as well as the gardener. Best results are obtained when orchid and gardener alike do their jobs well.

In addition to the orchid and the gardener, perhaps we might consider the source and creator of orchid and gardener alike. For the life and intelligence within both originates from the same higher source or intelligence, which some will call God.

Much of this applies to the relative role of the facilitator in pointholding. This person is like the gardener, responsible for providing the best possible conditions for each plant. These will include such factors as light, temperature, nutrients, water, and so on. And the best gardeners always use plenty of love as well. Pointholders as facilitators basically do the same thing. They provide the best possible conditions for the person on the table to flower. Love is a factor here as in the garden. Just as the conditions provided by the gardener can help or hinder the growth of the plants, so it is with facilitation. We can help or hinder the growth of the person on the table. And as any good gardener knows, timing and patience are important, as well as effort. It is not simply what is done, but when it is done.

The person on the table will flower in their own time: impatience or haste on the part of the facilitator will not speed this flowering up, and it may slow it down. We must also keep in mind that the person on the table and the facilitator also come from the same source and creator as orchid and gardener.

More on Individual Responsibility

UNDERSTANDING HOW TO BE A GOOD FACILITATOR MAY BE EASIER THAN realizing why it is so crucial for pointholders to play this role. There is much more than meets the eye concerning the vital point of individual responsibility. Many individuals with backgrounds in various types of counseling professions have been taught in therapist or practitioner centered modalities that the practitioner's responsibility is to move the person through their "stuff." However, in Body Electronics, there are no practitioners, but rather people trained in this field are educators who teach correct principles, set a good example by being present in their own lives, and let people govern themselves.

It is one thing to caution readers to avoid false concepts, but let us consider why such falsity has such an appeal not only for practitioners but for those they work with as well. Many people do not want to be responsible for their own progression. Thus, a teaching that places the responsibility outside of the individual (in this case, on the shoulders of the facilitator) has a great attraction for those who would not be responsible for themselves. However, central to Body Electronics is the principle that we are each individually responsible for our own situation. After all, how can we uncreate a given situation without first acknowledging that we created it? Dr. Ray notes that "responsibility is the willingness to be simultaneously cause and effect."[1]

Each is encouraged to take responsibility for their creations now and to acknowledge that they are now the effect of their previous creations. Body Electronics works best when we can work together cooperatively and interdependently. And as Stephen Covey correctly notes in *The Seven Habits of Highly Effective People,* interdependence is only possible once independence has been achieved. Without individual responsibility, cooperation is not really practical or possible.

On the other hand, some people aspire to the prestige and glory inherent in the role of practitioner in a practitioner centered modality. Some practitioners inflate the value of their role and revel in taking the credit for the progress of another. People play along, giving the facilitator credit for a breakthrough they have made in a session or becoming upset because they believe that their lack of progress is the practitioner's fault.

Let us always place the responsibility where it rightly belongs. This is not to say that the practitioner is of no consequence, but merely to place their role in proper perspective. Practitioners in the role of facilitator operate with the assumption that people are responsible for their own healing. The word facilitator means *someone who makes things easier* not someone who does it for us. A phrase I have coined that expresses much of the above is: Don't blame others for our success, or credit others with our failure.

DEPENDENCY RELATIONSHIPS

Some people seem to experience more on the pointholding table with certain facilitators than with others. It is possible for dependency relationships to be created such that the person believes that they can only have a good pointholding session with certain facilitators. However, while on the one hand it is good that they do have good results with this facilitator, ultimately it should be possible to get good results with others as well. Dependency relationships can become quite limiting in the end. It is like a plant that becomes convinced that it can only grow with a certain gardener. The plant should never forget, that as helpful as the gardener may be, it is perfectly capable of growing without any gardener at all.

What the Facilitator Works With

BODY ELECTRONICS WORKS BEST WHEN WE KEEP IT SIMPLE. SUCCESS comes from consistent application of the basics. A good example of this principle is the success of the Boston Celtics basketball team, which dominated the NBA from 1957 to 1969, winning the championship eleven times in thirteen seasons. Few teams in any sport anywhere have managed to succeed so consistently. While some attribute much of their success to leprechauns, certainly much of it was due to consistent application of the fundamentals of the game. While many other teams employed complex offenses, the Celtics stuck to the same few basic plays with options from one season to the next. Opposing teams were all familiar with the Celtics offense, but even when the opposition knew which play was coming, when a play was executed perfectly, it could not be stopped even with such knowledge.[2] In addition, the Celtics preseason training camp was particularly rigorous, long before this was common practice. Veterans from other teams who were traded to the Celtics were often shocked by the severity of training camp. While other teams "played themselves into shape" in the early part of the season, the Celtics were in top shape before the season began. Much of their undeviating attention to the fundamentals of the game was due to the influence of Arnold "Red" Auerbach, who was their coach during the first ten years of this period and their general manager throughout. I have read that Red began training camp each year by reminding his players that basketball is a simple game, and that "the floor is flat and the ball is round." Body Electronics also has some basic practices and principles that bring consistent good results, and in addition to making easier the work of the pointholdee, facilitators can lead the pointholding team in their task.

LOCATION, DIRECTION, AND PRESSURE COMBINED WITH ATTENTION AND INTENT

Chapter Sixteen explained that pointholders should take several factors into account in order to do an effective job on a point. The exact location is important, and sometimes minute changes in where the pressure is applied can make a huge difference as to how much pain is elicited. Similarly, the direction of pressure can make a big difference, and slight alterations in angle or direction can change the amount of pain elicited as well. (Remember: the amount of pressure applied should generally be as much as can be lovingly and willingly endured, but no more.) The three factors of location, direction, and pressure are the mechanical aspects of pointholding. And while each is important, it should be stressed that other factors are also important.

All pointholders should place attention both upon the points being held and upon the session itself, with a firm intent throughout. Pointholders will

---

be of much greater benefit to the person on the table if this is done: it is not enough just to do a good job with the physical mechanics of pointholding; all should put hearts and minds into it as well. When one is not facilitating but merely holding points, it is tempting to let the mind wander off. This is where firm intent must be maintained so that everyone's attention is upon the session.

Having all pointholders paying close attention to the person on the table as they repeat their word patterns may pay off handsomely. For as a person repeats a particular word pattern over and over, sometimes a slight variation will slip out just once. The person themselves may or may not even notice it. But often this is a prime opportunity to look at a much deeper resistance that has only briefly revealed itself.

Once in my experience a person was repeating the word pattern "I want to be loved" over and over for several minutes while intensifying the emotions involved and going through an associated memory. Just once, he said "I don't want to be loved." While he did actually hear this himself, as is so often the case when one is focusing on a particular word pattern intensely, he did not heed it. But when this was pointed out to him and he was asked to go into the "I don't want to be loved" word pattern, he was able to discover a huge and previously unrevealed area of resistance. One lesson in this is that each of us can potentially be of great assistance to each other through the simple discipline of paying close attention while we are holding points. Often when something like this slips out, many people present will actually hear it, but most will not truly notice it. Yet as soon as one person mentions it, others realize that they also heard it.

However, if the person on the table does not hear something themselves, and we are the only one who heard it, we must be absolutely certain we did hear it. Sometimes, especially when a person is face down in a face cradle, it is difficult to understand what they say. So it is wise to be aware of the possibility that we might simply have heard them wrong. But if two or more people heard it, or if the person on the table heard it themselves, this may be a great and not to be neglected opportunity to dig a bit deeper. Holding points with full attention can bring powerful results.

Privacy and Confidentiality

During pointholding sessions, many people may recall highly traumatic past events. (Some of these may be known or suspected already. Others will be quite surprising. With no coaching or suggestion, people do recall traumatic events that they had completely forgotten. When possible, the reality of events has repeatedly been confirmed by others still living.) For a person to get past their resistance within a given event, it may be necessary for them to regain clear and full memory of the event. So it is important that the pointholdee know what is happening. However, it is not necessary that anyone else know the details. It is quite possible (although tricky at times) to help facilitate a person without actually knowing what the memory is.

While in many cases it proves helpful for the person on the table eventually to speak openly about the event, they should do so only by their own choice. They should never be compelled, coerced or manipulated into divulging any details that they do not wish to share. Each person has the right to privacy. Further, whatever they do choose to share within the context of a pointholding session should not be talked about outside of this context without permission. We should treat all such information with strict confidentiality.

Reality and Surprises

With respect to remembering an event that had been totally suppressed, we should remain open to the possibility that a person may remember everything, but that much of what is remembered may be distorted. We should not be quick to jump to conclusions as a new memory slowly unfolds: we must be open but cautious.

Those facilitating must be careful not to suggest anything to the person on the table, draw conclusions for them, or otherwise influence them in any direction. We encourage them to repeat their own word patterns, but do not put words in their mouth. We encourage them to lovingly intensify the emotions they have themselves recognized, but do not suggest that they feel an emotion that we think they surely must have felt. And we encourage them to reexperience the thought pattern or sensory memory as far as they have remembered it, but do not suggest any details that they have no awareness of themselves. It is a process of discovering the truth, and the facilitator adding anything that does not belong will only make it harder to uncover what really happened.

STORY VERSUS EXPERIENCE

Body Electronics is meant to be experiential as opposed to intellectual. In terms of having a specific memory, there is a world of difference between a *story* and an *experience*. In a story, we are simply talking about a past event, rather than actually being there now. This is revealed by the fact that we are talking in the past tense, rather than the present tense. In an experience, we are ultimately experiencing the event as if it were happening. Such experiencing will not usually occur all at once: it may build slowly. Often the story will appear first. But we should always do our best to work for the experience rather than remain in the story, because people need to reexperience the thoughts, words, and emotions involved in order to release the resistance.

For the same reason it is not generally helpful to ask the person on the table why they feel a certain way or why a particular thing happened. For this simply encourages them to justify, rationalize, and analyze rather than to simply reexperience the thoughts, words, and emotions that are actually there to be handled appropriately. Asking why encourages the story rather than the experience.

In many instances we can come up with quite a sensible response why. But our answer to the question seldom has anything to do with reality. We will not truly come to why through any intellectual process or by reasoning. The why will reveal itself in the end once our resistance in this area has been resolved. Once our resistance is gone, the why is quite obvious to us. And it will be equally obvious to us that we could not have seen why so long as that resistance had remained in place, no matter how advanced our powers of reasoning.

The goal is not to steer the pointholdee through some sort of hypothetical or fictitious situation. Rather, we simply encourage them to experience what actually happened with love and forgiveness. The idea is not to try to rewrite or change history. For what has happened already is in the past. What we seek to change is not the past but rather our own resistance to it. That is, we change our attitude. In order to do this we must experience what actually did happen so that we may release ourselves from the bondage of our own resistance. "Ye shall know the truth and the truth shall set you free." To superimpose some fictitious version of history upon what is really there takes the individual further away from reality. The facilitator falling into the trap of attempting to analyze the experience for the person (particularly if the pointholdee falls in with them), will take the pointholdee further away from reality. Analysis of the experience, whether by the facilitator or the pointholdee as they experience it, removes the pointholdee from the experience and encourages rationalization, generalization, and justification.

THE LAWS OF LOVE AND LIGHT

As facilitators we encourage the person to hold the body and the tongue still, to search for the thoughts, words, and emotions, and to reexperience all these with unconditional love and unconditional forgiveness. We also encourage them to encompass rather than exclude, and to observe, receive, recreate, and release. In addition, the individual is taught to visualize the violet flame moving around and through them from the feet up through the top of the head as taught by Saint Germain in the books available from the Saint Germain Foundation.[3] For those unfamiliar with this concept, a brief explanation is offered. Love or enthusiasm transmutes the emotional body. This is also referred to as the Law of Love. The violet flame, properly applied, will transmute the mental body in a similar fashion. This is known as the Law of Light. Enthusiasm is the highest of the seven emotions, and when the individual is enthusiastic to the encompassment of all other emotions, this will automatically bring to the awareness any emotion less than enthusiasm. That is, the more enthusiasm we can generate, the more aware we become of the lesser emotions already there. The key is to encompass, not exclude. Similarly, the color violet is the highest of the seven colors of the visual spectrum (and vision is the highest of the five senses). When the violet flame is visualized to the encompassment of all else, it will naturally bring to the attention the rest of the visual spectrum and by extension all sensory experience. Again the key is to encompass, not exclude.

Native Language of the Pointholdee

It is often helpful to speak in a person's native language in order to help them get more fully into the experience rather than the story. It is not always needed; some people have no difficulty getting into the experience in a second language. But for others, speaking in a second language may hinder their getting into the experience, and so it is best to encourage them to say their word patterns in their native language. If somebody present speaks that language as well, it is generally preferable for them to facilitate or at least to translate for whomever is facilitating. Sometimes the best that can be done is for the facilitator to use the common language of both, and for the person to repeat their word patterns in their native language.

Attachments

Our own attachments large and small can hinder the progress of the person on the table. While our attachments can probably not prevent their progress, at times they may make it more of a challenge. Perhaps we are attached to being of help to the other person. This attachment on our part only makes it more unlikely that we will be of any help. Or perhaps we are attached to the other person being healed or resolving a particular resistance. Again, this attachment on our part only makes it more unlikely that either of these will happen. If we can let go of our own attachments, we can be part of the solution. Hanging on to these attachments makes us merely another aspect of the problem.

The essence of facilitation is to keep it simple. Just help the person to unfold in a quiet and unassuming manner. Be patient and nonresistant. Be okay with whatever happens. Disappointment can only grow where expectations have been planted. As a facilitator, if we are attached to a particular outcome we are resisting alternatives. Through our resistance, we become a part of the problem and not a part of the solution.

Resistance and Helping Others

In our sincere desire to be of service to another, we often find ourselves entertaining the thought that the other person is not doing it right. We may feel that they have lost their way, that they are somehow in error. And we may also sincerely believe that we know what they ought to do, the path the other should be following. We may easily fall into this trap, often precisely as a result of our sincere desire to help.

We can align ourselves with truth each moment, and allow others the freedom to do likewise. None of us can see another's path perfectly clearly; to believe otherwise is sheer delusion. Our own path is difficult enough to discern, as we must pass through the clouds of our own resistance to truly locate it. To find our own path is a tremendous challenge, and one that requires constant vigilance. A sure way to lose our own path is to allow judgment, criticism, or condemnation to enter into our own heart, even for an instant. Therefore, when we judge that another has lost their way or missed their path, or is in some way out of harmony with truth as we perceive truth, we make it more likely that we will lose our own path as we stumble in our own darkness. How can we discover and dispel the darkness within ourselves by fixating upon that which we, in our resistance and judgment, perceive in others? We slow down our own progression by judging that another has stumbled.

If we find ourselves disappointed in another, then perhaps we might consider that disappointment can only grow where expectations have been planted. There is no disappointment in the absence of expectation.

If we have any degree of resistance to another person being just as they are, then in reality we are resisting something within ourselves. This something may or may not be present in the other person, but it is surely present within us. "We do not see the world the way it is, we see it the way we are." Making judgments about another person, however slight, reveals far more about us than it does about them. If we allow our attention to become fixated upon the outer, which we do so long as we resist another person in any manner, we thereby avoid looking within. Thus, we perpetuate our resistance with resistance to the resistance.

We cannot truly serve others so long as we resist them. We must let them be; love them as they are, not as we wish them to be or think they should be. Each in their own unique manner can be a wonderful teacher to us, but only if we open the way through nonresistance. Those people whom we resist the most can be the best of mirrors for us in our own progression if only we can see them with love.

The only person we can truly resist is ourselves, and all we can really resist in the world around us is ourselves. For the world that we see is but a reflection of who we are. It is that simple.

POINTHOLDERS' HEALING CRISES

For those not familiar with Body Electronics, it is worth noting that not only can the people on the table go into healing crisis, but the pointholders may as well. There are a few considerations here. It is important for all concerned that pointholders continue to do the best job possible holding whatever points they are on. Partly this is due to consideration for the person on the table. But also, if we recall the principle that "whatever gets us into a healing crisis will be needed to get us through it," then for the benefit of the pointholder in healing crisis it will also be best for them to remain on the points. For holding these points is at least part of what brought on the healing crisis.

Nausea and vomiting are possible, so whenever pointholding is done it is a good idea to have buckets ready just in case. Pointholders in healing crisis have been known to faint. It is wise for anyone in this circumstance to give ample warning so someone can be prepared to catch or support them. When there are several tables at once, often someone will be the "floater." This person is not plugged in on any points, and is available to offer whatever assistance might be needed. With many tables, there may be a need for more than one floater.

It is entirely possible for both the person on the table and a pointholder to have good healing crises in the same session. The pointholder being in healing crisis need not adversely affect the experience of the person on the table. In many cases it seems to help trigger things in them, and is thus a bonus. However, there are times when it may be appropriate to postpone the pointholder's healing crisis until a later time and concentrate on the person on the table. Each situation will be unique; intuition and logic will reveal the appropriate course of action.

SYMPATHY VERSUS EMPATHY

Each of us will be faced with many circumstances where we are aware of another person who is either suffering in some manner, faced with a difficult situation, distressed, or basically in a position where it would be very normal to "feel sorry" for them. If we consider how our attitude towards their circumstances may impact upon them as well as us, then we will see the difference between sympathy and empathy. Briefly, we might define sympathy as having some awareness of another person's circumstances and having some resistance to these circumstances. Empathy might be defined as having some awareness of another person's circumstances and having no resistance to these circumstances. The major difference between sympathy and empathy is whether or not there is resistance involved on our part. Both sympathy and empathy are attitudes. They are not actions. So it is not a question of whether or not we offer assistance of some sort. We may or we may not. It is a question of what our attitude is towards the other person's circumstances.

The resistance that is present when we are in sympathy helps neither us nor the other person. In our case, this resistance harms us like any other resistance. When we fall into sympathy, we will tend to take upon ourselves the very thing that we resist in the other person. Perhaps this helps explain why so many healers become sick themselves. Not only are we harmed by our sympathy, however, but it really does no good for the other person. For one thing, the resistance that goes with our sympathy actually decreases our awareness of the situation itself. We see things less clearly as a result of our sympathy. Thus, if there is something we could do to assist, we are that much less likely to see what that might be. In addition, our resistance will make it harder for the other person to extricate themselves from their predicament, not easier. For we help to perpetuate their situation by resisting it. We are denying the God within that other person by resisting their circumstance, for every circumstance is, after all, a perfect outer manifestation of our inner creative efforts.

In contrast, when we feel empathy, we have no resistance to another person's circumstances. As a result, we have much greater awareness than we would in a state of sympathy. If assistance is appropriate and possible, we will be in an ideal position to offer it. Our lack of resistance means that we ourselves are not harmed, and just as importantly it places us in a better position to help if help is possible.

Suppose we are walking along and see someone stuck in a deep hole.

Sympathy is jumping in and being stuck with them. Empathy is finding a rope or other assistance, if possible. In Australia a few years ago, there was a fairly dramatic example of sympathy. A man down at the bottom of a pit was being asphyxiated by the fumes that had gathered there, and he did die as a result. At least one onlooker died from the same cause by jumping in to get the first man out. (Some accounts say that a second or even a third onlooker did the same and died as well.) With two or more men already dead, still another onlooker was ready to jump in and die as well. At this point, others interceded and nobody else died. This incident is a tragic illustration of the possible consequences of sympathy. While the effects of our sympathy will not usually be so dramatic or extreme, it is only a matter of degree.

Giving and Receiving Blessings

HEALTH IS ITSELF A BLESSING. AND HEALING, OR THE RESTORATION OF health, is a blessing as well. We have discussed the important role of gratitude in a person's own health and healing. But our attitude towards the health and healing of others is also of great importance and can have quite an impact upon our own health and healing, for better or for worse. Being grateful for the health and healing that others enjoy or receive opens up the door for us to receive the same or more. Yet when we are envious or jealous of the health or healing that others receive, this tends to prevent our own health or healing. Furthermore, it appears that our own quest for health and healing is greatly assisted by our willingness to assist others to do the same. Dr. Ray has phrased the following principles in this regard: "We will never receive a blessing that we are not willing to give to others." "We will never receive a blessing that we are not willing for everyone else to receive first."

Our willingness to assist others can play a great role in our own healing. Many people take this position: "Well, I'd love to help others, but I am too sick. After I get well, then I'll help others." It has been my observation that so long as this mental position is maintained, such a person will tend to remain too sick to help others. However, while there are certain exceptions, most of us are quite capable of assisting others to some degree.

It is not especially important how much we are able to give in comparison to anyone else. What is important is simply that we are willing to give whatever assistance we may. I have observed some seriously ill people being of great service to others. And in general, this benefits their own healing as well.

Certainly it is possible to go to the opposite extreme with these principles. However, we do not need to make everyone else more important than ourselves. Nor do we need to totally exhaust ourselves in serving others to the neglect of our own just needs. It is simply a question of coming to a happy medium of giving and receiving, and of being equally grateful for blessings no matter who receives them.

As we each work on our own path, and as we each put our focus on God from our own unique perspective, we may sooner or later come to a point where we consider how we may be of service to the God that exists in all life. Life involves both giving as well as receiving. Each of us has received to some degree. When we have received, there comes also a time to give to others what we have received. By giving, we also open the door to receive even more. Some would say that through giving we help to create the necessary space that receiving may take place. Thus, the cycle continues. A subtle but important consideration: are we able to serve without the need to serve, or are we attached to serving? Do we serve compulsively, or are we simply willing to be there without condition or expectation? Are we willing to be ready to serve if the opportunity arises, but equally willing to have no such opportunity? If we are truly willing to serve, the blessings of service will come, whether the chance to serve comes or not. And most likely it will come, if we are patient.

To extend this, please consider that blessings do not really come from us anyway. They come from God. Blessings may come through us, but not from us. (Alternately, we might say they come from the God within.) Similarly, blessings are ultimately received by us on behalf of God. (Or again, by the God within.) So in the end, it is really simply God giving to God, and God receiving from God. Perhaps if we see it that way, it may be easier to apply these principles.

PART FOUR

Outer Manifestation and Inner Essence

THERE IS A DANGER THAT THE AMOUNT OF DETAIL CONCERNING THE outer (nutrition, methods such as Body Electronics) will tend to direct people's attention towards the outer rather than to the inner essence that lies behind any and all outer manifestation. As Dr. Ray has commented: "We need to focus on the spiritual which transcends all material 'dogma.' The best scientific evidence still misses the boat as it focuses on the physical and misses entirely the spiritual. Man will wander around in the worldly darkness for millions of years if he only is obedient to all physical laws, nutrition, etc. The only way he can rise above and transmute the physical is to submerge himself in the Love of God and then all physical laws become play things to spirit that is still immersed in matter. It is primarily essential that we point to credibility in God consciousness rather than pay homage to the scientific mind."

Science as it now stands can merely view the outer manifestation, and this is not where truth is really to be found. No matter how sophisticated our capacity to measure and observe the outer manifestation may become, it is still the inner essence wherein truth is found. As Antoine de Sainte Exupery writes in his classic *The Little Prince,* "It is only with the heart that one can see rightly; what is essential is invisible to the eye."[1]

Many concepts that need to be understood are difficult to express adequately in words. "The Tao that can be spoken is not the Tao." The truth is not really to be found in the words, but perhaps these same words can nevertheless point to the truth. As it is said in Zen Buddhism, let us be careful then not to confuse the finger that points at the moon with the moon itself. If these words can point the way in some small measure to the truth, then their purpose will have been served. Part Four focuses on the movement from inner to outer, which is important not just in understanding how we create our reality and how we become ill in the first place but also for understanding how we heal.

Chapter Twenty

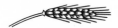

Iridology and Sclerology

The Iris, Sclera, and Pupil of the eye show the veil the soul has created, through consciousness (or forgetfulness), that reflects the illusion which prepares the soul for attaining the reality of full enlightenment.

David J. Pesek

Where there is no vision, the people perish.

Proverbs 29:18

IN THIS CHAPTER THE FIELDS OF IRIDOLOGY AND SCLEROLOGY WILL BE considered, with particular regard to their application to Body Electronics and the model of health and healing described in Part One. Iridology is the study of the iris of the eye and how from its structures, landmarks, and markings we can learn much about the condition of the various tissues of the body. A combination of iridology and sclerology developed by Dr. Ray and known as Iris-Sclera Integrated Diagnosis is commonly used in Body Electronics. Sclerology is a parallel science which concerns itself with the sclera or white of the eye surrounding the iris. It is a useful adjunct to iridology, especially when the two fields are correlated. While neither iridology nor sclerology is a method of treatment, both are often ideal for diagnosis. In the words of Dr. Bernard Jensen, who is considered to be one of the leading iridologists in the world:

The science of iridology is based on the analysis of one of the most complicated tissue structures of the whole body—the iris.

It is a method whereby the doctor or health practitioner can tell, from markings or signs in the iris, the reflex conditions of various organs and systems of the body. These markings present a detailed picture of the integrity of the body; its constitutional strength, areas of congestion or toxic accumulations and inherent strengths and weaknesses.[1]

Through the use of iridology and sclerology we can determine an appropriate program of nutrition (including supplements) and Body Electronics to meet an individual's particular needs. In addition to designing an initial program of nutrition and Body Electronics, subsequent reexamination helps establish the effectiveness of the program, as in some cases there will be improvement in the iris and/or sclera.[2] Many other methods of determining the condition of the body are helpful and may be employed as well, but Iris-Sclera Integrated Diagnosis is especially useful.

While the basic principles of iridology and sclerology are sufficiently simple and logical that most people can achieve a reasonable competency, most people will require considerable effort and much practical application to reach a level of more than minimal competence. Lectures by a trained iridology instructor and excellent books such as Dr. Bernard Jensen's *Iridology: The Science and Practice in the Healing Arts* are certainly a good way to begin. In the case of sclerology, there is little yet available in writing. But true understanding of iridology and sclerology will only come from extensive practical application of this information and lifelong study for anyone who truly intends to master these twin disciplines. However, an introduction here may shed further light on the mechanics of a process towards health.

Iridology

IRIDOLOGY IS A DYNAMIC DISCIPLINE WITH RESEARCH INTO IT STILL BEING carried out. Ultimately, of course, the understanding of the iris of the eye cannot be separated from the understanding of the physical body whose condition is represented therein. Truly mastering iridology requires the study of anatomy, physiology, nutrition, and a wide range of related disciplines. However, even a minimal understanding of iridology will be of great value not only in Body Electronics but in any field of health. With the exception of nutrition, there is probably no other body of knowledge which deserves more to be studied by every health practitioner.

SOME ADVANTAGES OF IRIDOLOGY

The advantages of iridology are numerous. It is inexpensive in that it requires a minimum of basic equipment: a powerful penlight and a 10X loupe for magnification to permit detailed viewing of the iris. For self-analysis, a concave radial mirror is employed. An iridology chart is also quite helpful, including a reverse or mirror image chart for self-analysis. Many iris charts are available, and while none are exactly the same, most are pretty close. A good iridology camera is useful but fairly expensive. It is quite possible to effectively practice iridology without the use of a camera, although the camera makes the process easier and more effective. I have had the opportunity to use certain accurate high-tech methods of diagnosis. The information which these vastly expensive machines has provided has tended to correlate to a high degree with that which could be discovered using iridology. While such machines may be wonderful and beneficial, their expense makes them far less practical for most practitioners and out of the question for virtually all lay people. The basic equipment for iridology fits in a pocket. Even an iridology camera is portable.

Another obvious advantage of iridology is that it is noninvasive, as nothing more is required than that the patient allow us to shine a light in the eye from the side and view the eyes through a magnifying loupe, as well as perhaps take eye photos. Iridology, unlike procedures such as x-rays and exploratory surgery, poses no health risks whatsoever to the patient other than the possibility of inadvertently poking them in the eye.

Beyond the simplicity, minimal expense, safety, and noninvasiveness of iridology, its main usefulness lies in its high level of accuracy, which many believe compares quite favorably with that of complicated, expensive, invasive, and potentially or definitely harmful methods. Jensen comments that "Iridology does not take the place of other methods of diagnosis or analysis; it has only added to those methods. When we stop to think that possibly we are only 25–30% correct in the diagnosing methods that we have today, it certainly behooves us to use every option possible to raise that percentage."[3]

WHAT IRIDOLOGY CAN DO

Iridology reveals the conditions of the various tissues of the body quite accurately. While the typical medical procedure of diagnosing a so-called disease basically amounts to naming and categorizing a particular group of symptoms, iridology is much better suited to determining the underlying causes. As Jensen notes, "grouping a list of symptoms into a disease name, in order to identify and administer the drug that will suppress these symptoms, is not a satisfactory solution to the problem of health care and maintenance. Iridology, in its basic philosophy, stresses the treatment of the patient, not the disease. By identifying the underlying imbalances in the body that produce the symptoms, it is an invaluable asset in the formulation of remedial therapies."[4] The chief applications of iridology in the field of Body Electronics are in determining an individual's diet and supplements, the particular points which need to be held, the need for various peripheral modalities in addition to nutrition and pointholding, as well as ascertaining other relevant physical factors which will influence the situation.

THE IRIS AS A MAP OF THE BODY

The mapping of the entire body onto the irides has been well documented and continually refined by numerous iridologists over the past one hundred and fifty years. By this mapping, each portion of the body is represented in a particular portion of one or both irides of the individual. This makes sense when we understand that the iris is the only exposed portion of the central nervous system.[5] Thus, the tissue condition of a given area of the body can be ascertained by examining the appropriate area of the iris.

Included here are three excellent eye charts, those of Bernard Jensen, Harri Wolf, and David J. Pesek.[6] In each of these eye charts, the iris is divided into concentric zones. These zones may be interpreted both structurally and functionally. That is, we may consider what structures of the body as well as what functions are represented in a given zone. Both the Jensen and Wolf charts have seven zones in them. The iris is divided into seven zones with Zone 1 being innermost and Zone 7 being outermost. Zone 1 is basically the stomach, Zone 2 the intestines; however, we may think of these two zones as also being the digestive system as a whole. Wolf relates Zones 1 and 2 to digestion and absorption respectively. Zone 3 is commonly thought of as showing the endocrine system. Wolf relates Zone 3 to transformation and distribution. Zones 4 and 5 contain muscle and bone structures in addition to organs and glands. Wolf relates Zones 4 and 5 to utilization and ultimate utilization, respectively. Zone 6 is the lymphatic and circulatory systems in many charts. Wolf relates Zone 6 to detoxification. And Zone 7 represents the body at a cellular level as well as the skin. Wolf relates Zone 7 to elimination.

The Pesek chart does not explicitly show seven zones as do those of Jensen and Wolf. If we compare it to these other two charts and use the same terminology as far as zones go, the basic difference is simply that there are no clear lines of demarcation to distinguish zones 3, 4, and 5 from one another. As in the other charts, however, the stomach is found in zone 1 and the intestines in zone 2. And the lymphatic and circulatory systems are found in zone 6, and the skin in zone 7, as in the Jensen chart. And despite the absence of actual lines to distinguish zones 3, 4, and 5, it is clear from comparing the charts that Pesek locates the various systems and organs similarly to Jensen and Wolf. The notable exception is that Pesek also locates the lymphatic system just outside the intestines, and the autonomic nervous system in zone 3.

While there are similarities between the charts, the differences are quite interesting. The iris is given further divisions as in a clock; thus, a particular organ is located in the eye by a zone and a time. The eye charts of Jensen and Pesek divide the iris up into twelve hours, while Wolf's chart divides it into sixty minutes. In the following discussion we will act as if Wolf's chart was divided into twelve hours rather than sixty minutes, as this will simplify our comparison of the charts.

CHART TO IRIDOLOGY

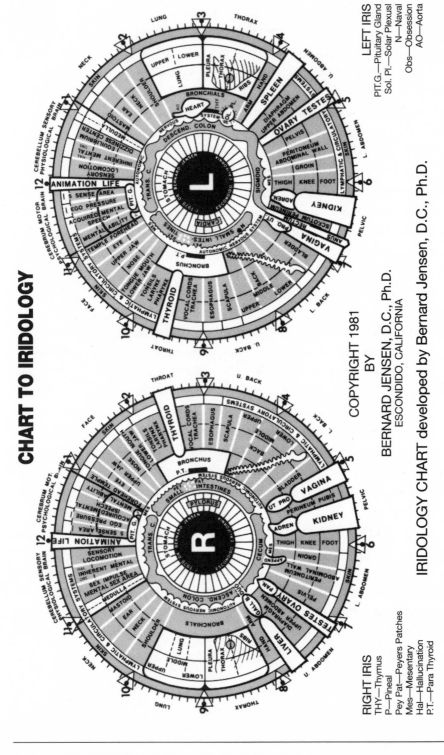

COPYRIGHT 1981
BY
BERNARD JENSEN, D.C., Ph.D.
ESCONDIDO, CALIFORNIA

IRIDOLOGY CHART developed by Bernard Jensen, D.C., Ph.D.

RIGHT IRIS
THY—Thymus
P—Pineal
Pey Pat—Peyers Patches
Mes—Mesentery
Hal—Hallucination
P.T.—Para Thyroid

LEFT IRIS
PIT.G.—Pituitary Gland
Sol. Pl.—Solar Plexusl
N—Naval
Obs—Obsession
AO—Aorta

FIGURE 16: BERNARD JENSEN, D.C.'s "CHART TO IRIDOLOGY." © 1981. REPRINTED WITH PERMISSION.

DIFFERENCES BETWEEN THE EYE CHARTS
OF JENSEN, WOLF, AND PESEK

Jensen shows the heart in the left eye in zone 3 from roughly 2:30 to 3:00 but does not show the heart in the right eye anywhere. While both Wolf and Pesek show the heart in the left eye in a similar position to Jensen's, they also locate the heart in the right eye in zone 3 between about 9:00 and 9:30. Jensen shows the thymus below the heart in zone 3 in the left eye but does not locate the thymus in the right eye. Pesek locates the thymus below the heart in zone 3 in both the left and right eyes. While Wolf also locates the thymus in both eyes, he locates the thymus in zone 3 directly across the pupil from the heart or at approximately 3:15 in the right eye and 8:45 in the left eye. Thus, while Jensen and Pesek locate the thymus in the lateral half of the iris, Wolf locates it in the medial half. (Lateral means away from the midplane of the body, while medial means towards this midplane. Thus, in the iris, the medial portion is towards the nose, while the lateral portion is towards the ears.)

Jensen locates the pancreas in zone 3 near 7:00 in the right eye but does not locate it in the left eye. Pesek shows the pancreas in roughly the same location as Jensen in the right eye but also locates the pancreas in zone 3 in the left eye at about 4:30. Both these locations are lateral. Wolf locates the pancreas in zone 3 both laterally as well as medially in both eyes, a total of four different pancreas locations. All three charts show the gall bladder in zone 3 between 7:30 and 8:00 in the right eye, with the liver found in a similar position from zone 4 outwards. Neither Jensen nor Pesek locate the liver anywhere other than this position in the right eye. Wolf also shows a medial location for the liver in both eyes, approximately 4:00 in the right eye and 8:00 in the left eye, a total of three different liver locations.

Jensen shows the adrenals just medial to 6:00 in zone 3 in both eyes. Both Wolf and Pesek show the adrenals in a similar position to Jensen but also extending across the midline to include a lateral position as well, with Pesek extending the adrenal area laterally even further than Wolf. All three charts show the kidneys just medial to 6:00 in both eyes from zone 4 outwards. While Jensen and Wolf do not show the kidneys elsewhere, Pesek

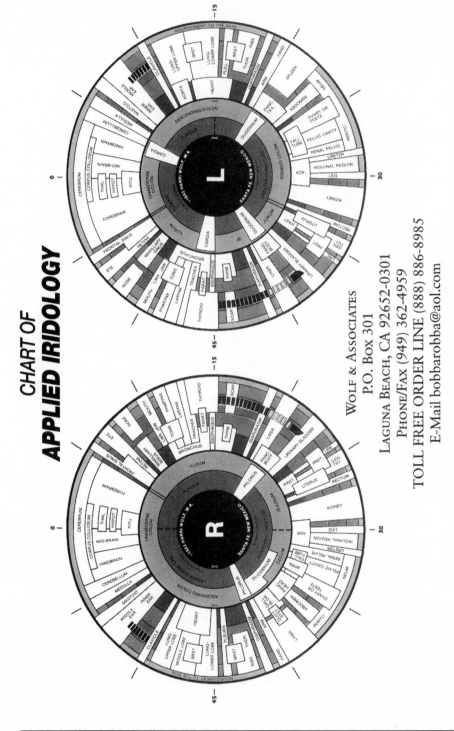

CHART OF
APPLIED IRIDOLOGY

WOLF & ASSOCIATES
P.O. Box 301
LAGUNA BEACH, CA 92652-0301
Phone/Fax (949) 362-4959
TOLL FREE ORDER LINE (888) 886-8985
E-Mail bobbarobba@aol.com

FIGURE 17: HARRI WOLF, M.A.'s "CHART OF APPLIED IRIDOLOGY." © 1983: REPRINTED WITH PERMISSION.

shows the kidneys as extending across the leg area and into a lateral position as well, covering an area from about 5:30 to 6:30 in both eyes.

All three charts show the pituitary gland in zone 3 slightly medial to 12:00 in both eyes, with slight variations as to how far the pituitary area extends. Both Pesek and Jensen show the pineal gland in zone 3 medial to the pituitary in both eyes. Wolf does not locate the pineal in either eye. Pesek locates the hypothalamus in zone 3 at 12:00 in both eyes. Wolf also locates the hypothalamus at 12:00 in both eyes, although he locates it above the pituitary in zone 4 instead. Jensen does not explicitly locate the hypothalamus in his eye chart. However, he does associate the hypothalamus with the Animation Life Center, which is found at 12:00 in both eyes in his chart. Thus, we might infer that he implicitly locates the hypothalamus at 12:00 in both eyes.[7] Both Jensen and Wolf show the medulla in a lateral position at about 1:00 in the left eye and 11:00 in the right eye. While Pesek does not actually show the medulla in his chart, he does label the corresponding area "Survival." And given that it governs many involuntary functions necessary for our survival, perhaps this may be considered an implicit location of the medulla.

All three charts show the lymphatic system in zone 6. As noted earlier, Pesek also shows the lymphatic system in zone 3. All three charts show the rectum at approximately 6:45 in the left eye. Wolf also shows the rectum in the right eye at about 5:15. Jensen locates the duodenum in zone 2 in the right eye at about 7:45. Both Pesek and Wolf show the duodenum in a similar position in the right eye. Both also show it in two positions in zone 2 in the left eye, approximately 4:15 and 7:45. All three charts show the stomach in zone 1, although there are slight variations as to where various portions of the stomach are located.

The other major difference between these eye charts is in what is commonly referred to as the brain area, or that portion of zones 3 through 7 that lies between about 11:00 and 1:00 in both eyes. Wolf divides this portion of the chart up structurally: pituitary, hypothalamus, thalamus, forebrain, mid-brain, hindbrain, corpus collosum, and cerebrum. Both Jensen and Pesek divide the brain area up into various functional divisions. These various areas are referred to by both Jensen and Pesek as *Brain Flairs*. Jensen offers a very comprehensive treatment of the brain area in his classic book

Chart of
HOLISTIC IRIDOLOGY®
© 1999 David J. Pesek, Ph.D.

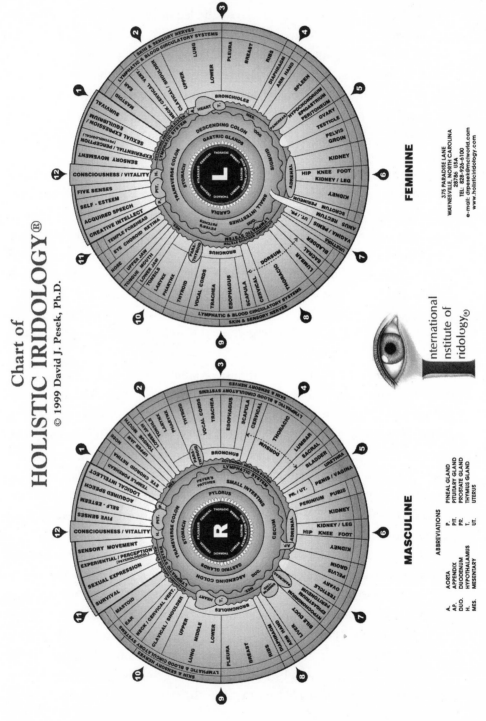

375 PARADISE LANE
WAYNESVILLE, NORTH CAROLINA
28786 USA
TEL: 828-926-6100
e-mail: drpesek@mchworld.com
www.holisticiridology.com

International
Institute of
Iridology®

FEMININE

MASCULINE

ABBREVIATIONS

A.	AORTA	P.	PINEAL GLAND
AP.	APPENDIX	PIT.	PITUITARY GLAND
DUO.	DUODENUM	PR.	PROSTATE GLAND
H.	HYPOTHALAMUS	T.	THYMUS GLAND
MES.	MESENTARY	UT.	UTERUS

FIGURE 18: DAVID J. PESEK, PH.D'S "CHART OF HOLISTIC IRIDOLOGY." © 1999. REPRINTED WITH PERMISSION.

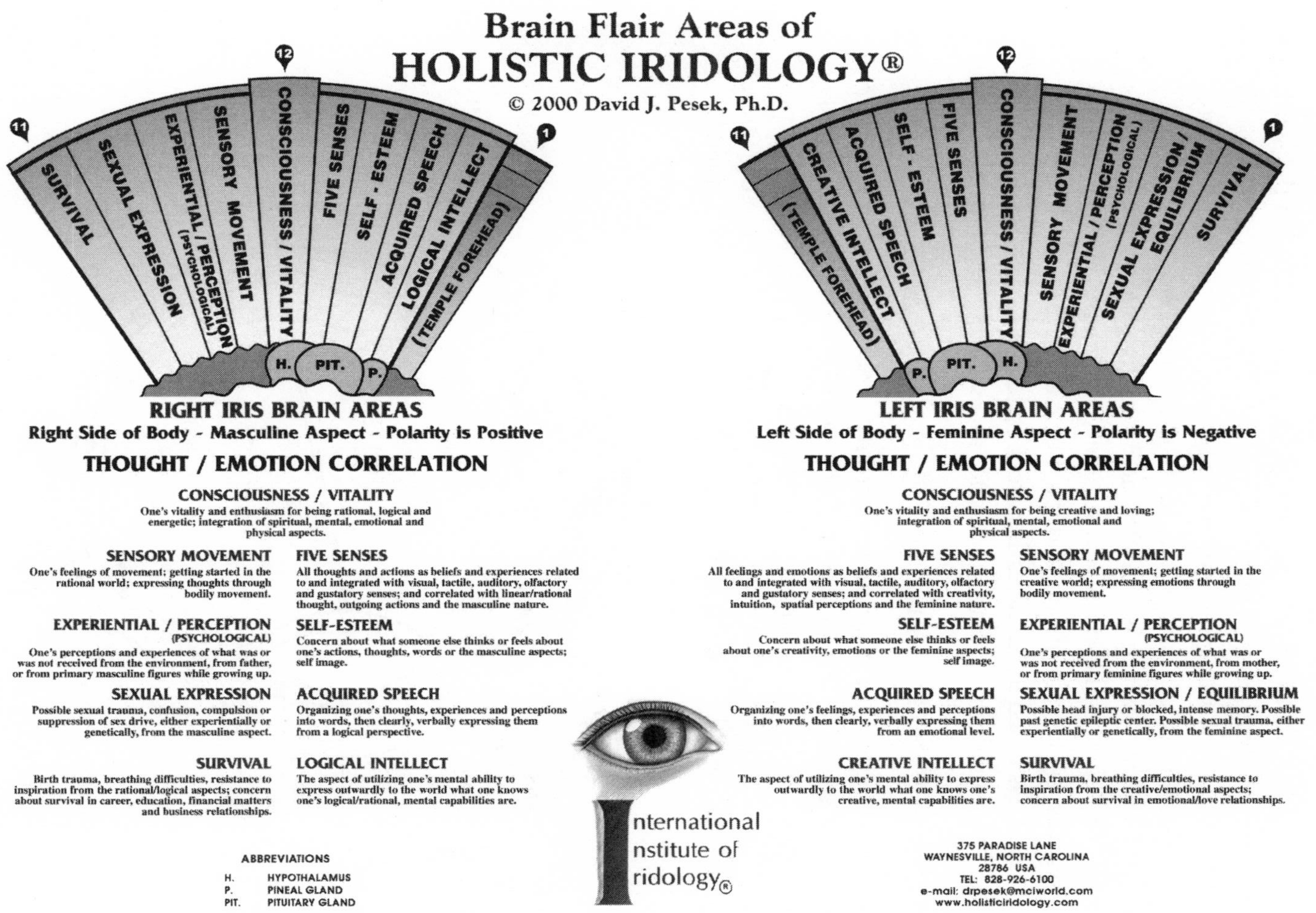

Brain Flair Areas of HOLISTIC IRIDOLOGY®

© 2000 David J. Pesek, Ph.D.

RIGHT IRIS BRAIN AREAS

Right Side of Body - Masculine Aspect - Polarity is Positive

THOUGHT / EMOTION CORRELATION

(Brain area labels: SURVIVAL, SEXUAL EXPRESSION, EXPERIENTIAL / PERCEPTION (PSYCHOLOGICAL), SENSORY MOVEMENT, CONSCIOUSNESS / VITALITY, FIVE SENSES, SELF - ESTEEM, ACQUIRED SPEECH, LOGICAL INTELLECT (TEMPLE FOREHEAD))

CONSCIOUSNESS / VITALITY
One's vitality and enthusiasm for being rational, logical and energetic; integration of spiritual, mental, emotional and physical aspects.

SENSORY MOVEMENT
One's feelings of movement; getting started in the rational world; expressing thoughts through bodily movement.

FIVE SENSES
All thoughts and actions as beliefs and experiences related to and integrated with visual, tactile, auditory, olfactory and gustatory senses; and correlated with linear/rational thought, outgoing actions and the masculine nature.

EXPERIENTIAL / PERCEPTION (PSYCHOLOGICAL)
One's perceptions and experiences of what was or was not received from the environment, from father, or from primary masculine figures while growing up.

SELF-ESTEEM
Concern about what someone else thinks or feels about one's actions, thoughts, words or the masculine aspects; self image.

SEXUAL EXPRESSION
Possible sexual trauma, confusion, compulsion or suppression of sex drive, either experientially or genetically, from the masculine aspect.

ACQUIRED SPEECH
Organizing one's thoughts, experiences and perceptions into words, then clearly, verbally expressing them from a logical perspective.

SURVIVAL
Birth trauma, breathing difficulties, resistance to inspiration from the rational/logical aspects; concern about survival in career, education, financial matters and business relationships.

LOGICAL INTELLECT
The aspect of utilizing one's mental ability to express outwardly to the world what one knows one's logical/rational, mental capabilities are.

ABBREVIATIONS
H. HYPOTHALAMUS
P. PINEAL GLAND
PIT. PITUITARY GLAND

LEFT IRIS BRAIN AREAS

Left Side of Body - Feminine Aspect - Polarity is Negative

THOUGHT / EMOTION CORRELATION

(Brain area labels: SURVIVAL, SEXUAL EXPRESSION / EQUILIBRIUM, EXPERIENTIAL / PERCEPTION (PSYCHOLOGICAL), SENSORY MOVEMENT, CONSCIOUSNESS / VITALITY, FIVE SENSES, SELF - ESTEEM, ACQUIRED SPEECH, CREATIVE INTELLECT (TEMPLE FOREHEAD))

CONSCIOUSNESS / VITALITY
One's vitality and enthusiasm for being creative and loving; integration of spiritual, mental, emotional and physical aspects.

SENSORY MOVEMENT
One's feelings of movement; getting started in the creative world; expressing emotions through bodily movement.

FIVE SENSES
All feelings and emotions as beliefs and experiences related to and integrated with visual, tactile, auditory, olfactory and gustatory senses; and correlated with creativity, intuition, spatial perceptions and the feminine nature.

SELF-ESTEEM
Concern about what someone else thinks or feels about one's creativity, emotions or the feminine aspects; self image.

EXPERIENTIAL / PERCEPTION (PSYCHOLOGICAL)
One's perceptions and experiences of what was or was not received from the environment, from mother, or from primary feminine figures while growing up.

SEXUAL EXPRESSION / EQUILIBRIUM
Possible head injury or blocked, intense memory. Possible past genetic epileptic center. Possible sexual trauma, either experientially or genetically, from the feminine aspect.

SURVIVAL
Birth trauma, breathing difficulties, resistance to inspiration from the creative/emotional aspects; concern about survival in emotional/love relationships.

ACQUIRED SPEECH
Organizing one's feelings, experiences and perceptions into words, then clearly, verbally expressing them from an emotional level.

CREATIVE INTELLECT
The aspect of utilizing one's mental ability to express outwardly to the world what one knows one's creative, mental capabilities are.

International Institute of Iridology®

375 PARADISE LANE
WAYNESVILLE, NORTH CAROLINA
28786, USA
TEL: 828-926-6100
e-mail: drpesek@mcIworld.com
www.holisticiridology.com

FIGURE 19: DAVID J. PESEK, PH.D.'S "BRAIN FLAIR AREAS OF HOLISTIC IRIDOLOGY."
© 2000. REPRINTED WITH PERMISSION.

Iridology: The Science and Practice in the Healing Arts,[8] and in this work he explores many physical, emotional, mental, and psychological aspects and how these may be represented in the brain area of the iris. Pesek presents these same aspects in an excellent chart entitled "Brain Flair Areas of Holistic Iridology" which is reprinted here with his kind permission (Figure 19). This chart makes particular reference to how the brain area of the iris may display certain of our emotional or reactive patterns quite accurately, and it is based upon the earlier work of Jensen and others as refined by Dr. Pesek in his many years of practice as a clinical psychologist.

Iris Anatomy and Eye Color

The iris is a fairly thin structure from front to back. According to *Gray's Anatomy*, "the iris is the circular muscular septum, which hangs vertically behind the cornea, presenting in its centre a large rounded aperture, the *pupil*."[9] It is also noted that "the posterior surface is of a deep purple tint, from being covered by two layers of pigmented, columnar epithelium."[10]

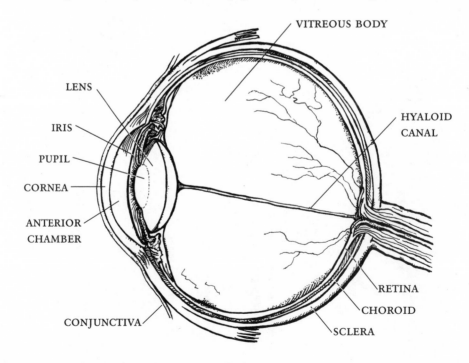

Figure 20: Cross Section of the Eye

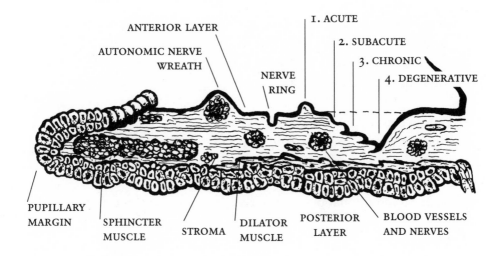

FIGURE 21: CROSS SECTION OF THE IRIS

1. In front is a layer of flattened endothelial cells placed on a delicate hyaline basement-membrane, and in men with dark-colored irides the cells contain pigment-granules.

2. *Stroma*—The stroma consists of fibres and cells. The former are made of fine, delicate bundles of fibrous tissue, of which some few fibres have a circular direction at the circumference of the iris, but the chief mass consists of fibres radiating toward the pupil. They form ... a delicate mesh in which the vessels and nerves are contained. Interspersed between the bundles of connective tissues are numerous branched cells. Many of them in dark eyes contain pigment-granules, but in blue eyes and the pink eyes of albinos they are unpigmented.[11]

With respect to the color of the iris, the following is noted:

The situation of the pigment-cells differs in different irides. In the various shades of blue eyes the only pigment cells are several layers of small round or polyhedral cells filled with dark pigment, situated on the posterior surface of the iris.... The color of the eyes in these individuals is due to this coloring-matter showing more or less through the texture of the iris. In the albino even this pigment is absent. In gray, brown, and black eyes there are, as mentioned above, pigment-granules to be found in the cells of the stroma and in the epithelial layer on the front of the iris; to these the dark color is due.[12]

Thus, we may consider three basic layers to the iris, which we'll refer to as the *anterior layer*, the *stroma*, and the *posterior layer*. Albinos will have pigment in none of these layers. A person with blue eyes will only have the dark purple pigment of the posterior layer. Any other eye color will be due to additional pigment in the stroma and the anterior layer.

IRIS LANDMARKS

Once this basic mapping is understood, we can look at the various landmarks of the iris. The border with the pupil, which may range in color from bright orange to black, has been referred to by various names, including the pupillary frill, pigment ruff, and pupillary margin. Here we will use *pupillary margin*. The outer margin of the iris also has various names. We will refer to it as the *limbus*. The next major iris landmark is the *autonomic nerve wreath*. Other names for this include collarette and ruff border. This will ideally be about one third of the way from the pupillary margin to the limbus and will form a symmetrical and gently scalloped circle. In practice it can be extremely distorted in shape and may be located both extremely close to the pupillary margin as well as near the limbus. In general, Zones 1 and 2 are inside the autonomic nerve wreath with Zones 3 through 7 outside. The autonomic nerve wreath (ANW) may in some instances touch either the pupillary margin or the limbus. It may also disappear in some places or even be almost completely invisible in a dark brown eye. Much

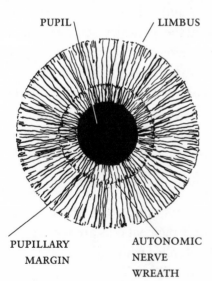

PUPIL   LIMBUS

PUPILLARY MARGIN   AUTONOMIC NERVE WREATH

FIGURE 22:

BASIC IRIS LANDMARKS

of iridology is concerned with observing with great exactness and precision these minute fiber structures, noting their relative straightness and density, their depth and color, and any abnormalities in their structure. In addition, typical iris markings include pigment spots or psora, lacunae, nerve rings, radii solaris, arcus senilus, anemia ring, lymphatic rosary, and scurf rim.

DEPTH AND COLOR OF IRIS FIBERS

One of the most important things to be aware of is the relative depth of the iris fibers. Jensen refers to various fiber depths as reflecting acute, subacute, chronic, and degenerative tissue conditions in the corresponding body areas. Dr. Ray expands upon this concept somewhat in describing seven basic fiber levels and their corresponding fiber colors which are referred to as levels one through seven. These seven levels of iris fiber color and depth are correlated with the seven levels of the scale of emotions as well. *Level one* is anterior in the iris, and the fiber color is white. This represents a normal or healthy tissue condition and relates to the level of enthusiasm. At *level two,* the iris fibers are bright white and have become more anterior. This indicates an acute or hyperactive condition in the tissues and corresponds to Jensen's acute level. This relates to the level of pain. If the body moves through the acute condition, then the fibers will eventually drop back to level one and return to a white color as a normal level of health is restored in the corresponding tissues. On the other hand, if the condition is suppressed or the body is for other reasons unable to maintain the acute condition any longer yet is also unable to overcome its cause, then the fibers will drop back to about the same depth as in level one but will become a light grey. This is referred to as *level three,* and relates to the level of anger. At *level four,* the fibers move further posterior and change to a grey color, a state corresponding more or less to Jensen's subacute level, and relating to the level of fear. At *levels five, six,* and *seven* the iris fibers move further posterior and change in color to a dark grey, a very dark grey, and finally to black. These levels coincide with the chronic and degenerative levels described by Jensen and relate respectively to the levels of grief, apathy, and finally unconsciousness. At level one, there is full sensitivity in the tissues and a basic absence of adverse symptomology as the tissues are at an

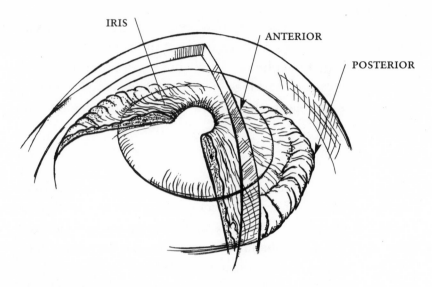

FIGURE 23: IRIS FIBER DEPTH

optimum level of health. At level two, there is a hyperactive condition in the tissues. There are numerous acute symptoms and much sensitivity in the tissues. At levels three through seven, the tissues become increasingly hypoactive and insensitive, and often there are virtually no symptoms due to the lack of sensitivity.

Hering's Law of Cure is well illustrated by the observation of the iris fibers. For as the fibers move from the lower levels back up to the higher levels, they pass through the various intermediate levels in reverse order, in much the same manner as symptoms are reexperienced in reverse order as health is restored to the body. If we are aware of symptoms only, then we are easily deceived. For symptoms can appear or disappear for completely opposite reasons. Supposedly negative symptoms are frequently the sign of a healing crisis, and thus, a positive sign. On the other hand the absence or disappearance of symptoms is not always a good sign but may simply be evidence of suppression. A person may feel good because they are truly in excellent health or else simply because all of the tissues of their body are in subacute stages or worse. A person may feel bad during an acute stage, yet this stage may be part of a process of degeneration towards the subacute or a process of healing, moving up towards level one. The former we shall refer to as a disease crisis while the latter is a healing crisis.

To distinguish between these two types of crises solely on the basis of symptomology is a tricky proposition. However, with the study of iridology, it may be possible to ascertain whether a particular condition is improving or worsening irrespective of the symptomology involved, for we can observe in which direction, whether anterior or posterior, the iris fibers are moving. When we observe new white fibers appearing where previously there has been only darkness, then we realize that no matter how awful the symptoms may be, healing is taking place and the body is simply coming back to life in this area.

Careful observation of iris fiber level also allows us in some cases to predict and anticipate healing crises in advance. This can help us to be better prepared for these inevitable experiences along the path to higher health both physically, and more importantly, psychologically. As the vibratory rate of the tissues increases and the iris fibers move further forward, it is to be expected that the same symptoms which were suppressed on the way down will be reexperienced in reverse order on the way back up. (Changes in iris fiber color and depth can be incredibly subtle, so it must be emphasized that it is not always possible to track changes in health in this manner.)

CONSTITUTION AS INDICATED BY IRIS

The constitution of the individual is revealed by the relative density and straightness of the iris fibers. Densely packed and straight fibers indicate a strong constitution, while wavy and loosely packed fibers show a weak constitution. Between the two extremes are numerous gradient levels of variation within the category of a mixed constitution. Even in the same iris there is often tremendous variation in the inherent strength of the tissues. A strong constitution indicates greater stamina and vitality, increased ability to resist any type of disease process, more rapid healing rate, greater recuperative abilities, and in general the ability to withstand more abuse. A weak constitution indicates lesser stamina and vitality, lesser recuperative abilities, less rapid healing, and in general a greater need to take better care of the body we have been given. Individuals with excellent constitutions may enjoy apparently excellent and vigorous health to an advanced age despite a lifetime of poor nutrition, alcohol, cigarettes, and

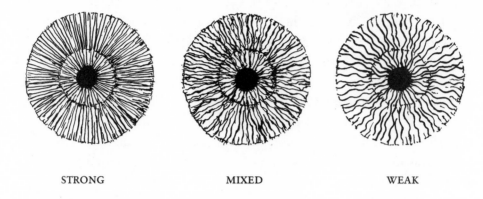

STRONG   MIXED   WEAK

FIGURE 24: STRONG, WEAK, AND MIXED CONSTITUTIONS

other destructive habits. Individuals with weak constitutions may be forced at an early age to take excellent care of their body and yet still be possessed of only minimal vitality despite their good habits.

It is wise to consider our constitution, for it greatly influences how rapidly we may be capable of going through the healing crises necessary to restore full health. People with weaker constitutions will generally require more effort to get the same results. It is often advisable for the person with a weaker constitution to make improvements in diet and supplements less rapidly so the initial healing crises are not too severe to be tolerated. Naturally, the attitude of the individual will also play a major role here in determining how quickly to proceed. The role of attitude is at least as significant as that of constitutional makeup.

LACUNAE

Lacunae (or lesions) in the iris represent inherited weaknesses in the given area. The location of the lacuna will indicate which area of the body is inherently weak. There may be considerable variation from the iris chart in the location of various body parts from iris to iris. Just as a surgeon will find that no two people's organs are placed in the exact same location, so too will the iridologist find that locations in the iris may vary as much as a half hour from the chart. This means that other factors such as symptoms past and present, medical history, family history, and other methods of diagnosis may often be needed to determine which body part is represented. Even then it is wise to consider that there may be several possibilities in the given situation.

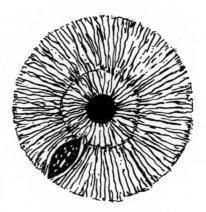

The size of a lacuna is not related to its severity. Factors which need to be considered include its shape, its relation to the ANW, and the fiber level within the lacuna itself. The fiber level will tell much as to whether the condition is acute, chronic, or otherwise. The presence of an inherited weakness does not guaran-

FIGURE 25: LACUNAE

tee that there is a problem but shows that there is a predisposition to a problem in this area. With proper care, problems need never develop in these inherently weak areas. However these are the most likely areas for problems to develop when we live our lives in such a manner as to violate natural laws of health. In many cases it is found that lacunae which are relatively narrow and which indent deeply into the ANW indicate a more serious condition than a wider lacuna where the ANW is less indented.

PIGMENT SPOTS OR PSORA

We must also carefully consider pigment spots or *psora* in the iris, also known as metabolic pigmentation or foreign body pigment. At the very least, these indicate areas of relative weakness within the body where tissue is underactive and toxins have begun to accumulate. Again, the size of the pigment spot is of little importance; the most important factor is the color. In general, the darker the spot the more severe the condition. A black or very dark brown pigment spot will generally indicate a potentially serious problem. In some cases no obvious accompanying symptoms are involved, and the condition, as well as the pigment spot, may remain relatively unchanged for decades. Location is also important. When the location is determined with respect to the eye chart (note that up to a half hour variation from the chart is possible), other factors must be taken into account in determining which area of the body is indicated by the pigment spot. It is possible that the individual will not currently be experiencing any noticeable symptoms in any of the possible areas and may not even recall ever having done so. Hence, in some cases while the extent of the problem may be known, the exact location may not be completely certain. Other methods of analysis may be used in conjunction with iridology for improved accuracy.

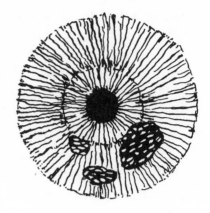

FIGURE 26: PSORA

RADII SOLARIS

Radii solaris (or radial furrows) are another major iris landmark often present. They resemble spokes radiating out from the pupil or the ANW towards the limbus. These are sometimes referred to as parasite lines. However, while there may be parasites present in the indicated areas, parasites cannot themselves be seen in the iris as they are not a part of the body. What is indicated by the radii solaris is tissue of diminished electrical potential or lessened vitality. Such tissue is said to be a host condition for parasites. Just as a sufficiently healthy plant is virtually immune to pests, so too is healthy tissue far less susceptible to bacteria, viruses, and parasites. In addition to the location of the radii solaris, the color and length are carefully noted. The darker and longer the radii solaris, the more severe the condition. As the condition improves, the radii solaris will often grow lighter and shorter from the periphery of the iris inward. Radii solaris which originate at the pupil may indicate reflex problems from the intestines out into the other tissues of the body.

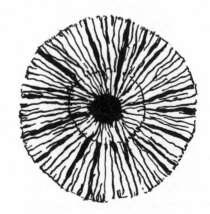

FIGURE 27: RADII SOLARIS

Nerve Rings

Nerve rings are another major landmark. Nerve rings look somewhat like rings in a tree, although they usually are portions of circles rather than complete ones. They are also referred to as contraction furrows or as stress rings. Here is indicated the tendency for the individual to experience stress or tension to a significant degree. As Dr. Jensen puts it, "nerve rings show stress and imply a need for relaxation."[13] Of particular interest are the beginning and end points of the nerve

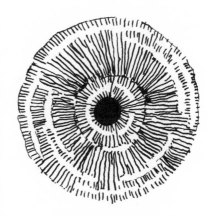

FIGURE 28: NERVE RINGS

rings, the areas through which they pass, fiber level, and the zone in which they are located, all of which indicate potential problem areas in the body. These will be some of the primary areas where the body will experience stress. The zone in which the nerve ring is located will also indicate where the body may experience stress. A nerve ring in Zone 7, for example, may indicate a tendency towards skin problems. The fiber level of the nerve ring will indicate whether the condition is chronic, acute, or otherwise.

Other Landmarks

Other major iris landmarks to check for include arcus senilus, scurf rim, anemia ring, mineral ring, and lymphatic rosary. The *arcus senilus* "is a sign of cerebral anemia."[14] The *scurf rim* "reflects the condition of the skin as an eliminative organ."[15] The scurf rim also reflects the overall condition of the body at a cellular level. The *anemia ring* is a sign of anemia, while the *lymphatic rosary* indicates a congested lymphatic system. The *mineral ring* may be a sign of inorganic min-

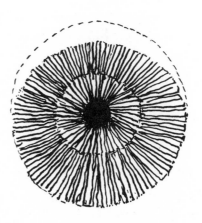

FIGURE 29: ARCUS SENILUS

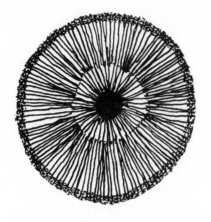

FIGURE 30: SCURF RIM

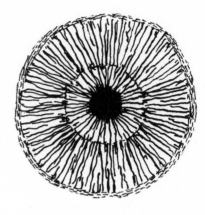

FIGURE 31: ANEMIA RING

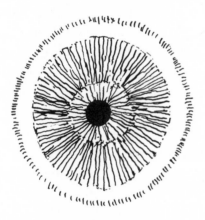

FIGURE 32: MINERAL RING

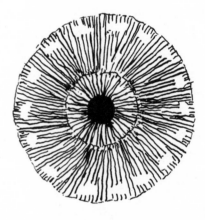

FIGURE 33: LYMPHATIC ROSARY

erals, including sodium or calcium, settling out in the tissues as well as a buildup of cholesterol. Other names for a mineral ring include *sodium ring* or *cholesterol ring*. Any deviation or abnormality in iris fiber structure should also be carefully noted.

CHANGES IN IRIS STRUCTURE AND COLOR

As discussed earlier, the iris has three basic layers: the anterior layer, the stroma, and the posterior layer. Albinos will have pigment in none of these layers. A person with blue eyes will only have the dark purple pigment of the posterior layer. Any other eye color is due to additional pigment in the stroma and/or the anterior layer. With some exceptions, most babies are born with deep blue eyes. This deep blue color indicates that the pigment in the stroma and in the anterior layer is not present. For those whose eyes stay blue, this pigment does not appear. Pigment in the stroma and the anterior layer will gradually appear in some people's eyes over time. As a result, the eye color will change from blue to gray, green, brown, black, and so on. Much of this pigmentation will be a brown color and referred to as melanin, and most iridologists will readily acknowledge its gradual appearance. Yet there is some dispute as to its significance as well as disagreement about whether or not it is possible for it to diminish or disappear once it is present. However, in my experience and that of others, color changes can be in response to either physical healing of some sort, consciousness change, or more likely both. In that context, the eye color change has invariably been in the direction of lighter eye color or less brown. (There are no instances to my knowledge where eye color has become darker as healing or consciousness change has occurred.) If the amount of dark pigmentation were to diminish, then clearly a brown eye would begin to look lighter in color. Were the dark pigmentation to disappear entirely, then a formerly brown eye would be blue. Again, bear in mind that the posterior layer is a dark purple color in brown as well as blue eyes. The color difference is simply a result of the presence or absence of dark pigment in the stroma and anterior layer.

I have seen dark eyes get somewhat lighter in color as some of the melanin pigmentation has disappeared. My own eyes have gotten lighter, and my father's eyes also changed, this happening when he was past sixty years of age. His formerly brown eyes are now quite green in the outer half or more. Such iris color changes are not uncommon, yet they do not happen to everyone.[16]

Eye color would appear to be only one of numerous factors in the iris, and not necessarily any more important than constitution, fiber structure, symmetry of the ANW, radii solaris, nerve rings, lacunae, pigment spots, fiber color and depth, and so forth. A person with dark brown eyes may have an excellent constitution and a fundamentally sound iris structure. A person with blue eyes might have an extremely poor constitution and numerous other indications of problems. We should not make sweeping generalizations about people with brown eyes versus people with blue eyes insofar as overall health or amount of resistance are concerned. Changes in iris fiber structure (which might include constitution, fiber structure, symmetry of the ANW, radii solaris, nerve rings, lacunae, pigment spots, fiber color and depth, and so forth) are generally extremely subtle at best.

REFLEX CONDITIONS

In addition to iris signs, another thing to check for when observing the iris is reflex conditions. Here, a problem in one portion of the body will have a direct bearing on a problem elsewhere. One situation in which this reflex concept will be especially helpful is when there are severe symptoms experienced in a body part that does not show anything out of the ordinary in the iris itself. In many such instances, the real physical source of the problem is somewhere other than where the major symptoms are being experienced.

A major reflex to consider is the *zero degree reflex*. This is where two body parts are found in the same eye at the same time but in different zones. The transverse colon and the brain would be a prime example of a zero degree reflex, as would be the heart and lungs, or the liver and gall bladder. The reflex activity from various areas of the colon to the rest of the body on a zero degree reflex must always be considered, as well as numerous other zero degree reflexes. (It is important to note that reflex activity is in both directions.) To say that reflex activity is taking place between two body parts does not mean that one is necessarily the cause of problems in the other. It means that the condition of one will influence the condition of the other. When we look upon the body as a whole and realize that no one part can suffer without having a detrimental effect on the rest of the body, and that no one part of the body can be absolutely healthy if any other part is not, then the concept of reflex activity seems pretty sensible. When we view it in terms of practical experience and see it in action, then it becomes undeniable.

Besides the zero degree reflex, other prominent reflexes which have been observed are at 180 degrees, 90 degrees, 60 degrees, and 120 degrees. Reflex activity also appears evident at 30 and 150 degrees. Examples of 180 degree

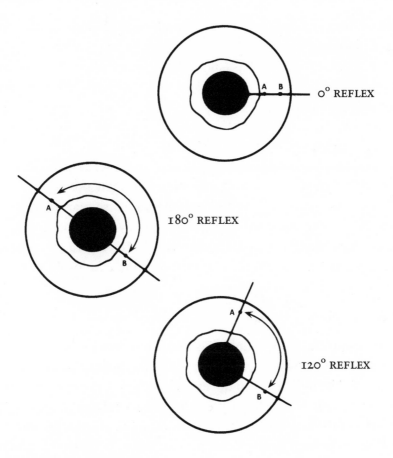

FIGURE 34: REFLEX CONDITIONS

reflexes include pancreas and eyes, bronchus and bronchials, thyroid and breast, thyroid and thymus, and ears and bladder. Examples of 90 degree reflexes include adrenals and thyroid, heart and pituitary, and liver and bladder. Examples of 60 degree reflexes include prostate and testes, uterus and ovary, heart and medulla, lungs and medulla, and pituitary and thyroid. Examples of the 120 degree reflexes include the medulla and ovary/testes, heart and anus/rectum, and bladder and pineal. Examples of 30 degree include pituitary and medulla, and thymus and spleen. Examples of 150 degree reflexes include liver and thyroid, and pituitary and adrenals. There is still a great deal that is not understood about reflex activity, but many previously confusing situations become much more understandable when we begin to understand and apply this concept. A simple example: the eyes and the pancreas are a 180 degree reflex to each other. Thus, a person with pancreatic problems (such as a diabetic) might develop problems with the vision as a result. And indeed, it is observed that many diabetics eventually go blind.

Uses of Iridology in Healing Work

A GOOD METHOD OF THOROUGHLY EXAMINING THE IRIS IS TO BEGIN WITH the pupil and work out through the pupillary margin, then Zone 1 out to Zone 7, noting what is observed and paying attention to the interrelationships between various body parts. In Iris-Sclera Integrated Diagnosis the sclera is also closely observed as is the relationship between the sclera and the iris.

DETECTING PROBLEMS EARLY

One great advantage of iridology is that a problem may be fairly obvious in the iris many years in advance of any clinical symptoms. This early detection allows the individual to do something about the condition before it becomes extremely serious or life threatening. Individual weaknesses are also evident through iridology, again even in the absence of symptoms. It can be quite helpful to the individual to be aware of weaknesses so that these areas can receive the special attention they require. In many cases there may be a number of problem areas in the body, and iridology can often make clear their relationship as well as indicating which is the most serious and should receive first attention.

It is extremely common for obvious problems to be indicated in the iris with complete absence of symptoms in the corresponding area of the body. On many occasions I have seen this only to hear from the individual some time after the eye reading that they have since experienced serious symptoms in the indicated areas during healing crisis, many times also getting the memory of when they had felt that way before. Within the context of the healing crisis, wherein the individual will have the opportunity to reexperience all symptoms, both physical and psychological, the question of when they have felt this way before is always pertinent, especially when we consider the importance of memory. Indeed, often the physical symptoms help to trigger the memory, thus revealing the underlying patterns of thought, word, and emotion that are the root of the situation.

IMPROVING DIGESTION

As the body heals from the inside out, improving the digestion is a major priority for many people. Many of the initial symptoms of healing crisis will tend to involve the digestion. Dietary changes, enzymes, friendly microbes, mature green papaya, and other supplements will all assist in improving the digestion and elimination immensely. To see what is needed the fiber structure and color within the ANW must be carefully scrutinized and the various portions of the intestines checked in the iris. The presence of diverticuli, outpouchings, and strictures is noted as well as the overall pattern of the ANW, wherein a constricted, tight ANW indicates a spastic colon and a loose ANW indicates a sluggish or atonic colon. Variations in the recommended program may be suggested, depending on these particular individual conditions. A person with a sluggish colon relatively free of strictures might well benefit from the use of psyllium, for example, whereas for a person with strictures in the sigmoid area, the use of psyllium is frequently counterproductive as there may be a tendency for it to further constipate the person.

SUPPORTING OTHER CHANGES

The endocrine system is also checked, and in many cases certain of the glands will require some assistance from an appropriate herb. The lymphatic system is checked, and in the event of lymphatic congestion, lymphatic enzymes are utilized to help clear this out. Mature green papaya may be used to insure proper protein digestion so that the lymphatic congestion does not get any worse. The skin is assisted in its eliminative capacity by various supplements such as Schweitzer fluid and niacin as well as dry brushing. For parasitic involvement herbs which are often effective at eliminating parasites may be used. Nerve rings require more of an attitude adjustment than a nutritional one, although extra calcium and magnesium may be helpful. The individual with nerve rings should be advised to work on "lovingly and willingly enduring all things." Major organs such as the kidneys, liver, lungs, and heart are checked and appropriate supplements may be taken as needed.

Numerous other supplements might be recommended for an individual on the basis of what is observed in the eyes, and many are commonly indicated. When doing an eye reading, in addition to indicating which supplements would be beneficial, I usually indicate which of these would be of highest priority and which of a lesser priority, as most people's willingness to expend time, money, and so forth is limited. One job of the iridologist is to help them do the best and most effective job they can within these limitations. Another might be to instruct them in basic principles of health in the hopes that many of these limitations will eventually disappear.

CHOOSING POINTS IN BODY ELECTRONICS

With the help of iridology and sclerology, individual needs for Body Electronics are determined, though they could be useful with other healing methods as well. In addition to suggesting need for dietary changes and supplements, the condition of the iris will also reveal which points would need to be held and especially which would be top priorities. The endocrine system as well as all major organs should be checked thoroughly. In determining which points to hold on the spine there are two ways to proceed. We can determine weaknesses in organs and glands using iridology and then hold points on the vertebra associated with these organs and glands. The alternative is to go directly to the spine and manually locate the areas that need work. In my experience the same vertebra tend to be selected using both methods, which should hardly be surprising.

Being able through iridology to spot potentially serious problems in advance and thus to take appropriate corrective measures is also quite advantageous. For instance, it is not uncommon for tumors to be present without a person knowing it. If a tumor does exist, points must not be held anywhere near it at first, as this might break up the tumor. An intense nutritional program must be followed in such cases before any pointholding should be attempted in the area of the tumor. Even then no pointholding should be done without a qualified iridologist who is thoroughly trained in Body Electronics to ascertain that there is no danger. For this reason alone, we perform at least a cursory eye reading on everybody before holding points on them. Generally when there is a tumor present and it is in an advanced stage where it is no longer contained and is beginning to spread into the surrounding tissue, the prime avenue of approach will initially be nutritional. In this manner integrity can be restored to the surrounding tissues, and the tumor may be contained. This will occur as a necessary step prior to the tumor eventually shrinking and disappearing, in accordance with Hering's Law. Possible iris signs of tumors include black or extremely dark brown pigment spots; black holes in the iris fiber structure surrounded by white swollen fibers; extreme distortions in fiber structure; and heavy dark red transversals which are blood vessels which have risen up and moved anterior to the iris fibers. There is no universal "tumor" sign in the iris, but each of the signs mentioned above has been associated with tumors which were verified medically.

The degree of severity of any problems which might exist in the body is important, and iridology can help determine this. When more severe degenerative conditions exist, generally a stricter dietary regimen and a more intense program of supplementation will be necessary if progress is to be made. This will be especially true if the individual also has a somewhat weak constitution. By contrast, a person with no major problems and a strong constitution can expect improvement with a less drastic program of diet and supplementation. In the latter case, Body Electronics can begin fairly quickly. In the former, it is best to allow the body chemistry to change for a longer time to insure that a condition of nutrient saturation is well established in the tissues prior to pointholding. For most people, however, a gradual approach is best, and part of the job of the iridologist will be to recommend where in their nutritional program to place priorities. For example, a typical eye reading may uncover the need for dozens of supplements. Few people, other than those with serious problems or ample time and finances, will be willing to immediately begin taking forty or fifty supplements. Thus, the iridologist may recommend all these items but also mention a much smaller number as being the items of greatest priority. Rather than second guess the patient, I often simply ask them how much they are willing to do. Iridology, after all, is not a method of treatment, and if the patient is unwilling or unable to follow any of the recommendations, then improvement cannot be expected.

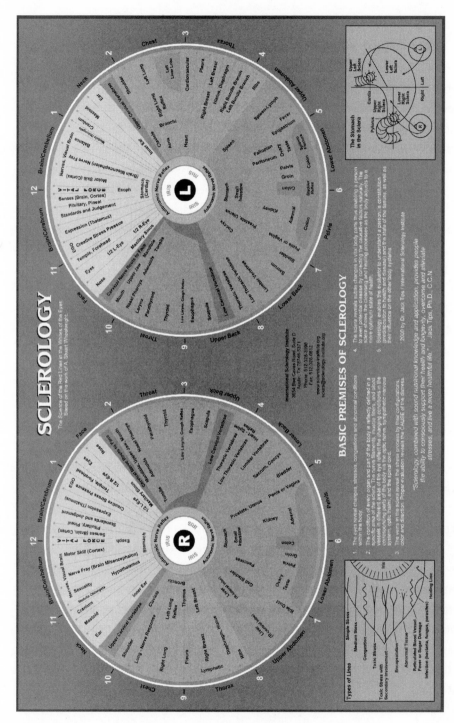

FIGURE 36: JACK TIPS'S EYE CHART

Sclerology

MUCH VALUABLE INFORMATION CAN ALSO BE ATTAINED THROUGH sclerology, either on its own or used along with iridology. Sclerology has received nowhere near the amount of attention iridology has, little has been written on the subject, and there are far fewer practitioners. It is much younger as a discipline than iridology. Yet it has much to offer.

Included here is an excellent sclerology chart developed by Jack Tips.[17] What follows here are some basic principles of sclerology. For more detailed treatment readers are referred to *Insights in the Eyes* by Jack Tips.

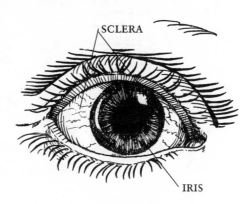

FIGURE 35: THE SCLERA

The amount of information revealed through sclerology is usually less than that gained through Iridology, for the sclera is not as complex as the iris.[18] Yet much can be discovered, and it is quite a reliable form of analysis. In addition it is beneficial to use sclerology in some particular cases: for instance, when analyzing an extremely dark brown iris, often relatively little can be readily observed. It is also useful in cases where all or a portion of the iris has been surgically removed, as well as other conditions which obscure the iris.

CORRELATING IRIS AND SCLERA

The map of the body found in the iris has been discussed previously. A location in the iris is precisely defined by three things: which eye, left or right; what time, as in hours of a clock; and which zone, which is related to distance out from the pupil towards the limbus. The sclera appears to offer a similar map, and basically, the sclera and iris correlate in a simple manner. For the most part, the left iris will relate to the left sclera, while the right iris will relate to the right sclera. A given time in the iris will relate to the

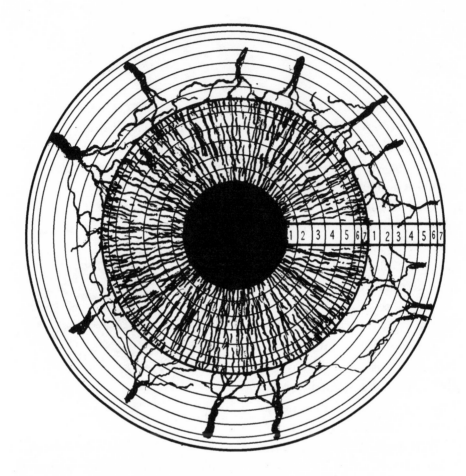

FIGURE 37: CORRELATING IRIS AND SCLERA

same time in the sclera. As far as iris zones go, distance from the pupil in the iris will correspond to distance from the iris in the sclera. For example, zone 1 in the iris would correspond with the part of the sclera nearest to the iris. And zone 7 in the iris would correspond to a portion of the sclera that is roughly as far away from the iris as zone 7 is from the pupil.

INDICATING LINES

Virtually all scleras will display fairly obvious blood vessels that point more or less towards the iris. These are referred to as indicating lines. Much of the time they will be pointing towards a particular endocrine gland or major organ. Hence, the time at which they are located will indicate to which gland or organ they are related. Some will be quite dark and thick, while others will be lighter in color or fainter. Some will be quite straight, while others will be wavy or crooked. Some will fork. Some may have red, blue, brown, or black dots on their ends. Some will approach the iris closely or even touch the iris. Others will not come very close to the iris. All of these factors have significance. These indicating lines can change gradually or in some cases quite rapidly. Changes in these indicating lines can show improvement or worsening of various situations.

The presence of an indicating line shows a certain degree of stress on a particular gland or organ. This is not necessarily a bad thing. (In fact, the total absence of all indicating lines would be much more serious. For when the sclera goes totally white, this is a sign that the body is essentially no longer responding to stress. It tends to happen shortly before death, and sometimes in cases of severe shock or substantial blood loss, and is always a serious indication.) In general, thick or dark indicating lines show a more significant degree of stress. When indicating lines come closer to the iris or touch it, this also shows a higher level of stress on the gland or organ in question. A wavy or crooked indicating line tends to show a more chronic situation. It also tends to show poor circulation to the gland or organ in question. The wavy indicating line might be compared to a stream that meanders along at a slow rate, whereas a straighter indicating line would be like a more vigorous stream with better flow. This is a simple overview of indicating lines, and certainly there are subtleties and exceptions that are beyond the scope of this presentation.

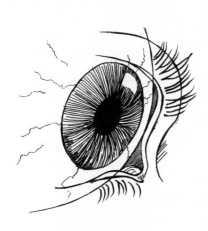

FIGURE 38: INDICATING LINES

Degeneration Lines

There are also blood vessels known as degeneration lines which run more or less parallel to the circumference of the iris, which might also be expressed as perpendicular to the indicating lines. If present they always signify some sort of problem in the corresponding tissues, although their exact interpretation can vary depending upon several factors. A degeneration line crossing an indicating line can often indicate a potentially serious problem in the corresponding tissues, for example. A common type of degeneration line is found in the medial inferior portion of the sclera, which corresponds to the spinal area. These are often referred to as spinal degeneration lines. They can be associated with scoliosis and various other spinal problems. Careful study of the spinal degeneration lines can in some cases indicate a specific area of the spine as a problem area.

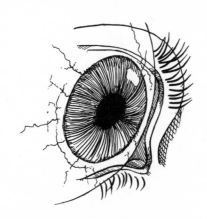

FIGURE 39: DEGENERATION LINES

Red, Blue, Brown, and Black Spots

Spots or dots of various colors can be found at the end of indicating lines as well as on their own. Depending upon their number and color, they often indicate problems of varying degrees of severity. Their order of increasing severity would typically be from red to blue to brown to black. They can be associated with a variety of situations including tumors, leukemia, and stroke.

Blue Blotches

In some cases a large blue blotch may be seen in the sclera that looks some-

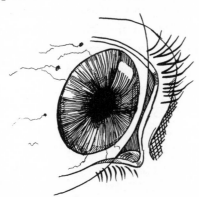

FIGURE 40: RED, BLUE, BROWN, AND BLACK SPOTS

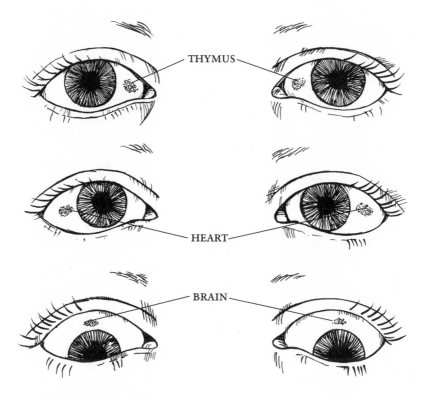

FIGURE 41: BLUE BLOTCHES

thing like a bruise. This can vary widely in color. The darker and more prominent it is, the more severe the condition indicated. When it is found laterally in the sclera, it is commonly associated with degeneration of the heart. When it is found medially in the sclera, it is commonly associated with a breakdown of the thymus and immune system. These blue blotches can also be located elsewhere in the sclera. Blue blotches between 11:00 and 1:00 pertain to the brain, and indicate a relative lack of circulation to the brain. This may be related to numerous factors, including problems in the upper cervical spine.

THE HEART

Several indications of heart problems or stress may be seen in the sclera. Recall from the iris charts that the heart is laterally at approximately 3:00

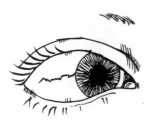
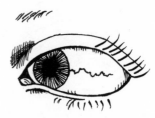

FIGURE 42: HEAVY HEART INDICATORS TOUCHING IRIS

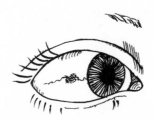
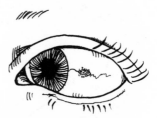

FIGURE 43: HEART INDICATORS WITH RED BLOTCHES

in the left eye and about 9:00 in the right. It will be the same relative position in the sclera. A dark heavy indicating line at either of these approximate positions shows heavy stress on the heart. An indicating line at either of these approximate positions that touches the iris or comes close to doing so also shows such stress. In some cases, along such indicating lines in the heart area will be found red blotches. These often show some previous damage to the heart, as from a heart attack, for example.

BLUE RINGS

Several types of blue rings may be seen in the sclera. A narrow one immediately surrounding the iris is known by some as an *anemia ring*. A broader blue ring that extends out approximately three-eighths of an inch or one centimeter or so from the iris is also sometimes seen. Both of these blue rings indicate that the body is poorly oxygenated. How dark blue these rings are will show the extent of the problem.

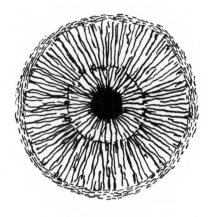
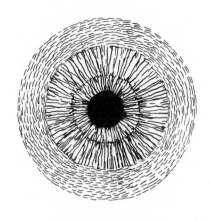

FIGURE 44: THIN BLUE RING   FIGURE 45: WIDE BLUE RING

ARCUS SENILUS AND ANEMIA IN THE EXTREMITIES

In many eyes the sclera will be seen to actually overlap or obscure the outer portion of the iris. When the sclera moves across the superior portion of the iris, it is called *arcus senilus* (or "arc of senility") and shows poor circulation and nutrient supply to the brain. (See Figure 29.) It can be found in people of all ages, despite its name. When the sclera overlaps the iris all the way around, this is known as anemia in the extremities. This would indicate poor circulation to the body as a whole.

OTHER SCLERA SIGNS

Brown pigmentation in the sclera refers to problems with the digestion, liver, and gall bladder. Dr. Ray has coined the term *hamburger* to refer to this brown pig-

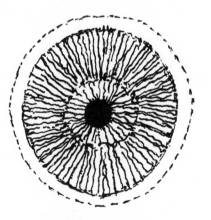

FIGURE 46: ANEMIA IN THE EXTREMITIES

mentation in the sclera. Yellow throughout the sclera is a sign of problems with the liver. Localized yellow deposits in the sclera are associated with cholesterol buildup and poor fat metabolism in general.

TIE-INS

When two or more indicating lines are joined by a common degeneration line, this is called a tie-in. We might recall that these indicating lines are typically associated with endocrine glands, and that each endocrine gland is associated with a specific emotion. (See Figure 3 in Chapter Two.) A problem in a given gland will have

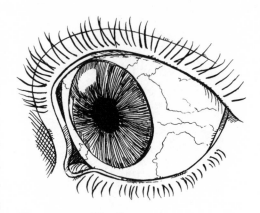

FIGURE 47: TIE-INS

some relationship to resistance with respect to the associated emotion. Thyroid problems, for example, are often related to anger; pancreas problems are often related to grief. When we have a tie-in, there is some relationship between the various glands that are on the tie-in. If we consider the emotions associated with these glands, it might be said that there are resistance patterns that involve more than one emotion. For example, a pituitary-thyroid tie-in might involve simultaneous pain and anger. In Body Electronics, when a tie-in is present it is common practice to hold all points on the tie-in at the same time in a pointholding session. It is also the convention in this unique case to stay plugged in on all these points until all are done.

Iridology and Sclerology

FAR MORE COULD BE WRITTEN ON THESE TWO AREAS, BUT MUCH MORE than this is beyond the scope of this present work. These two fields, and especially their interconnection, would require quite a lengthy book to address sufficiently, and numerous color photos would also be required to really do the job justice. This is not my intention here. Rather, a few of the basics have been presented so these can be related to the overall principles of health and healing we have been discussing. Both of them are useful for diagnosing and also for keeping track of progress as we go along on a path toward a state of perfect health. Both can give some outer indication of what is happening on an inner level and how it relates to our physical health.

Chapter Twenty-One

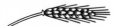

Biological Transmutations

The only constant in the outer universe is change.
Anonymous

THE PROCESS OF HEALING, WHETHER ASSISTED BY BODYWORK, IM-
proved nutrition or other means, will involve biological transmutation. To better understand its mechanics, we can consider the work
of Louis Kervran, as discussed in his book *Biological Transmutations*.
Kervran may be considered the pioneering researcher in the field of biological transmutations, and in this book is found a tremendous amount of
vital information upon the subject. Biological transmutations may be considered to be atomic reactions that take place within living organisms under
certain circumstances. In other words, there is a transmutation of elements,
not merely a chemical reaction. Kervran offers ample evidence of this phenomenon from his many years of research in the field. (A listing of some
of the specific biological transmutations noted by Kervran is included in
Appendix Two.)

Endothermal and Exothermal Reactions

TRANSMUTING SIMPLER ELEMENTS INTO MORE COMPLEX ELEMENTS RE-
quires an input of energy. Such reactions are known as *endothermal
reactions*. When an individual undergoes an endothermal reaction, they

typically feel cold in some part or all of their body. This cold may be quite extreme. In an extremely hot room, the individual may shiver despite being covered by many blankets. Typically the individual will also feel cold to the touch. In more extreme endothermal reactions, this cold may be felt at quite a distance from the individual.

Transmuting more complex elements into simpler elements appears to liberate or release energy. Such reactions are known as *exothermal reactions*. When an individual undergoes an exothermal reaction, they typically feel heat in some part or all of their body. This heat may be quite extreme. Some individuals have described it as feeling like a blowtorch. Typically the individual will also feel hot to the touch. In more extreme exothermal reactions, this heat may be felt at quite a distance from the individual.

In an endothermal reaction, as simpler elements are transmuted into more complex ones, some of the electrons which begin at a lower energy state (that is, closer to the nucleus) must move further out to higher energy states. Thus, an input of energy is required, and cold is experienced as this energy is pulled in from the surrounding environment. In an exothermal reaction, as more complex elements are transmuted into simpler ones, some of the electrons which begin at a higher energy state (that is, further from the nucleus) must move closer in to lower energy states. Thus, an output of energy is produced, and heat is experienced as this energy is released into the surrounding environment.

In the regeneration of the human body, these endothermal and exothermal reactions may play an extremely significant role. In many cases their presence is accompanied by obvious regeneration of the physical body. There are a number of factors, nutritional and otherwise, that are necessary in order for these reactions to occur.

Hormones and the Endocrine System

ONE FACTOR THAT MAY BE NECESSARY FOR THESE ENDOTHERMAL AND exothermal reactions to take place is the presence of appropriate hormones. Kervran mentions hormones as being necessary for several specific biological transmutations. For example, the transmutation of sodium into potassium was demonstrated to be dependent upon the presence of the hormone aldosterone from the adrenal glands.[1] Several transmutations involving calcium are said to be related to hormones from the thyroid gland.[2] Kervran himself does not state that all transmutations are dependent upon the presence of specific hormones. However, a wealth of experience supports this concept.

Since the endocrine glands secrete the various hormones, their full function is extremely important. Within many healing modalities, great emphasis has been placed upon restoring the full activity of the endocrine system, and it has consistently been observed that the endocrine glands play a vital role in the regeneration of the body. Their involvement in these biological transmutations would further underscore the necessity of restoring endocrine function if the body is to regenerate.

Amino Acids and Protein Digestion

HORMONES ARE SUBSTANCES THAT ARE IN PART COMPOSED OF AMINO acids. Certain hormones require a broad variety of amino acids for their production, in some cases as many as twenty different amino acids for a single hormone. Some amino acids are considered essential amino acids because the body either cannot produce them itself or does not produce them in sufficient quantities. Thus, the essential amino acids must come from the diet. Of the essential amino acids, there are two (lysine and tryptophan) that are denatured at a fairly low temperature of approximately 43 degrees Celsius or 110 degrees Fahrenheit according to Dr. John Whitman Ray. When protein is heated above this temperature, these two amino acids are no longer available to the body. For this reason, we must regularly consume a good source of raw protein containing these two amino acids to assure the abundance of all essential amino acids. Otherwise, we will be unable to form all of the various hormones the body requires.

It is not enough merely to ingest appropriate protein, but rather that this protein must be digested and assimilated. Many people have very poor protein digestion. In iridology, this may be evidenced by the degree of lymphatic congestion indicated in zone 6 of the iris. An obvious remedy would be to consume protein along with appropriate proteolytic enzymes to assure its digestion. In addition to various types of enzyme supplements, we might note that certain fruits are rich sources of various proteases. These include the papain in the pawpaw or papaya, the actinidin in the kiwi fruit, the ficin in the fig, and the bromelain in the pineapple. (See Chapter Nine for more information on amino acids, enzymes, and protein digestion.)

Louis Kervran makes abundant mention of enzymes as being necessary for the various biological transmutations to occur. Kervran notes that "nature has many ways to prevent a deficiency resulting not from the lack of an element but from an insufficient production of the enzyme that carries out the transmutation."[3] Kervran further notes that "enzymes, which are a kind of biological catalyst, are no doubt responsible for making this *in vivo* reaction possible at low temperature."[4] We might consider at this point that in addition to the many previously known roles of enzymes in human health and in the regeneration of the physical body, enzymes also play a vital role in the initiation of the biological transmutations.

Bacteria, Algae, and Mushrooms

IN ADDITION TO ENZYMES AND HORMONES, KERVRAN MAKES SPECIFIC mention that various bacteria, algae and mushrooms are also capable of performing biological transmutations. In particular, Kervran mentions that bacteria within our intestines may play quite a significant role in the biological transmutations. That is, many of the biological transmutations that take place within us may in fact be performed by our friendly bacteria rather than ourselves. For this and many other reasons, it is imperative that the individual establish and maintain a robust colony of friendly microbes throughout the digestive system. (See Chapters Nine, Twelve, and Thirteen for more on this.)

On this topic, the following was related to me by Dr. John Whitman Ray. A scientist in Michigan performed an interesting experiment. Upon observing the incredible power of certain microbes in their ability to break down cellulose through the secretion of enzymes, he wondered what other substances these microbes might be able to break down. A site was selected where the soil was highly contaminated with various toxic wastes. A thick layer of rotted wood was spread over this soil. After this rotted wood had been broken down further by microbial action, the soil was analyzed once more. The microbes had not just broken down the wood chips, but at the same time the toxic wastes had been broken down into harmless substances. This may have been accomplished by the microbes and their enzyme secretions through biological transmutations. Again, Kervran specifically mentions bacteria, algae and mushrooms as being capable of biological transmutations. Kervran also speculates in his book that radioactive wastes might perhaps be neutralized by biological transmutations as well.[5]

Minerals

ABUNDANT EMPHASIS HAS BEEN PLACED UPON THE MANY ROLES OF MINerals in health and regeneration. (See Chapters Nine, Ten, and Thirteen.) Biological transmutations appear to be a means for the body to provide itself with a given mineral. Indeed, there are often a number of options that the body has to produce a given element. Calcium, for example, can be derived from magnesium, or from silica, or from potassium. Both potassium and magnesium can in turn be derived from sodium. So by a two-step process calcium could also be produced from sodium, either via magnesium or via potassium. There are endless examples, but the basic point is that the body has any number of ways of manufacturing the various minerals it requires. However, Kervran does note that despite this vast ability of the body to manufacture the elements that it requires, nonetheless, it often appears that some of the desired element must be present already in order for more of it to be produced.[6] Perhaps some of the desired element must be present to serve as a pattern or template in order for more to be formed.

The body requires a large number of minerals for many purposes, and often these minerals must be in specific ratios to each other. Many nutritionists have placed a great emphasis upon the need to correctly balance the ratios of minerals that are ingested. Similarly, in agriculture many farmers have placed a great emphasis on balancing the minerals applied to the soil. However, often this is done with no awareness of the reality of biological transmutations. What must be considered is that the final balance that is achieved within the body (or in the soil) will not be the same balance that is applied from the outside. Rather, through the mechanism of biological transmutations, a proper balance will be reached naturally given the presence of all necessary factors. Within the body, some of these factors will include minerals, enzymes, hormones, amino acids, proper function of the endocrine glands, and the activity of friendly microbes. There are probably others as well. Kervran also notes that in many instances where the body needs a certain element for a specific purpose, all evidence suggests that it actually prefers to make that element rather than simply ingest it. For example, the silica in horsetail, which can be transmuted into calcium, seems to bring about healing of bones far more rapidly than the ingestion of any type of calcium.[7]

Monopoles

ANOTHER FACTOR WHICH RELATES TO BIOLOGICAL TRANSMUTATIONS IS the activity of structures known as monopoles, which occur within the mitochondria (as the next chapter explains). According to Dr. John Whitman Ray, it is through the proper activity of these monopoles that the biological transmutations are activated.[8] While the activity of the monopoles appears to be necessary to trigger the biological transmutations, it also appears that the presence of the melanin-protein complex will interfere with or prevent this activity. Thus, the resistance of the human mind must also be considered as a powerful factor with regard to biological transmutations. Indeed, it is upon the release of this resistance that such transmutations often occur, as is quite extensively noted within the field of Body Electronics.

Hydrogen and Oxygen

KERVRAN STATES AS A GENERAL PRINCIPLE WITH REGARD TO BIOLOGICAL transmutations that "a law now emerges. Reactions at the nuclear level of the atom always involve hydrogen and oxygen."[9] A great many of the reactions noted by Kervran are indeed the addition or subtraction of either hydrogen or oxygen. It should be noted, however, that of the reactions described by Kervran, a few do not involve hydrogen or oxygen.

Many individuals who were quite poorly oxygenated have been able to rapidly build up the ability of their blood to carry oxygen through the ingestion of large quantities of chlorophyll. There is a strong similarity between certain portions of the hemoglobin molecule, which carries the oxygen, and chlorophyll. A major difference is the iron in the hemoglobin as opposed to the magnesium in the chlorophyll. It has been speculated that this consistently observed phenomenon may be related to a biological transmutation of magnesium to iron. If we follow Kervran's rule regarding oxygen or hydrogen as being probable elements in such a transmutation, it might be noted that $2Mg + 2H >> Fe$ is one possible scenario. (That is, two atoms of magnesium plus two atoms of hydrogen might transmute to one atom of iron.) Kervran himself notes the frequent transmutation of manganese to iron, that is $Mn + H >> Fe$. (One atom of manganese plus one atom of hydrogen transmuting into one atom of iron.) There may, of course, be an entirely different process involved as well.

The Role of Consciousness

SO FAR, WE HAVE PRIMARILY CONSIDERED A FEW OF THE MANY PHYSIcal factors pertaining to these biological transmutations, although the role of consciousness has been alluded to briefly. The relationship between the biological transmutations and the human mind, and in particular to the scale of emotions (enthusiasm, pain, anger, fear, grief, apathy, and unconsciousness, as well as the seven levels within each level), is explored in considerable detail in the second and third books in the *Logic In Sequence Series* by Dr. John Whitman Ray. He explains in considerable detail that there are various cycles within cycles of endothermal and exothermal reactions which vary according to the position along the scale of emotions as well as the direction of motion (involutionary or evolutionary). It should be noted that as there are cycles within cycles, there are many places along the scale of emotions where both endothermal and exothermal reactions may occur simultaneously. This phenomena has indeed been observed on many occasions in Body Electronics.

Conclusion

THE STUDY OF BIOLOGICAL TRANSMUTATIONS OFFERS MANY FASCINATing insights into our understanding of health and healing, and it would be wise for each of us to consider it more closely. The following chapter further clarifies the process of healing by means of biological transmutations.

Chapter Twenty-Two

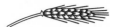

Back to Health:
Monopoles, Melanin, and Uncreation

*All forms of resistance build a wall of separateness which turns
life into a battlefield. . . . To walk through life without resistance
is to be free. . . .*

J. Krishnamurti

BIOLOGICAL TRANSMUTATIONS ARE ACTIVATED THROUGH THE PROPER
activity of monopoles. This is a part of the process of *uncreation* of
patterns of resistance held within the melanin-protein complex or
crystal. Let's see how this process works.

Inner Essence and Outer Manifestation

BEFORE ANY OUTER MANIFESTATION IN THE PHYSICAL UNIVERSE OCCURS,
there must first exist its corresponding counterpart which springs from
the inner essence. This inner essence does not exist in the physical universe,
and does not involve wavelength, frequency, or vibration as we normally
consider them. The inner essence is *still*. Consider: "Be still, and know that
I Am God." From this inner stillness or inner essence come the thought,
emotion, and word patterns which will eventually exist in time and space.
Through the exertion of desire and will these patterns spring into what we
know as reality which we term the outer manifestation. It must be fully

understood that all outer manifestation eventually arises from the inner essence.

The act of creation is fundamentally an act of faith. "Faith is the great prime motivating force behind any outer activity." Only through faith can the intelligence exercise will and desire. Or as Dr. Ray has also expressed it, "Faith can exist without Thought, but Thought can never exist without Faith."[1]

Thought, Word, and Emotion

BEHIND ANY OUTER MANIFESTATION LIES A COMBINATION OF THOUGHT, feeling, and spoken word, expressed as thought patterns, emotional patterns, and word patterns. From the inner essence, the outer manifestation is expressed or reflected simultaneously with the expression of will and desire acting upon the thought, emotion, and word patterns which originated in the inner essence. Before the thought, word, and emotion come into existence in the mental body in the outer manifestation, there must have existed the prototype in the inner essence. As Dr. Ray has expressed it, "Thought is the vehicle through which Faith expresses itself. Words give power to Thought which brings the creative action to manifestation in physical reality. Emotion in its various stages of consciousness and intensity moulds creative action into distinct and individual designs and manifestations."[2]

The thought pattern may be considered to be the sensory aspect of creation, that is, time, place, form, and event. The emotional pattern would be the associated feelings or emotions: enthusiasm, pain, anger, fear, grief, apathy, unconsciousness. The word patterns would be the associated verbal expressions or mental utterances. These three together comprise the composite pattern behind any outer manifestation. These three together remain in the inner essence until desire and will bring them into a pattern of duality which simultaneously becomes an inner and outer creation.

HOLDING PATTERN IN A CONTINUAL STATE OF CREATION

In order for a given composite pattern of thought, feeling, and spoken word to result in a corresponding outer manifestation, the combination of thought, word, and emotion must be held in a continual state of creation by the intelligence. This can be done in several different ways: consciously by choice or unconsciously through resistance. When done consciously, this is an act of will and desire. But even when the creation is held in place unconsciously through resistance, it was already there before it was resisted. We have each set many creations into existence. And in many cases we have then viewed our own creations with resistance or denial of our own responsibility for that which we have set in motion. This resistance traps our attention upon that which we resist, thus perpetuating the very thing we resist. As we enter into a state of resistance, we are no longer capable of seeing things as they really are. Rather, we see only in part, and that which we do see is distorted. Thus, resistance always contains a lie. For if we see things only in part and with distortion, then we do not really see the truth. "Truth is the knowledge of the way things are, the way things were, and the way things are to be." Only a state of unconditional love contains no lies, for in such a state, and only then can we see truly.

Faith, Will, and Desire

THROUGH FAITH AND THE ACTIVITY OF THE INTELLIGENCE, WHEREBY will and desire are exercised, the inner essence is reflected into outer manifestation in the physical universe. As Dr. Ray has expressed it, "Until desire and will are expressed, the thought, feeling and spoken word remain in the mental body. When the thought, feeling and spoken word remain in the mental body they are considered to be an informational field or a scalar wave."[3] And as amplified by Dr. Ray in unpublished writings:

> In any creation wherein there is resistance, as soon as the desire and will are withdrawn from the creation, the creation immediately or gradually goes into dissolution and returns to the void.
>
> There does indeed exist another level of duality wherein the mental body which exists within time and space has its prototype outside of time and space. It is the desire and will which when exercised cause that which is in the mental body outside of time and space in the inner essence to be manifested within time and space or the outer manifestation.[4]

Scalar Waves and Composite Waves

OUTSIDE OF TIME AND SPACE WE HAVE THE INNER ESSENCE. THAT WHICH is created in the inner essence outside of time and space can be considered to be an informational field or scalar wave. This informational field or scalar wave is not a vector, consisting of magnitude and direction; therefore, it exists outside of time and space, in the inner essence. When will and desire act upon this informational field in the inner essence, giving this scalar wave a vector quality of magnitude and direction, it then exists within time and space in what we can call the mental body. We now find that the outer is a reflection of the inner. It is through this reflection from the inner essence that the creative force is brought into time and space. Through will and desire the scalar waves from the inner essence are actually converted into a composite wave or morphogenetic field. The morphogenetic field or composite wave, which exists in time and space, in turn then determines the structure of physical matter. As Dr. Ray has expressed it: "The scalar wave is not a vector. The will and desire give it a vector quality which brings it into activity in time and space. A scalar wave is an indication of an informational field existing outside of time and space. It has not yet been brought into creation in the physical universe as we know it through the mechanism of desire and will."[5]

Again, the great prime motivating force behind any such activity is always faith. If we think of will and desire in mathematical terms with analogy to a vector, we might compare these two to the qualities of magnitude and direction.

Monopoles

IN ORDER TO UNDERSTAND HOW THE SCALAR WAVE OR INFORMATIONAL field is converted into the composite wave or morphogenetic field, or vice-versa, we must consider the existence of *monopoles*. Dr. Ray states:

In the human body, a monopole is a helix formation, a spiral of DNA like material composed of seven turns in a spiral. One spiral turns to the left surrounded by another spiral which turns to the right, thus comprising a monopole. The cytoplasm of the human cell has within it a sphere-like or rod-like material which we call mitochondria. Each healthy mitochondrion has a triple axis of monopoles, each having the capacity to become perpendicular to each other and each able to vary their axis slightly such as the triple axis found in a crystalline formation....it will vary in positioning according to its restrictions and limitations which are determined functionally and hereditarily by the melanin-protein complex.[6]

This monopole or spiral within a spiral is one continual strand.

FROM INNER TO OUTER AND FROM OUTER TO INNER

It is the monopoles that operate as the interface or converter between the reflection of the inner and the outer, converting scalar wave to composite wave and vice-versa. In converting the scalar waves into composite waves, they are involved in the process of creation, and in converting the composite waves back into scalar waves, are equally involved in the process of uncreation. The monopoles are essential both for sending and receiving information. As Dr. Ray states:

> When a wave frequency resonates within the monopole ... it converts the composite wave into a scalar wave (informational wave) which will then be interpreted by the intelligence. This is the receptive portion of the monopole(s). Please consider that if the triple axis of monopoles cannot adjust themselves to resonate with the energy pattern of the external stimulus there will be no conversion into an informational wave or scalar wave. Now, on the other hand, a scalar wave created by the intelligence and sent forth with desire and will shall be converted by the resonating monopole complex to a composite wave. The thought, feeling and spoken word are therefore combined with desire and will and the process of creation is underway. The composite wave is the result of the transmission activity of the monopoles working collectively together as a triple axis complex.[7]

It is the proper activity and function of the monopoles that triggers the biological transmutations which are experienced in part as endothermal and exothermal reactions. (See Chapter Twenty-One.) These endothermal and exothermal reactions have been widely experienced by many individuals, and have been observed to play a significant role in the regeneration of the physical body. They cannot take place without the proper activity of the monopoles. It should again be noted that the presence of sufficient hormones (as catalytic agents), enzymes, minerals, and other nutrients (nutrient saturation) are also necessary for these biological transmutations to take place. However, the proper activity and function of the monopoles can be hindered by the presence of the melanin-protein complex.

The Melanin-Protein Complex

THE *melanin-protein complex* HAS OFTEN BEEN DEPICTED AS AN ORGANIC computer chip. It displays semi-conductive properties, in much the same manner as a computer chip. "Melanin has been shown *in vitro* to have semi-conductive properties and to respond to photic, acoustic and electrical stimulation. The known semi-conductive properties of melanin include the ability to threshold and memory switch, photo-conductivity, and piezo-electric responses. Recently a significant correlation between pH changes and melanin's semiconduction properties has been discovered. Specifically, during the 'on' state, *in vitro* melanin develops a pH gradient proportional to the amount of the current times the duration of current. Reversing the current for an equal time cancels this pH gradient."[8]

Melanin is a molecule that appears to be present in virtually all life forms today, to have been present far back in time, and to become more concentrated in higher life forms, reaching its peak concentration in mankind. "Melanin is an ancient pigment which was present at the inception of 'life' and which appears to have a nearly ubiquitous distribution within and among living organisms. Melanin's long evolutionary history, its hormone-like transport throughout the entire body via the vascular system, the strategic location of neural-crest derived melanin in areas such as the autonomic and sensory ganglia and diffuse neuroendocrine loci, and increasing concentrations of neuromelanin in the brains of higher animals all point to a highly significant functional role."[9]

Melanin is found in the greatest concentration in some of the most metabolically active tissues. Much of it is located in the brain, and it can be related not just to physical functions, but to emotions and consciousness as well. "Most neuromelanin is located in the brain in a region that functions as a '*gate*' or '*filter*' system for all sensory input and all motor output, all emotional and motivational input and output, as well as a region that provides *conscious awareness* in general."[10]

Dr. Ray has suggested that our reactive mechanisms are self-perpetuating, and that the melanin-protein complex may be inherited. It is interesting to note that exactly how melanin is produced is not yet known, but it appears to be capable of manufacturing itself. "We suggest that neuromelanin is a self-organizing biopolymer which can organize as well as derive itself. The exact synthesis and structure of melanin remain unknown because of its resistance to analysis . . . a closer examination of its synthetic mechanisms suggests that (neuro)melanin may actually be capable of *self-synthesis*."[11]

Reactive mechanisms are highly varied, and the unconscious or reactive mind would seem to be quite unique to the individual. If the melanin-protein complex is indeed the physical storehouse of this reactive mind, it is interesting that it too is quite unique. "It is likely that each neuromelanin molecule (like each person's 'mind') is structurally and functionally *unique*. We may tentatively hypothesize that each individual's unique mental capacity (i.e. one's 'mind') is directly correlated with his/her unique melanin-monoamine configurations and interconnections."[12]

Existing scientific research distinguishes between the melanin found in the central nervous system (which includes the iris) and that found in the skin. To date there does not appear to be research to support the concept that the melanin found in the skin is related to the neuromelanin or that found in the central nervous system. "One's neuromelanin does not correlate clearly with one's skin melanin, in either known formative mechanisms, gross amounts, or major functions. While the internal molecular arrangements and diffuse interconnections of one's neuromelanin-monoamine network may vary uniquely with each individual, such variations in one's neuromelanin do not correlate (in any obvious way) with one's skin color (whether white, red, yellow, black, brown, or albino)."[13]

It has been observed by many people involved in Body Electronics that some of the melanin (brown) pigmentation in the iris of the eye will gradually or even suddenly disappear upon the release of various reactive mechanisms or resistance patterns. In other words, the reduction in iris melanin seems to be directly related to consciousness change on the part of the individual. There have been a large number of people throughout the world over the last few decades who have personally observed this phenomena in themselves as well as others. This would suggest that the melanin in the iris might be considered *neuromelanin,* or at least closely related to it. It is sensible to relate the iris to the central nervous system if we consider that "the eye develops in the embryo as a protrusion of the forebrain."[14] This would also support the thesis that the melanin functions as a storehouse for our reactive patterns. We do not at this time have any way of ascertaining whether there is also an internal reduction of the melanin in the body that might occur simultaneously with the reduction in iris melanin, although this might be inferred. Perhaps at some future time we may be able to investigate this more directly. There is certainly room for much further study in this area.

What Melanin Does

MELANIN RECEIVES AND RESPONDS TO MANY STIMULI

The melanin-protein complex functions as a sort of *black box,* whereby various stimuli are received and various responses are then accordingly sent out. There is an impressive amount of scientific research to support this theory. It has been shown, for example, that melanin responds directly to many types of external stimuli, including the entire spectrum of visible light (as well as that above and below this spectrum), electromagnetic fields, and sound or acoustic fields, as well. "Melanin is *black* because its absorbed light is not re-radiated, but is instead captured and converted into rotational and vibrational energy (i.e. heat). The relatively 'featureless' spectrum of melanin, from the far ultraviolet spectrum through the visible and into the infra-red spectrum, means that such photon capture is available for any photon wavelength (and energy) between these spectral limits. Hence, melanin can be thought of as 'black' over a larger range than just the visible spectrum. Melanin responds with conductivity changes to *electric* and *acoustic* fields as well as direct *photic* stimulation...processing all three sources of energy input."[15] Thus melanin can be seen to respond directly to light, sound, and electromagnetic fields. Melanin may well respond to many other types of stimuli as well, including conceivably all external stimuli. For example, melanin "exhibits extraordinary binding of aromatic and lipid-soluble compounds,"[16] which suggests that it may respond to olfactory stimuli (or smell) also.

Melanin Can Regulate Numerous Processes

Having established that melanin responds to a broad range of external stimuli, we might consider how this information may then trigger various responses. According to Barr et al., melanin is capable of regulating a staggering array of physiological processes, having the potential both to receive diverse stimuli and then to trigger a broad range of responses:

> Melanin ... functions as the major organizational molecule in living systems. Melanin is depicted as an organizational "trigger" capable of using established properties such as photon-(electron)-phonon conversions, free radical-redox mechanisms, ion exchange mechanisms, and semiconductive capabilities to direct energy to strategic molecular systems and sensitive hierarchies of protein enzyme cascades. Melanin is held capable of regulating a wide range of molecular interactions and metabolic processes primarily through its effective control of diverse covalent modifications.[17]

Melanin seems also to influence physiological function in much the same manner as hormones, that is via the blood, and even a small quantity of melanin can have a significant effect.[18] Readers are referred to the work of Barr and his colleagues, which provides even more detail about the characteristics and functions of melanin.[19]

How Melanin-Protein Complex Interferes with Monopoles

WE MUST NOW CONSIDER HOW THE MELANIN-PROTEIN COMPLEX MAY interfere with the activity of the monopoles. As stated above, when the monopoles are properly functioning, they are able to convert scalar waves to composite waves and vice-versa. However, in the presence of the melanin-protein complex, this normal conversion process does not happen. Rather, the information that would normally be received by the monopoles is intercepted by the melanin-protein complex, the predetermined response is set in motion, and the monopoles are never activated. The monopoles can never be activated fully as long as the corresponding melanin-protein complex is present. This predetermined response can be understood from the standpoint of stimulus-response mechanisms, wherein a given stimulus will trigger the melanin-protein complex to bring about a certain response. As Dr. Ray states:

> The monopole fields in a healthy, normal body are found in triplicate, each axis basically perpendicular to each other with some variation including opportunity for appropriate flexibility. The monopoles in coordination are then capable of receiving information in the form of wavelength and amplitude as part of the electromagnetic spectrum and then are capable of converting the incoming information to scalar waves which then can be interpreted by the intelligence on the mental body level outside of time and space. One must then understand that the function of incoming information will be determined by the presence or lack of presence of the melanin-protein complex which determines the stimulus-response mechanism based on incoming information which we will call sensory experience. In other words, if there does exist the melanin-protein complex, then any sensory information may be converted immediately to a preprogrammed response to the given stimuli as determined by the structure of the organic computer chip of melanin-protein.[20]

In this manner, not only are the monopoles never activated, but the intelligence of the individual never becomes aware of the sensory information. Thus, the individual's response simply perpetuates the stimulus-response mechanism involved. Without awareness, no free choice exists.

Perception and Reality Altered

IN SCRIPTURE IT IS STATED THAT "WE SEE THROUGH A GLASS DARKLY." THIS inability to see reality clearly is directly related to the melanin-protein complex, which may be thought of as an organic computer chip. The melanin-protein complexes throughout the physical body represent all of the suppressed or resisted patterns of thought, feeling and spoken word. Thus, the melanin-protein complex may be viewed as a storehouse of reactive patterns. These reactive patterns might include those on the Hereditary Level, the Soul Level, and the Entity Level as well as the various resisted traumas of this particular lifetime. All of these and perhaps more can be encoded in the melanin-protein complex. As stated above, the presence of the melanin-protein complex interferes with the activity of the monopoles, and prevents the intelligence from directly receiving information.

In addition to altering the way in which we see things, the melanin-protein complex has a tremendous effect upon what we actually create in our lives. For the reactions which are locked within the melanin-protein complex (or crystal) act like a beacon, whereby these stored suppressed energy patterns are continually emitted and so are held in a continual state of creation. Thus, by the Law of Attraction, the outer universe simply reflects back to us the very resistances that are being constantly emitted from the melanin-protein complexes. "What we resist, persists."

The melanin-protein complex is considered to be virtually indestructible. According to Dr. Ray, it is only broken down by a certain hormonal substance secreted by the pineal gland. As the pineal gland resonates to the emotion of enthusiasm, this hormonal substance that transmutes the melanin-protein complex could be considered to be dependent upon enthusiasm or unconditional love. Thus, it is only through love or nonresistance that the melanin-protein complex may be broken down. Melanin is not only extremely stable, but as a result of this stability, its exact composition and origin remain elusive.[21]

Process of Creation

MONOPOLES SERVE AS AN INTERFACE BETWEEN SCALAR WAVES AND composite or sine waves. According to Dr. Ray, this process also involves the activity of the corpus callosum. He states that the corpus callosum, which interconnects the two hemispheres of the brain, functions like a mobius strip and plays an integral role in this process. Through the activity of will and desire, the scalar waves are converted into composite waves. This is part of the process of creation.[22]

For the sake of simplicity, all such wave forms within time and space may be considered to be in the form of sine waves. There is a branch of mathematics known as Fourier analysis which shows that all wave forms, no matter how complex, can be reduced to the sum of a series of sine waves of varying amplitudes, frequencies, and phases. Thus, all vibration is reducible to sine waves. The mathematical equations to do this are known as *Fourier transforms,* after their inventor Jean Fourier. They were first formulated in the eighteenth century. In the 1940s, Dennis Gabor used these Fourier transforms to come up with the theories necessary to develop the hologram. Gabor was eventually awarded a Nobel Prize for this work.[23] When the scalar wave is converted into a composite or sine wave, and this sine wave is held in a state of creation, then a corresponding outer manifestation will arise and persist. It will persist so long as the sine wave continues to be held in a state of creation, whether consciously or unconsciously. When done consciously, we would refer to this as the *vibration of creation.* Once this is denied or resisted, it may then be locked in unconsciously, through resistance.

Process of Uncreation

THROUGH BODY ELECTRONICS, OTHER HEALING, OR AWARENESS WORK, the composite waves or sine waves are released from the melanin-protein complex, which allows the stored patterns of thought, word, and emotion to be considered so that they may then be transmuted. To the extent that we are able to lovingly and willingly re-experience these patterns, the sine waves are able to be received through the monopoles. When operating properly, the monopoles and the corpus callosum would appear capable of taking each sine wave and recreating it exactly 180 degrees out of phase. From a mathematical point of view, two equal sine waves that are 180 degrees out of phase will cancel each other out. That is, the sum of two such waves is everywhere zero. Thus, through the activity of the monopoles and the corpus callosum, these sine waves which had previously been held in a state of creation now disappear or return to the void. Thus, we have the process of uncreation.

It is frequently observed that when an individual is able to experience this release and transmutation of stored suppressed patterns of thought, word, and emotion, they often experience a very fine vibration in the body. This may be referred to as the *vibration of regeneration*. As this is essentially the healing crisis sparked by release of the original resisted vibration of creation, we might also term it as the *vibration of uncreation*. For example, when an individual's scar disappears in such a fashion, this may be understood as a process of uncreation rather than a process of creation. When the area that formerly had the scar returns to its scarless state, this scarless state has not been created, for it truly was always there. What has happened, rather, is that the scar has been uncreated, thus allowing the original underlying state to reappear. Perfection is everpresent; it is only the overlays of our human creation (which are themselves also perfect) that obscures perfection from our view.

The Overhead Projector Revisited

TO EXPLAIN THIS PROCESS OF UNCREATION WE CAN GO BACK TO THE analogy of an overhead projector and how it projects an image upon a screen, which we first presented in Chapter One. When a transparency with a drawing on it is placed upon the overhead projector, an image of this transparency is thereby projected onto the screen. We might consider this image on the screen to be akin to the physical body, while the transparency whose image is projected onto the screen is like the morphogenetic field or composite wave that determines the structure of the physical body. Imagine that we place an initial transparency upon the projector depicting a body without any imperfection. Upon the screen we would see then the image of a perfect body. Imagine that we leave this initial transparency upon the projector but place various other transparencies on top of this initial transparency, each one containing one or more imperfections. These transparencies would then represent sequential distortions to the morphogenetic field, the product of resistance. As each successive transparency was placed upon the stack, the image projected upon the screen would take on more and more imperfections. Similarly, as our resistance accumulates, our own body becomes more and more imperfect. Although the underlying transparency with no imperfections was still there at the bottom of the stack, as more and more transparencies containing imperfections were placed on top of it, this would become less and less apparent.

Now consider what would happen if we removed one or more of these transparencies. The image on the screen would change immediately. Any imperfections that were the result of a given transparency projected onto the screen would disappear from the screen as soon as that transparency was removed from the stack. And as this was done, the initial transparency of perfection would become more and more apparent in the image projected upon the screen, even though it had been there at the bottom of the stack the whole time.

In a similar fashion, if we release the resistance that has been reflected in a particular scar, that scar will disappear. We need not create the scarless area any more than we need to redo the initial transparency, for both have always been there. Just as we need only remove the distorted transparency to allow the underlying pattern of perfection to be more apparent upon the screen, so all we need to do is uncreate the resistance that lies behind the scar.

Free within the Hologram

EACH OF US, AS AN INTELLIGENCE WITHIN A PHYSICAL BODY, IS CONstantly exposed to a vast sea of information or vibration. Resounding throughout the physical universe there are a multitude of frequencies or vibrations. We may also consider these to be thought patterns (or sensory information), word patterns, and emotional patterns. The entire physical universe is a hologram: within each part of the whole is contained all the information of the whole. Thus, each of us, wherever and whenever we may be, is ultimately exposed to all the information that is. Yet it appears that in general only a tiny portion of this vast sea of information or vibration ever reaches the conscious mind. Furthermore, much of what we appear to be aware of is in reality a distortion.

If our monopoles were fully functioning, with no interference from the melanin-protein complex, our ability to receive and respond to this vast sea of information would increase tremendously. The vibrations that resound throughout the cosmos would be observed, then received through the monopoles, then recreated 180 degrees out of phase, then released. There would be no residue, no resistance left behind to obscure our ability to receive. Each creation would simply disappear back into the void immediately when the attention was withdrawn from it. Only when this creation was resisted or denied would there be this "residue." On a moment to moment basis we would be able to observe each outer manifestation and immediately see the reflection of the inner essence within it—thus perfect receptivity. Simultaneously, we would be able to convert each reflected inner essence into the corresponding outer manifestation in an ongoing process of creation without resistance. We would be simultaneously yin and yang, with no resistance to either. Such a state would persist unless we allowed ourselves to enter into resistance in the first place.

Bound within the Hologram

YET FOR EACH OF US NOW, THERE IS THE REALITY OF THE MELANIN-protein complex. We exist within a vast sea of information, which may also be considered "light" in the sense that "light is the law that governs all things." In an area where we have resistance, we will have encoded within the melanin-protein complex various patterns of thought, word, and emotion. These patterns will each exist at specific frequencies. Exposure to these same frequencies from the universe around us will cause the melanin-protein complex to resonate or activate it to send out the preprogrammed response to the stimulus received. Thus, we have the stimulus-response mechanism. If the monopoles are never activated, the information never makes it to the conscious mind. Rather, it is intercepted by the melanin-protein complex, which triggers the stimulus-response mechanism. Thus, in an area of resistance, encoded within the melanin-protein complex, we will have an inability to receive or be yin. (Please consider also that these frequencies coming from the universe around us are in reality a reflection of the resistance patterns already within us). In an area of resistance we will be unable to receive information consciously, for without the activation of the monopoles, we will remain incapable of converting the outer manifestations (or manifestation) into the reflection of the inner essence. Let us also consider our ability to create or be yang. We will be unable to visualize in an area where we are simultaneously resisting. That is, in an area of resistance, we will not be able to convert the reflection of the inner essence into the outer manifestation, for due to the resistance in this area we will not be able to view the reflected inner essence clearly in the first place. Thus, we will have a lack of creativity as well as a lack of receptivity within the given area as long as this information remains locked within the melanin-protein complex.

If through healing work or awareness practices we are able to receive a given area of resistance locked within the melanin-protein complex, and if we are able to recreate this information as it is received, then it may be transmuted and released. In so doing, we restore to ourselves within this given area of resistance the ability to receive as well as the ability to create. Clearly for each of us, there are numerous areas of resistance. As each of these is released, we thereby restore to ourselves a degree of freedom.

Melanin–Protein Complex an Effect of Our Resistance

A FINAL NOTE: WE HAVE RELATED THE PRESENCE OF THE MELANIN-PROTEIN complex to the resistances of the human mind, and we have considered how the melanin-protein complex will interfere with the activity of the monopoles. It must be clearly understood that the melanin-protein complex is in no way the cause of our resistances, but rather it is an effect of our resistances. The cause of our resistances lies outside of time and space within ourselves. The melanin-protein complex is simply the storehouse of this information within the physical body. Some may view it as a hindrance to spiritual progression, due to its ability to short-circuit our awareness. Yet there is another perspective: if we are indeed to progress spiritually, then surely we must view (with unconditional love and unconditional forgiveness) and release these patterns of resistance within ourselves. And none of us can truly see ourselves clearly enough to know exactly what we need to look at. Yet by simply applying various levels of law, the melanin-protein complexes throughout the physical body will gradually yield up the information encoded within them. This gives us an opportunity to release these resistances as they are brought to view. But as this release of information occurs, will this automatically help to free us from the snares of our own resistances, or may we still remain enmeshed in darkness? Dr. Ray has noted that "if we focus on the melanin-protein complex, we focus on untruth—hopefully we will be able to see the truth under the untruth. The focus on the truth will lead us back to the cause. One cannot comprehend truth by focusing upon untruth. This is why the scientist who focuses upon matter will miss the boat, as our focus should be on God—especially the attributes of God."[24]

Encompassment and Exclusion

IF WE ARE TO RELEASE OURSELVES FROM THE SHACKLES OF OUR OWN RESISTANCES and judgments, we must learn to focus our attention to the encompassment of truth, rather than to the exclusion of truth. This concept of focusing our attention to the encompassment rather than exclusion is difficult for the linear mind to grasp. It may help to understand that it is possible on the one hand to focus attention upon something to the exclusion of all else. This type of activity most certainly has its proper time, place, and purpose. Yet, on the other hand, we can also learn to discipline the mind such that we become gradiently more and more capable of focusing our attention upon something while encompassing all else. As we focus attention in this manner, we become not only more aware of that which we are focusing upon, but simultaneously more aware of all else, for our attention is both focused and diffused. This can only happen as we move beyond linear thinking and into holographic thinking. It should be noted, so that there is no misunderstanding, that holographic thinking is also a necessity in order to master focusing our attention upon something to the exclusion of all else. Both activities, focusing with exclusion as well as with encompassment, are equally necessary to master on the pathway to perfection. If our attention remains focused only upon the resistance or darkness, then surely we will continue to perpetuate this resistance or darkness. We must, therefore, learn to focus our attention in such a manner that we may encompass not merely the resistance or untruth, but the truth behind it simultaneously. We must encompass the truth behind the untruth. Resistance traps our attention upon that which we resist. Therefore, as our resistances are gradiently released through obedience to law, we must encompass them with love and forgiveness; otherwise, we merely compound these resistances with more resistance. Untruth must be encompassed with truth, resistance with love, and darkness with light. If these principles can be applied without deviation, then we can indeed free ourselves from the shackles of our own resistance.

Chapter Twenty-Three

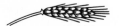

The Possibility of Healing

What lies behind us and what lies before us are tiny matters compared to what lies within us.

Oliver Wendell Holmes

HEALTH IS INDEED A PRECIOUS GIFT, AND TO REGAIN OR MAINTAIN our health, we should understand as many of the factors involved as possible. This book, based on my own experience and research, presents many of these in such a manner that they may be practically applied.

It is worthwhile to be reminded of the possibility of healing. Our bodies are marvelous, really, and given the chance they can heal. But all too often, through our fixation upon disease and deterioration, we forget the enormous capacity that we all possess for healing and regeneration. If we wish to access and maximize this capacity, we might consider just what are the principles that govern health and healing, for then we can be in a position to apply them to our advantage.

In this book, many levels of principle or law have been presented: for example, various laws pertaining to the physical body—nutrition, exercise, sleep, and so forth. Laws pertaining to the emotional body have been presented, and many others as well. In order to explain some of these other laws, various models or analogies have proven useful.

If we wish to regain or maintain our health, it may be necessary for us to understand and apply many different levels of law, for these levels will interact with one another. We might consider progressively higher and lower levels of law. If we consider two levels of law, the relatively higher level could be considered a relative level of light in comparison to the relatively lower level of law which would be a relative level of darkness. It is said that "light comprehends darkness, but darkness does not comprehend light." In a similar fashion, the lower level of law can be comprehended or understood from the higher level, whereas the higher level cannot be understood from the lower level. In fact, the higher level of law will often appear to be quite a contradiction from the vantage point of the lower law. This principle is exemplified in the following Zen story. Two monks, a senior monk and a young novice, had taken strict vows in many areas of life. One of these was a vow of celibacy, no contact with women. As they were travelling one day, they came to a river in flood. A beautiful prostitute was afraid to cross the river, so the elder monk carried her over on his back, at which point she went one way and the monks went another. The novice monk was greatly confused by his mentor's behavior, for it was a clear violation of their vows. He walked along in silence for several hours, wrestling with his own increasing confusion and annoyance at the inappropriate behavior of the other monk. Finally, unable to contain himself a moment longer, he angrily confronted his mentor, demanding to know how he could behave in such a fashion. The elder monk responded simply, "I left her by the side of the river. Why do you still carry her on your back?"

In the same way, higher laws are often hard to comprehend from the vantage point of a lower law. Nutrition is a certain level of law, for example. According to nutritional laws we might eat in certain ways, and refrain from certain foods. For example, we do not eat pork. Yet perhaps we are travelling in another part of the world with different customs than our own, and invited into somebody's home for a meal, which might be a great honor. If pork is served and we eat the pork, we break one level of law. Yet, if under these circumstances we refuse to eat it, other levels of law might be broken. If we must choose between several levels of law which conflict, it is best to obey the higher law. So to honor the hospitality of our host, we might eat the pork. When we break a lower law to obey a higher law, we are not completely exempt from the consequences of the broken lower law. (In this example, we still have to digest the pork.) But the consequences of breaking a lower law are mitigated to a great extent if we break it in order to obey a higher law.

There is another aspect of these levels of law. In general, a higher level of law is at once harder to live by yet simpler to express. In other words, the law is briefer yet more difficult. The laws of nutrition, for example, are numerous and lengthy, as lower laws generally are. Yet take a much higher set of principles such as "Love thy neighbor as thyself" and "Love the Lord thy God with all thy heart, might, mind and strength." This is certainly easier to express than the laws of nutrition, and yet at the same time a far greater challenge to obey.

If we consider the many laws or principles presented in this book, for many the best approach may simply be to start with the basics and gradually incorporate higher levels as deemed appropriate. Nutrition and various other principles pertaining to the physical body are a good starting point. When we do a reasonable job of meeting our body's needs for nutrition, sleep, exercise and so forth, we place ourselves in a position where it is more likely that we will be successful in regaining or maintaining our health. Yet there are many other factors involved as well. If we wish to be healthy, it is not enough to take care of the body alone: we must also take care of the heart and the mind, for in the end it is simply not possible to be healthy on any one level without also being healthy on all other levels as well. Each of the many levels of our existence—physical, emotional, mental, spiritual—exerts a powerful influence upon all others, as has been expressed by countless teachers through the ages.

Whatever is "true" in this book is neither new nor unique, for what is true now has always been true and will continue to be true. The intention of this book is to help express these truths in such a manner that they may be received and applied. For only through its application can truth be of any value to us. Truth does not come from any of us, but merely through us, for truth can come only from God. Whenever any of us expresses truth, this expression comes from the God within us, which is the same God that is within all life. And whenever any of us is able to receive truth, this receiving is also by God, or by the God within us. Truth, then, comes from God and is received back unto God. And hopefully somewhere along the way, it is acted upon, at which point we are God in action.

Much more could be written on most of the topics presented, but let this suffice for now. May each of you who read these words be blessed always by all that life has to offer.

Appendix One

On Enzymes:
Condensed Summary and Conclusions

by Edward Howell
(reprinted with permission from *Food Enzymes
for Health and Longevity* by Dr. Edward Howell)

1. Enzymes are normal constituents of all cellular matter.

2. Enzymes are far more thermo-labile than vitamins.

3. All wild animals live exclusively on raw food including a full quota of enzymes. So did an early type of man.

4. Modern cookery destroys more enzymes than in primitive times.

5. The enzyme complex is a biological entity composed of corporeal and incorporeal fractions. Enzymes and catalysts do not display all features in common.

6. Behavior of the dead intestine as regards permeability to enzymes is no criterion as to absorbability of enzymes by the living intestine.

7. Extensive absorbability of enzymes is proved by the following evidence:

   (a) Yeast cells, bacteria, and unsplit proteins are absorbed.

   (b) Orally administered enzymes are recovered in the urine.

   (c) Large quantities of enzymes are secreted into the gastrointestinal tract, but only a small amount is recovered in the feces.

   (d) Loss of the pancreatic enzymes by experimental or human pancreatic fistula is rapidly fatal, invalidating the supposition that extensive fecal secretion of enzymes is tolerable. On the contrary, death is not inevitable in experimental or human biliary fistula where no enzymes are sacrificed.

(e) Oral administration of enzyme extracts to human patients results in improvement in systemic disease.

8. Enzymes in raw foods take priority in digestion over secreted enzymes. Exogenous or food enzymes become active the moment the cell wall is ruptured by mastication and before endogenous or secreted enzymes have made an appearance.

9. Endogenous enzymes are secreted in response to specific stimuli by starch, protein, fat, etc.

10. Metabolism and digestion exact a toll resulting in a depreciation of the enzyme potential and the excretion of "spent" enzymes in the urine, feces, and sweat.

11. If some digestion is performed by exogenous enzymes, the stimulus to secretion of endogenous enzymes is less intense. Consequently, there is less drain on the enzyme potential.

12. While the enzyme value of raw food is small, the sum total of enzymes available in a raw food diet consumed in a period of years far exceeds both the enzyme value of digestive secretions and the whole body.

13. Experimental evidence indicates that food enzymes do a measurable amount of digestive work in the test tube and in the organs of living animals.

14. The technique of vitamin essaying fails to indicate that a diet which may be effective in maintaining health in the early life of the experimental animal will be equally effective in conserving health and preventing disease in the period of middle life and old age.

15. The pancreas of herbivorous animals is relatively only about one half as large as that of American adults and their salivary glands do not secrete enzymes, while human salivary glands are highly active. The fact that herbivorous animals using enzyme-containing raw food can digest much carbohydrate food with only a small pancreas and no

salivary enzymes, while man, on a heat treated enzyme deficient diet requires a large pancreas and active saliva, offers convincing testimony on the utility of food enzymes.

16. The pancreas of Orientals on a heat-treated, high carbohydrate rice-type diet is relatively about 50 per cent heavier than that of Americans, and their salivary glands are also heavier. This hypertrophy of the pancreas and salivary glands in response to higher intake of enzyme-deficient carbohydrate foods has been confirmed experimentally in animals.

17. Increase in metabolic activity such as muscular work, pregnancy, fever, and increased food intake is paralleled by rise in the enzyme content of blood serum and increased loss of "spent" enzymes in the urine.

18. Observed subnormality in enzyme content of body fluids in disease cannot ultimately be relegated to failure of pancreatic function since it is traceable to a fundamental default, i.e. failure of a heat-treated diet to supply the enzymes necessary to maintain the enzyme potential of the tissues.

19. The white blood cell is endowed with a greater diversity of enzymes than other cells. The digestive action characteristic of phagocytosis is thereby better defined.

20. The protective value of fever is illustrated by the fact that bacterial activity decreases with increase in fever while enzyme activity actually increases with increase in fever.

21. Available evidence is interpreted as signifying that the animal organism can sequester and utilize the enzymes of bacteria when food enzymes are not available. The innocuousness of such behavior is open to serious doubt.

22. Of ten species of animals examined, human blood serum contained the smallest quantity of enzymes and yet the excretion of "spent" enzymes in human urine was about as great as in the animal urine. Considered together with other evidence, there is an implication that the discrepancy is related to man's ingestion of a heat-treated enzyme-deficient diet.

23. Maintenance of a normal blood serum enzyme level after experimental pancreatectomy supported by insulin medication emphasizes the subordinate role played by the pancreas and other enzyme secreting organs as assembling, conditioning, and disbursing organs and points to the tissues as the ultimate reservoir of enzymes.

24. The synonymity of the subtle power operating in the organism with the vital factor of the enzyme complex, enzyme energy, enzyme activity, metabolic activity, vital energy, nerve force, resistance, and life force is rendered probable by the nature of the evidence. Enzymes, being capable of exact measurement, are the true yardstick of vitality.

25. That the enzyme potential, vitality, and "resistance" are one and the same entity is emphasized by the following evidence. The length of life is held to be inversely proportional to the rate of energy expenditure.

(a) Influence of temperature.

(1) Higher temperature increases the speed of enzyme reactions in vitro but brings about a correspondingly speedier inactivation of the enzyme.

(2) The higher temperature of fever causes extra loss of enzymes in the urine.

(3) Higher temperature increases the tempo of life in fruit flies and water fleas, measured by quickened movement, but also shortens the life span correspondingly.

(4) Evidence of approaching senility such as loss of hair, weight loss, decrease in length, wrinkling of the skin, sluggish movements, and failure of reproduction can be made to appear sooner or later in life depending on the rate of energy dissipation which is influenced by the temperature.

(5) Higher temperature increases frequency of the heart beat and CO_2 production in cold-blooded animals.

(6) Higher temperature increases the velocity of germination of seeds.

(7) Higher temperature increases the velocity of incubation of eggs.

(b) Influence of food.

(1) The amount of food consumption regulates the quantity of enzymes engaged and consequently determines the daily urinary toll. The amount of enzymes the organism must sacrifice daily through the urine is influenced by the meals, there being a regular cycle of rise and fall with an immediate rise after a meal.

(2) Greater food consumption markedly decreases the life span in fruit flies, water fleas, rats, and trout.

(3) Greater quantity or variety of food increases the height of college students and increases the weight of albino rats. More organic defects appear in school children with the better physical development.

(c) Influence of heredity.

(1) A long-living type of fruit fly has a considerably higher content of esterase and protease than a short-living type.

(2) The hereditary influence in human longevity is generally recognized.

(d) Both enzyme content and viability in seeds diminish with age.

(e) Enzyme content of the whole macerated bodies of fruit flies, grasshoppers, beetles, and rats is greatest in early maturity, decreasing to a minimum in old age.

(f) Enzyme content of human saliva and urine becomes markedly decreased in old age.

(g) Enzyme content of body fluids is diminished in many diseases.

(h) Basal metabolism decreases in old age.

(i) There is incompatibility between maximum growth and physical development on the one hand, and maximum length of life, good health, and freedom from physical defects on the other.

(j) Changes in the chemical composition of the tissues in disease are similar to the changes occurring in old age.

26. Jungle animals are free from degenerative disease. The formerly high mortality and morbidity in zoo animals has taken a steep downward turn with the advent of the raw food diet.

27. Changes in weight of organs occasioned by disease are accompanied by compensatory weight alterations of all of the organs and the development of related symptomatic phenomena.

28. The appearance of disease in long-term, vitamin-supplemented diet experiments utilizing heat-treated food presages the need of the organism for all food constituents, including food enzymes.

29. Differences in the health, physical condition, and life span between animals maintained on a heat-treated, vitamin-supplemented diet, and animals maintained on a raw, unheated diet can only be ascribed to extremely heat-labile factors of which enzymes are the outstanding representatives.

30. There is a striking contrast between cooking tribes, such as the primitive American Indian, requiring a comprehensive materia medica and the raw diet consuming Eskimo with no medicines or apparent need for them.

31. The legendary longevity of Bulgarian peasants, ascribed by Metchnikoff to innocuous intestinal bacteria, can be more satisfactorily explained on the basis of the enzymes contained in the predominantly raw diet of dairy products.

32. Discrepancies between breast-fed and bottle-fed babies in mortality and morbidity, and incidence of caries and the differences in hemoglobin content and bone content of calcium and phosphorous of rats fed on raw or pasteurized milk can be considerably ascribed to the moderate quantities of several enzymes contained in raw milk but which are almost completely lacking in pasteurized milk.

33. The high health standards of the primitive isolated Eskimo contrasted with the soaring morbidity of the modernized Eskimo offers an unparalleled example of the utility of enzymes in the food supply. The diet of the primitive Eskimo contains large quantities of whole fish including all of the enzymes of gastric juice, pancreatic juice, and intestinal

juice; liver and stomach contents of animals including gastric juice and its enzymes; and great amounts of raw meat. The remarkable absence of ketosis on a diet high in protein and fat and low in carbohydrate is probably related to the ingestion of enzymes with the food including lipase in seal fat.

34. The therapeutic efficacy of several types of raw food diet has been established and its unique value found to reside in its enzyme content.

35. Universal craving for salt on a heat-treated diet is thought to be actuated by the necessity for increased enzyme activity which is stimulated by salt. A possible obnoxious influence of salt ingestion is indicated by the fact that on a raw food saltless diet the urinary elimination of chlorides is very low while the blood chlorides remain exceptionally high.

36. The hypoglycemic or hypoglycosuric action of enzymes has been demonstrated by oral or intravenous administration of enzyme preparations, by consumption of enzyme-containing raw foods, and by increasing the serum-enzyme level through experimental pancreatic or salivary duct ligation.

37. Successful enzyme therapy of a number of ailments has been reported. Orally administered, enzymes perform efficiently in the digestive tract and display considerable digestive activity even in the presence of a normal concentration of endogenous enzymes.

Biological Transmutations

SOME ELEMENTS INVOLVED IN BIOLOGICAL TRANSMUTATIONS:

Symbol	Atomic Number	Element
H	1	Hydrogen
Li	3	Lithium
C	6	Carbon
N	7	Nitrogen
O	8	Oxygen
F	9	Fluorine
Na	11	Sodium
Mg	12	Magnesium
Al	13	Aluminum
Si	14	Silicon
P	15	Phosphorous
S	16	Sulfur
Cl	17	Chlorine
K	19	Potassium
Ca	20	Calcium
Mn	25	Manganese
Fe	26	Iron

TRANSMUTATIONS INVOLVING POTASSIUM (K)

- Na + O >> K
- Ca – H >> K
- K + H >> Ca
- Ca >> K + H

TRANSMUTATIONS INVOLVING MAGNESIUM (Mg)

- Mg + O >> Ca
- Na + H >> Mg
- Mg + Li >> P
- P – Li >> Mg

TRANSMUTATIONS INVOLVING CALCIUM (Ca)

- Ca – H >> K
- K + H >> Ca
- Ca >> K + H
- Mg + O >> Ca
- Si + C >> Ca

TRANSMUTATIONS INVOLVING SILICON (Si)

- Si + C >> Ca
- Cl >> C + Na >> C + (Li + O) >> 2N + Li >> Si + Li

TRANSMUTATIONS INVOLVING SODIUM (Na)

- Na + O >> K
- Na + H >> Mg
- Na >> Li + O
- Na – O >> Li
- Cl >> C + Na >> C + (Li + O) >> 2N + Li >> Si + Li

TRANSMUTATIONS INVOLVING ALUMINIUM (Al)

- Al + H >> Si

TRANSMUTATIONS INVOLVING PHOSPHOROUS (P)

- Mg + Li >> P
- P + H >> S
- P >> C + F
- P – Li >> Mg

TRANSMUTATIONS INVOLVING CHLORINE (Cl)

- N+ C >> Cl
- Cl >> C + Na >> C + (Li + O) >> 2N + Li >> Si + Li
- Cl – O >> F

TRANSMUTATIONS INVOLVING NITROGEN (N)

- 2N >> C + O or CO
- C + O >> 2N
- N+ C >> Cl

TRANSMUTATIONS INVOLVING MANGANESE (Mn)

- Fe – H >> Mn

TRANSMUTATIONS INVOLVING IRON (Fe)

- Fe – H >> Mn

TRANSMUTATIONS INVOLVING SULFUR (S)

- 2O >> S

TRANSMUTATIONS INVOLVING OXYGEN (O)

- Na + O >> K
- 2N >> C + O or CO
- Mg + O >> Ca
- Na >> Li + O
- Cl – O >> F
- Na – O >> Li
- C + O >> 2N
- 2O >> S
- Cl >> C + Na >> C + (Li + O) >> 2N + Li >> Si + Li
- Cl – O >> F

Transmutations involving
CARBON (C)

- $2N \gg C + O$ or CO
- $Si + C \gg Ca$
- $P \gg C + F$
- $C + O \gg 2N$
- $N + C \gg Cl$
- $Cl \gg C + Na \gg C + (Li + O)$
  $\gg 2N + Li \gg Si + Li$
- $C + Li \gg F$

Transmutations involving
LITHIUM (Lɪ)

- $Na \gg Li + O$
- $Mg + Li \gg P$
- $P - Li \gg Mg$
- $Na - O \gg Li$
- $Cl \gg C + Na \gg C + (Li + O)$
  $\gg 2N + Li \gg Si + Li$
- $C + Li \gg F$

Transmutations involving
FLUORINE (F)

- $P \gg C + F$
- $Cl - O \gg F$
- $Cl - O \gg F$
- $C + Li \gg F$

Transmutations involving
HYDROGEN (H)

- $Ca - H \gg K$
- $K + H \gg Ca$
- $Ca \gg K + H$
- $Na + H \gg Mg$
- $Al + H \gg Si$
- $P + H \gg S$
- $Fe - H \gg Mn$

Chapter Notes

PART ONE: HEALTH AND HEALING

CHAPTER 2: A BASIC MODEL TO CONSIDER

1. This particular scale was introduced to me by Dr. John Ray. It is closely modeled upon, in fact virtually identical to, a scale originally presented by L. Ron Hubbard in Scientology. Some say the scale was developed by Hubbard; others say he adapted it from an old Tibetan text or elsewhere. Regardless of its origin, I have found it to be an extremely useful tool for understanding self and others.

2. It must be stressed that the kundalini experience as we rise through the level of pain involves an intensely physical component which can best be described as the experience of burning, searing pain in the physical body from the inside out. Any who have experienced this will note that it is unforgettable. If we are not sure we have experienced it, chances are we have not, for its intensity is beyond words. It is often accompanied by dramatic, profound and apparently miraculous changes in the structure of the physical body such as spines straightening out or calcifications, scar tissue, tumors, and other abnormalities dissolving and disappearing, as well as regeneration of damaged or surgically removed tissue. This will seem an incredible assertion to many. I can only state that among people who have put the principles outlined in this book into practice in their own lives, such "miracles" occur frequently. Indeed, they are seen as being the inevitable consequence of the correct application of these principles. It should also be noted that under most circumstances, the fire of the kundalini will only be released when we are thoroughly prepared nutritionally, having achieved the state of nutrient saturation which is covered in Part Two.

3. Several points should be noted here with reference to "past lives." When a memory of an experience comes up that is clearly not from this lifetime, it may not be possible to distinguish whether it is on the Hereditary or Soul Level. If we

accept these concepts, a given memory could conceivably be both. For perhaps we actually were our own ancestor a few generations before our own current lifetime. Thus, there may be considerable overlap between Hereditary and Soul Levels in many instances.

4. Keyes, *The Hundredth Monkey,* pp. 11–18.

5. Sheldrake, *A New Science of Life.*

6. A branch of mathematics known as Fourier analysis shows that all patterns, no matter how complex, can be reduced to the sum of a series of sine waves of varying amplitudes, frequencies, and phases. Thus, all patterns are reducible to sine waves. The mathematical equations to do this are known as *Fourier transforms,* after their inventor Jean Fourier. They were first formulated in the eighteenth century. In the 1940s, Dennis Gabor used these Fourier transforms to come up with the theories necessary to develop the hologram. Gabor was eventually awarded a Nobel Prize for this work. All the information that is stored on the holographic plate and used to project the hologram will be in the form of these sine waves (Talbot, *The Holographic Universe).*

CHAPTER 3: THE GREAT PARADOX OF HEALING

1. Camus, *The Myth of Sisyphus & Other Essays,* p. 88.

2. Ibid., p. 89.

3. Ibid.

4. Ibid., p. 91.

CHAPTER 5: THE REQUIREMENTS OF HEALTH AND HEALING

1. Dement, *The Promise of Sleep,* pp. 324–325.

2. Ibid.

3. Ibid.

4. Ibid., p. 363.

5. For those who use eyeshades to go to sleep in a room that is not dark, the following is noted by Dr. Dement. Studies have clearly demonstrated that our daily cycle of sleep and wakefulness can be shifted to some degree by exposing the eyes to sufficiently bright lights at appropriate times. Interestingly enough, the same effect can be produced by shining the light on the back of the knees instead of the eyes. Assuming that the skin on the back of the knees is not unique, this would suggest that bright light anywhere on the skin can interrupt rest in much the same fashion as it would if shining on the eyes.

6. Batmanghelidj, *Your Body's Many Cries for Water,* p. 19.

7. Dr. Batmanghelidj found that the majority of cases of dyspeptic pain would disappear completely within eight minutes simply by drinking one or two glasses of water! In fact, in this manner he treated 3000 persons with dyspeptic pain and certain related conditions with 100% success. His report on this was published in June 1983 in the *Journal of Gastroenterology*.

8. Batmanghelidj, *Cries for Water*, p. 72.

9. Ibid., p. 158.

10. Ibid., pp. 68–69.

11. Ibid., pp. 25–40.

12. Flanagan and Flanagan, *Elixir of the Ageless*, p. 6.

13. Ibid., p. 7. Flanagan arrives at his estimate by noting that H_2O is similar in structure to H_2Te, H_2Se, and H_2S, molecules containing tellurium, selenium, and sulfur respectively. Based on known rules, the heaviest of these four substances H_2Te should have the highest boiling and freezing points, followed by the next heaviest H_2Se, then the next heaviest H_2S, with the lightest substance, H_2O, having the lowest boiling and freezing points. The other three substances do indeed follow this rule, and by comparing molecular weights, Flanagan makes his estimates for the boiling and freezing points of H_2O as indicated.

14. Kronberger and Lattacher, *On the Track of Water's Secrets*, p. 157.

15. Ibid.

16. Ibid., pp. 157–158.

17. Morell, "The Bio-Electronic Method of Prof. Vincent."

18. Ibid.

19. Flanagan and Flanagan, *Elixir*, pp. 7–8.

20. Ibid., p. 8.

21. Ibid., p. 83.

22. An ion is a charged particle formed when a neutral atom or group of atoms loses or gains one or more electrons. An anion would be an ion with a negative charge, while a cation would be an ion with a positive charge.

23. Kronberger and Lattacher, *Secrets*, pp. 155–156.

24. Ibid., pp. 156–157.

25. Ibid., pp. 158–159.

26. Ibid., p. 159.

27. Ibid., pp. 159–160.

28. Ibid., pp. 161–162.

29. Ibid., p. 160.

30. Archer, *On the Water Front*, p. 35.

31. Currently, there are many devices that purport to alter the structure of water in such a way as to make it more healthy and otherwise beneficial. Many of these devices are marketed with some pretty impressive claims. Yet few of these devices come with descriptions of rigorous scientific proof of any such claims. While it is possible that some of these devices may indeed work as well or even better than the Grander devices, I have yet to see any such evidence.

32. This was reported in *Krone* 14 Sept. 2000 [translation given in material provided by Grander Water Technologies (Australia) Pty Ltd].

Chapter 6: The Healing Crisis

1. In many cases a skilled iridologist can be quite accurate in predicting certain of the symptoms that may arise, and there are doubtless other methods of ascertaining this. Certainly the past health history is a good indication of what may lie ahead in eventual healing crisis.

2. Szekely, *The Essene Gospel of Peace, Book One*, p. 24.

3. Ray, *Logic In Sequence: Book Two: The Healing Crisis*.

PART TWO: NUTRITION

Chapter 7: Dietary Reform: Some Basic Concepts to Master

1. D'Adamo, *Eat Right For Your Type*.

2. See Cousens, *Conscious Eating* and also Chopra, *Perfect Health*.

Chapter 8: Passing the Test of Reality: the Work of Dr. Weston A. Price, D.D.S.

1. *Nutrition and Physical Degeneration* is available through the Price-Pottenger Nutrition Foundation (PO Box 2614, La Mesa, CA 92044 USA; fax 1-619-574-1314; *info@ price-pottenger.org*; *www.price-pottenger.org*) along with much other valuable information. I consider this to be one of the most important books ever written on the subject of nutrition. And as my friend Dr. Roy Kupsinel M.D. has noted, this book should be required reading at all medical schools, and dental schools as well. When I first came across this book in 1994, I found that it challenged and contradicted some of my own beliefs as to what constituted a proper diet for human beings. This was particularly so with regards to the efficacy of a pure vegan diet. If any read this book with an open mind, they may find themselves blessed in a similar fashion.

2. On the topic of root canals, see also Meinig, *Root Canal Cover-Up* and Price, *The Price of Root Canals*.

3. Price, *Nutrition and Physical Degeneration,* p. 495.

4. On the bright side, it has been demonstrated with animals that while severely deformed offspring could readily be induced through inadequate parental nutrition, these same deformed animals could produce apparently normal offspring if they were properly fed. This was done, for example, with pigs. Entire litters of pigs were born without eyeballs through feeding their parents a diet devoid of vitamin A. Yet these same eyeless pigs could produce offspring with normal eyeballs and fine vision if they were properly fed themselves. It's possible that these apparently normal pigs were not completely free of *all* the adverse effects experienced by their parents due to the faulty nutrition of their grandparents. Nevertheless, clearly there is at least the possibility of normalcy despite the deformities of the parents, which is good news for modern people. For it shows that if we return to an obedience to natural law, the results of previous violations may be overcome. Dr. Francis M. Pottenger, Jr. M.D. experimented with cats on healthy and deficient diets over a ten year period. He found that for the kittens of cats in the second generation of degeneration due to a deficient diet, it took four generations to bring them back to normal. More on Pottenger's work can be found in his book *Pottenger's Cats—A Study in Nutrition,* also available from the Price-Pottenger Nutrition Foundation.

5. Many authorities in Price's day had also observed that at the point of contact between isolated populations and "civilization" many of the children born subsequently experienced various cranial, in particular facial, deformities not previously apparent in these populations. A common explanation of the day was that these deformities were the result of interbreeding between these previously isolated populations and the Western people entering these areas. That is, these deformities were considered by many to be a phenomena of the intermingling of different racial stocks. Price was aware of this argument, and it is indeed mentioned numerous times in his book. He refuted this explanation with a simple observation: such cranial and facial deformities as others attributed to interbreeding were also found in children of "pure blood" who were conceived after one or both of their parents changed over to a Western diet and away from their native diet. Thus, changed diet was responsible for these deformities and would fall under the category of *intercepted heredity.* Pottenger also noted similar deformities in the offspring of cats on a deficient diet, and in the offspring of various other animals, such as cows, pigs, and dogs, when they were on a deficient diet.

6. Price, *Nutrition and Physical Degeneration,* pp. 286–288.

7. Page, *Degeneration—Regeneration,* pp. 222–223.

8. There is no indication either way in his book as to whether improved nutrition also resulted in ability to meet the remaining four criteria or not. With analogy to Pottenger's cats, however, it would not be surprising if the return to our full genetic potential takes several generations or more. The reader is referred to *Pottenger's Cats: A Study in Cat Nutrition* for further specific information on these studies. Besides all of the obvious degenerative changes Francis Pottenger noted and quantified in the cats fed various deficient diets, it is significant that within a span of four generations these cats on deficient diets died out completely. Each generation on such diets was worse off than the preceding generation, which would certainly support Weston Price's concept of intercepted heredity. Eventually a point was reached where the final generation was no longer even fit enough to successfully reproduce. This would suggest that the inability to reproduce on a widespread basis is a sure sign of degeneration. But it would not appear to be one of the initial signs. (The initial signs would include dental decay followed by dental, cranial, and skeletal deformities in the succeeding generation.) Rather, widespread reproductive failure would be one of the more advanced or perhaps final signs of demise. There have doubtless always been individuals who were not capable of reproducing for various reasons. Yet as birthrates continue to decline in "developed" countries, as sperm counts continue to decline, and as infertility clinics blossom into thriving enterprises over the past few generations, one can only wonder how rapidly the human race is approaching its own demise. Perhaps we will not wipe ourselves out with a nuclear war. Maybe we'll manage to do it through faulty nutrition. Pottenger also conducted experiments to return cats who had been degenerating for one or more generations back to full health. He found that with those cats in the second generation of degeneration, four generations were required in order to produce once again cats that he considered normal. It would appear that on the one hand, so long as we can reproduce effectively there is hope that health can be restored. Yet it would also appear that for many of us the improvements involved in the return to our full health potential may be spread out over a few generations.

9. Price, *Nutrition and Physical Degeneration*, p. 279.

10. Fallon, *Nourishing Traditions*, p. 422.

11. Price, *Nutrition and Physical Degeneration*, pp. 282–283.

12. *PPNF Fundamentals*, as reprinted in the Price-Pottenger Nutrition Foundation Resource Catalog–Fall/Winter 1998.

13. Hamaker and Weaver, *The Survival of Civilization*

14. It is certainly possible to make spiritual progress while the physical body

is itself deteriorating. A person might, for example, be held in a concentration camp or as a political prisoner for many years under harsh conditions, and their physical body would likely decline in such a circumstance. Yet if they were able to apply various higher laws, as for example the Laws of Love and Forgiveness, certainly they could simultaneously progress on other levels. But consider: there may be a significant difference between a situation leading to physical decline that is to some degree beyond our obvious control (such as the above example) and a situation leading to physical decline that we do in general have control over (our own diet.) Most of us do have many options available as to what we eat. If we choose, whether in ignorance or otherwise, a diet that leads to physical degeneration, is this in general compatible with spiritual progression?

15. A simple example that illustrates the above is that according to many authorities the requirement for vitamin B_{12} is increased by fifty to one hundred times during pregnancy.

16. Szekely, *Medicine Tomorrow,* pp. 26–27.

17. Price, *Nutrition and Physical Degeneration,* p. 495.

18. Ibid., p. 433.

CHAPTER 9: GETTING THE MOST OUT OF OUR FOOD

1. Given the steady depletion of soil minerals and the obvious fact that where these minerals tend to end up is in the ocean, the mineral content of the ocean is probably increasing year by year.

2. Hamaker and Weaver, *The Survival of Civilization,* p. 4.

3. Ashmead, *Chelated Mineral Nutrition,* pp. 6–7.

4. I once lived for six months on an island with a substantial deer population. There were no predators for these deer, as the sheep farmers on this small island shot any wild or even wandering dogs on sight. Hunting by humans, while it does reduce the deer population, does not remove the least fit animals in the same way a natural predator would. Many deer are also killed by automobiles, which is also unlikely to selectively target the less fit deer. One of the island veterinarians told me that as a result of this, the population contained a greatly disproportionate number of deformed deer. The gene pool of the deer suffered due to a lack of predation.

5. Levy, in "The Challenge of Antibiotic Resistance," states that "the same drugs prescribed for human therapy are widely exploited in animal husbandry and agriculture. More than 40 percent of the antibiotics manufactured in the U.S. are given to animals. Some of the amount goes to treating or preventing infection,

but the lion's share is mixed into feed to promote growth. . . . In agriculture, antibiotics are applied as aerosols to acres of fruit trees, for controlling or preventing bacterial infections. . . . The aerosols also hit more than the targeted trees. They can be carried considerable distances to other trees and food plants."

6. *PPNF Fundamentals,* p. 17.

7. Ibid., p. 5.

8. McDougall and McDougall, *The McDougall Plan,* p. 100.

9. Ibid., p. 104.

10. Ibid., p. 100.

11. Ibid.

12. Ibid., p. 101.

13. Ibid., pp. 101–102.

14. Ibid., p. 102.

15. Ibid.

16. Ibid.

17. Ibid.

18. See Nelson, *Food Combining Simplified.* and Shelton, *Food Combining Made Easy.*

19. Nelson, *Food Combining Simplified,* p. 20.

20. Ibid.

21. Ibid., p. 21.

22. Ibid., pp. 21–22.

23. Ibid., p. 23.

24. Ibid.

25. Ibid., p. 24.

26. Howell, *Food Enzymes for Health and Longevity.*

27. Enzymes can only work when in contact with whatever they are meant to break down, and the enzymes found in most plant foods need to be released by the rupturing of the cell wall. Hence, proper chewing of food is essential, and often neglected.

28. Tietze, *Papaya: The Medicine Tree.*

29. Ibid. While papaya seeds are used as a form of birth control in some cultures, they are not a contraceptive, for they do not prevent pregnancy. Rather, they induce an abortion. Some anecdotal evidence suggests that young women who use papaya seeds on a continual basis may risk permanent infertility. While I do not pretend to offer the final word on papaya seeds, to women I would advise caution for this reason.

CHAPTER 10: ESSENTIAL NUTRIENTS AND THEIR SOURCES

1. While Erasmus' *Fats that Heal, Fats that Kill* is mainly about fats and oils, it is one of a handful of books on nutrition that truly deserves to be called a classic. In addition to the thorough presentation of many highly technical areas, Erasmus has succeeded in writing a book that can be understood by everyone.

2. Ibid., pp. 207–208.

3. Jensen, *Tissue Cleansing Through Bowel Management*, p. 29.

4. With respect to "foreign proteins" and "synthetic compounds" entering our bodies, Erasmus, notes in *Fats that Heal, Fats that Kill*, p. 352: "the most common route of their introduction is through our digestive system. It has been estimated that over a normal lifespan, our body processes 10,000 kg (22,000 pounds) of antigens from foods, compared to 200 to 400 kg (440 to 880 pounds) from water, and 400 to 600 kg (880 to 1320 pounds) from air." In other words, the amount of antigens we introduce into our bodies from food is ten to sixteen times as much as the amount from air and water combined.

5. Individual needs for specific essential nutrients can vary tremendously, at least by a factor of ten in most cases.

6. Ashmead, *Chelated Mineral Nutrition* and also Rodale, et al, *The Complete Book of Minerals for Health*.

7. In recent years some individuals have found that colloidal minerals derived from finely ground rock dust can be quite effective when prepared properly despite the fact that they would not be chelated. These minerals are decanted one or more times. This means the rock dust is stirred into water and allowed to settle over night. Only the portion that remains in suspension is ingested. It is extremely important to note that such nonchelated minerals must be prepared properly so as to ensure that they are colloidal, for the possibility exists that minerals that are neither chelated nor colloidal may be harmful to the body. Nevertheless, some individuals have gotten good results with a colloidal but nonchelated mineral prepared from fine rock dust. An advantage of this is that it is quite inexpensive when compared to a chelated colloidal mineral supplement. The disadvantage is that in this form it is difficult to consume large amounts as we can only drink so much of this cloudy water daily. While some have done it with apparent good results in the short run, I cannot recommend the practice of consuming such rock dust without decanting, as I have doubts as to its safety in the long run.

8. Weston Price noted that without exception all of the peoples he studied

consumed at least some of their animal protein in a raw form.

9. Erasmus, *Fats that Heal,* p. 263.

10. An excellent source of information including recipes and methods of preparation is *Nourishing Traditions* by Sally Fallon. This is a combination recipe book and reference book that is in keeping with the research of Weston Price, Francis Pottenger, Edward Howell, and others.

11. The hemp plant is also known as the marijuana plant. It should be noted that the psychoactive parts of this plant are not found in the oil, which is made from the seeds only. Were hemp production legalized, we would have a superior source of oil as well as hemp seed butter, which is a good protein source. Hemp also makes superb and durable clothing, sturdy rope, and fine paper. Its use for paper would certainly save many trees. Hemp is apparently easy to grow without pesticides. If we consider that roughly one quarter of the yearly use of pesticides worldwide is for cotton, the use of hemp for clothing would have enormous environmental benefits. Lest this sound like a plug for marijuana, let me state for the record that I consider the use of marijuana to be detrimental physically, emotionally, mentally and spiritually. And I respect anyone else's right to have a contrary opinion.

12. Gerson, *Healing Newsletter.*

13. Erasmus, *Healing Newsletter.*

14. Budwig, *Flax Oil as a True Aid Against Arthritis, Heart Infarction, Cancer, and Other Diseases,* p. 10.

15. Erasmus, *Fats that Heal,* p. 187.

16. Please note that in no cases were both the milk and meat altered. All cats on a deficient diet received either raw milk or raw meat. And all received cod liver oil as well.

17. Such light bulbs are not always easily available, and they are more expensive, but if they can obtained they are well worth the extra cost. This subject is covered in great detail in the books *Health and Light* and *Light, Radiation, & You* by John Ott.

18. More information can be found in the short book by Dr. Budwig: *Flax Oil as a True Aid Against Arthritis, Heart Infarction, Cancer and Other Diseases.*

19. Budwig, *Flax Oil,* p. 41.

20. Ibid., pp. 54–55.

21. Erasmus, *Fats that Heal.*

22. Ibid., p. 190.

23. As both the essential fatty acids and chlorophyll are related to light, this also suggests a relationship of some sort between light and oxygen.

24. Budwig, *Flax Oil,* pp. 10–11.

25. Ibid., p. 35.

26. Finkel, *Fresh Hope With New Cancer Treatments,* p. 53.

27. Ibid., p. 49.

CHAPTER 11: AVOIDING DETRIMENTAL FOOD CHOICES

1. Meinig, *Root Canal Cover-Up,* p. 23.

2. Ibid.

3. Page, *Degeneration—Regeneration.*

4. Ibid.

5. Page also found that the certain people required additional methods he developed to correct fundamental endocrine imbalances that were also involved. While the correct nutrition would improve the situation, it would not always be sufficient by itself. He used a method now referred to by some as *microendocrinology* where minute quantities of certain hormones were administered. He also developed his own unique method of body measurement by which he was able to determine the precise nature of the endocrine imbalance. His methods appear to have been quite successful.

6. Page, *Degeneration,* p. 57.

7. Page, p. 81.

8. Ibid., pp. 82–83.

9. An extremely thorough explanation of margarine and hydrogenation can be found in *Fats that Heal, Fats that Kill* by Udo Erasmus.

10. Erasmus, *Fats and Oils: The Complete Guide to Fats and Oils in Health and Nutrition,* pp. 98–100.

11. Budwig, *Flax Oil,* p. 11.

12. Ibid., p. 20.

13. Ibid., pp. 15–16.

14. *PPNF Fundamentals.*

15. Oster and Ross, *The XO Factor,* p. 26.

16. What got Dr. Oster interested in finding the cause was pretty simple. He had a heart attack. He then followed quite diligently the basic recommendations of the cholesterol myth. A few years later, he had another heart attack.

17. This enzyme is also produced naturally in the body. Apparently the endogenous form is not found in the circulatory system under normal circumstances.

18. Dr. Oster had a number of patients from India in his Connecticut practice. He found that those who had only recently arrived from India had few problems in their blood vessels despite a high consumption of dairy products. In India, these dairy products would have been unhomogenized. However, within a few years in the United States and consuming large amounts of homogenized dairy products, many of these same patients would have extensive arteriosclerosis. It was also noted that those who had only consumed the raw dairy products would be lacking the antibody for XO from cows. This would indicate that when raw cow's milk was consumed, the XO was not absorbed. Yet after a period of consuming the homogenized cow's milk, the antibody for the XO from cow's milk would appear. This indicates that after milk is homogenized, the XO can now be absorbed and thus cause damage to the arteries. It should also be noted that XO is an enzyme that readily survives the low heat of conventional pasteurization. It is only destroyed by boiling or by ultra-pasteurization.

19. If we have a garden and we have more produce than we can possibly use at the time, it is relatively simple to ferment many vegetables and fruits. These fermented foods from our own garden will be inexpensive, highly nutritious, and will keep for extended periods of time.

20. Fallon et al., p. 30.

21. For the present and future health of all children, breastfeeding is essential. The nutrition of the mother must be adequate as well; otherwise her milk will be inadequate in quality. For further information on breastfeeding, contact your local chapter of La Leche League, an international organization designed to encourage breastfeeding.

CHAPTER 12: PRINCIPLES OF EATING WISELY AND WELL

1. Page, *Degeneration—Regeneration*, p. 84.

2. Price, *Nutrition and Physical Degeneration*, p. 265.

3. Refer to *Enzyme Nutrition* and *Food Enzymes for Health and Longevity* by Edward Howell for more detail.

4. Unlike the enzyme inhibitors, phytic acid is not neutralized by cooking. Thus, a yeast bread made from whole grain flour would interfere with mineral absorption due to the phytic acid.

5. Numerous recipes for preparing grains in these ways can be found in *Nourishing Traditions* by Sally Fallon et al.

6. PPNF Fundamentals, p. 8.

7. Ibid.

CHAPTER 13: THE USE OF SUPPLEMENTS

1. See the *Resources and Suppliers* pages for information on how to obtain the various supplements mentioned in this chapter. Most are available from Enzymes International in Wisconsin, USA, with the exception of the Grainfields products from AGM Foods in Brisbane, Australia.

2. Howell, *Food Enzymes,* p. 122.

3. Numerous mineral supplements are quite ineffective and quite a few are actually damaging to the body. Particular emphasis should be placed upon using mineral supplements that are colloidal and naturally chelated.

4. See the *Resources and Suppliers* pages for information on AGM Foods and Grainfields products.

5. Erasmus, *Fats that Heal,* p. 326.

6. Levy, "The Challenge of Antibiotic Resistance."

7. See *Resources and Suppliers.*

8. See *Resources and Suppliers* for information on Enzymes International and various supplements, including the mature green papaya products developed by Dr. Koesel.

9. Microscopes which are designed to permit live blood cell analysis make it possible to examine a small drop of blood straight from the body, and note its activity and composition. Many people's blood can be observed to have large amounts of "debris" of various sorts present. In many cases, if protease is ingested orally and the blood is reexamined a short time later, much of this debris has been removed.

10. In extreme situations, people have been known to ingest six ounces (180 ml) or more per day. This tends to bring about good results but will almost inevitably bring about severe healing crisis in the process. Beware!

11. A word of warning is that a blood cholesterol count only measures the amount in the blood stream and does not measure that on the vessel walls. In some instances it will indicate the true extent of the problem. However, a person may have a relatively normal reading and yet have tremendous buildup. This same person can then begin an extensive program of lecithin and lipase and, as the cholesterol is gradually disappearing, have a tremendous blood cholesterol count increase temporarily. Thus, while they are actually getting better, their reading will appear to show the opposite.

12. Available from Enzymes International. See *Resources and Suppliers.*

13. Finkel, *Fresh Hope With New Cancer Treatments* and McCabe, *Oxy-*

gen Therapies: A New Way of Approaching Disease.

14. Available from Enzymes International. See *Resources and Suppliers.*

CHAPTER 14: DEGENERATIVE DISEASES

1. Airola, *There Is A Cure For Arthritis,* pp. 25–26

2. Finkel, *Fresh Hope with New Cancer Treatments,* p. 3.

3. While all such incidents may be a result of a combination of our own free choices as exercised within the limits of our reactive patterns, and thus, within our control to a certain degree, in the treatment of a degenerative condition, incidents which have already occurred are now beyond our control.

4. Finkel, *Fresh Hope,* p. xv.

5. Ibid., p. v-vi.

6. Airola, *Arthritis,* p. 52.

7. This study was conducted by the United States Public Health Service in the 1940s. The full data from the study were never made available to the scientific community for review or analysis. It took a Freedom of Information Act lawsuit by Dr. Yiamouyiannis to secure the data from the Justice Department.

8. Finkel, *Fresh Hope,* p. 95.

9. Fluoride is strongly correlated with increases in birth defects, hip fractures in the elderly population, skeletal deformities, immune system disorders, cancer, and much else as well. More information on the political and economic interests behind fluoride may be found in an excellent chapter on fluoride in *Murder By Injection: The Story of the Medical Conspiracy Against America* by Eustace Mullins. Sodium fluoride, as noted previously, is a toxic by-product of the fertilizer and aluminum industries.

10. As discussed in Chapter Five, most, if not all, methods of filtration, including reverse osmosis, may cause some degree of energetic damage to the water. The Grander units can help reverse such damage, and so Grander treatment of the water should ideally follow any type of filtration that might be used to reduce the level of physical contaminants found in water.

11. George Meinig spent much of his professional life performing root canals. He was a founding member of the American Association of Endodontists. (Endodontists are dentists who specialize in root canals.) Meinig is on the Board of Directors of the Price-Pottenger Nutrition Foundation. After his retirement from dentistry, he discovered some of Price's research on root canals in their archives. Disturbing as this must have been to someone who had performed thousands of root canals, Dr. Meinig had the courage to write a book on the subject

and help prevent much future suffering from root canals.

12. *The Price of Root Canals* is a compilation of Weston Price's own writings on the subject which has been assembled by Hal Huggins. Hal Huggins has also repeated and verified quite a number of Weston Price's experiments on root canals.

13. Meinig, Cover-Up, pp. 1–2.

14. Page, *Degeneration,* p. 250.

15. Airola, *Arthritis,* p. 57.

16. Finkel, *Fresh Hope,* p. 63.

17. Page, *Degeneration.*

18. Finkel, *Fresh Hope,* p. 55.

19. Ibid., p. xiv.

20. Ibid., p. 101.

PART THREE: BODY ELECTRONICS FUNDAMENTALS

CHAPTER 15: BASIC THEORY OF BODY ELECTRONICS

1. Ray, *Logic In Sequence: Book One: The Laws of Perfection.*

2. In some cases a state of nutrient saturation sufficient for some several hours of Body Electronics will already exist without any dietary modifications or the addition of any supplements. This readiness results from a combination of factors, including the individual's constitution and prior dietary habits.

3. It has been convincingly demonstrated over many years that the successful application of Body Electronics is simply not possible without an abundance of minerals as well as enzymes circulating in the tissues of the individual. This is not to say that these nutrients must come from any specific source, rather that, whether these come from the diet or from appropriate supplements, they must be there for Body Electronics to succeed.

CHAPTER 16: THE PRACTICE OF BODY ELECTRONICS

1. Houston, *The Healing Benefits of Acupressure,* p. 18.

2. Kervran, *Biological Transmutations.*

3. Dr. Ray suggests that this is the pulse rate of the universe.

4. Some points may finish well after others, even an hour or more after. There is an exception known as a *tie-in* which is indicated by particular signs in the sclera of the eye. (See Chapter Twenty.) The convention with a tie-in is to stay plugged in on all points involved in the tie-in until they are all finished.

5. In situations where it is deemed necessary, several points may be held in advance of the typical sequence of endocrine points. These will be points relating to the pancreas, the heart, and the heart firing mechanism. Reasons to jump ahead to the pancreas might include diabetes or cancer, since the pancreatic secretion of chymotrypsin helps to digest abnormal tissue. Also with reference to the pancreas, Melvin Page notes a strong connection between sufficient insulin secretion and the ability to heal. In the case of the heart and heart firing points, many people will have either a genetic weakness in the heart, evidence of significant stress on the heart, or a history of heart problems.

6. Francis Pottenger does mention that children who had various deformities such as overbites as a result of faulty nutrition had these deformities corrected simply with a return to proper nutrition. However, such correction had to occur at a sufficiently early stage.

7. Magoun, *Osteopathy in the Cranial Field.*

8. With respect to these reflexes between muscles and organs or glands, it might be noted that some individuals have experimented quite successfully with techniques such as sustained yoga postures or numerous repetitions of a certain motion against resistance to help bring out the traumas and resistances locked within these muscles. When done in conjunction with a state of nutrient saturation and with an understanding of the various principles involved, this can be quite effective.

9. Some anecdotal evidence suggests that tumors and other abnormal tissue may grow or increase in size initially as the body begins to regenerate. Should the process of regeneration continue, this initial stage would be followed by the decrease and eventual disappearance of the tumor or abnormal tissue. The concern is that if one does enough of a program to enter into this early stage of regeneration but not enough to pass through it, then the tumor or abnormal tissue may end up larger, which poses an obvious risk. Hence, it is strongly advised that if there is any possibility of a tumor or other abnormal tissue, that Body Electronics only be undertaken by those on a thorough nutrient saturation program as outlined extensively in this book.

CHAPTER 17: INDIVIDUAL RESPONSIBILITY AND THE POINTHOLDEE

1. Ray, *Book One*, pp. 284–288.

2. Also, beyond the persistence of the person on the table in hanging in there and sticking with the same memory, in many cases the perseverance of the facilitator will also play a big role.

CHAPTER 19: CONSIDERATIONS FOR BODY ELECTRONICS FACILITATORS

1. Ray, *Book One,* p. 111.

2. Hall of Famer Bill Russell was the pivotal player on those Celtic teams, and the eleven league titles won by his Celtics teams during his thirteen year career arguably make him the greatest team sports athlete in modern history. "The Celtic offense, seven plays with options, was so basic that everybody in the league had it memorized. 'I was on an All-Star team with guys like Bob Pettit, Jerry Lucas, and Oscar Robertson that went behind the Iron Curtain in 1964,' Russell said. 'When we got to Poland,' Red says, 'I don't know what kind of plays we're going to use. We've got guys from five different teams here.' Pettit says, 'Let's use the Celtics' plays. Everybody knows them.'" *The Boston Globe,* 23 December 1999.

3. These books are available from the Saint Germain Foundation, 1120 Stonehedge Drive, Schaumburg, IL 60194; (847) 882-7400 or (800) 662-2800.

PART FOUR: OUTER MANIFESTATION AND INNER ESSENCE

1. de Sainte Exupery, *The Little Prince,* p. 87.

CHAPTER 20: IRIDOLOGY AND SCLEROLOGY

1. Jensen, *Iridology: The Science and Practice in the Healing Arts,* p. 1.

2. Changes in the iris and sclera can be extremely subtle, so in many cases it will not be especially easy with iridology and sclerology to ascertain whether improvements are being made. Certainly there are instances where despite obvious improvements in health there may be no obvious change in the iris or sclera.

3. Jensen, *Iridology,* p. 222.

4. Ibid., p. 1.

5. The direct connection between the iris and the entire body is exhaustively detailed by Jensen (pp. 133–150). This amounts to a structural method of iris analysis in that various areas of the iris will represent the corresponding areas of the body.

6. Bernard Jensen's eye chart is available from Bernard Jensen International, 24360 Old Wagon Road, Escondido, CA 92027; ph: (760) 749-2727; fax: (760) 749-1248. Harri Wolf's eye chart is available from Harri Wolf, c/o Healthbuilders, 23232 Paseo De Peralta, suite 205, Laguna Hills, California 92653; *Wolf1Angel@aol.com.* David Pesek's eye chart is available from David J. Pesek, Ph.D., International Institute of Iridology, 375 Paradise Lane, Waynesville, NC

28785; ph: (828) 926-6100 fax: (828) 926-6084; e-mail: *drpesek@holisticiridology.com, www.holisticiridology.com.*

7. Jensen, *Iridology,* p. 471.

8. Ibid., pp. 453–496.

9. Gray, *Gray's Anatomy,* p. 828.

10. Ibid., p. 831.

11. Ibid.

12. Ibid., p. 832.

13. Jensen, *Iridology,* p. 104.

14. Ibid.

15. Ibid.

16. In my estimation, the degree and frequency of eye color change has often been exaggerated. I do not wish to imply that such changes happen either readily or frequently. And with a few exceptions most such changes that I have personally observed have been pretty subtle. There is certainly no consensus within the international iridology community as to whether or not such color changes do take place. I have met many iridologists who acknowledge having seen such changes, and many others who report never having seen them. In my estimation, however, the proportion of iridologists who acknowledge color changes is far higher than it was fifteen years ago when I began studying iridology.

17. This eye chart is © 2000 by Jack Tips/International Sclerology Institute, 3654 Bee Caves Road, Suite D, Austin, TX 78746; ph: (512) 328-3996; fax: (512) 328-0812; e-mail: *apple-a-day@jacktips.com www.sclerology-institute.com.* For further information on sclerology, please consult *Insights in the Eyes* by Jack Tips.

18. To be perfectly accurate anatomically, the structures being examined in the field of sclerology will include both the sclera as well as the conjunctiva as well as possibly other adjoining tissues.

CHAPTER 21: BIOLOGICAL TRANSMUTATIONS

1. Kervran, *Biological Transmutations,* p. 29.

2. Ibid., pp. 146–149.

3. Ibid., p. 45.

4. Ibid., p. 3.

5. Ibid., pp. 110–113.

6. Ibid., p. 115.

7. Ibid., p. 143.

8. Extensive information on this may be found in Dr. Ray's first three books in the *Logic In Sequence Series*.

9. Kervran, *Biological Transmutations*, pp. 11–12.

CHAPTER 22: BACK TO HEALTH: MONOPOLES, MELANIN AND UNCREATION

1. Quotation taken from my lecture notes taken while in attendance at a seminar with Dr. Ray in September and October 1985.

2. Ibid.

3. Ray, *Book Three*, p. 890.

4. From personal correspondence with Dr. Ray.

5. Ray, *Book Three*, p. 890.

6. Ibid., pp. 899–900.

7. Ibid., p. 904.

8. Barr et al., "Melanin: The Organizing Molecule," p. 28.

9. Ibid., p. 44. Author's note: However, while it was stated that melanin was probably present at the inception of life, if we consider that the melanin-protein complex is an outer manifestation of resistance, it would seem that the melanin would not have appeared until resistance first entered the picture.

10. Ibid., p. 7.

11. Ibid., p. 21.

12. Ibid., pp. 18–21.

13. Ibid., p. 6.

14. Jensen, *Iridology*, p. 133.

15. Barr et al., "Melanin," pp. 10–12.

16. Ibid., p. 24.

17. Ibid., p. 1.

18. Ibid., p. 5.

19. In the words of Barr et al., Melanin functions in many ways:

1. As an amorphous semiconductor, may regulate neuronal firing.

2. May function as an organic superconductor at room temperature.

3. As a melanosome, may store and release energy in a manner similar to mitochondria.

4. May direct embryological tissue differentiation as well as tissue regeneration.

5. May direct mast cell functioning.

6. May direct homeostatic regulation of neuroendocrine functioning, immune

response, tissue repair/regeneration, and the autonomic nervous system.

7. May play both a cytoprotective and a cytotoxic role through its photon-phonon and free radical properties and its strong binding of lipid-soluble molecules.

8. May regulate enzyme and membrane activity via its control of metal ions functioning as cofactors or activators.

9. May regulate the various vitamins and cofactors involved in metabolism ("Melanin," p. 24).

Furthermore, they state:

... that melanin is the basic organizing molecule within *in vivo* systems can be supported by ... major lines of research and argument. *First* are its remarkable set of properties as a unique biopolymer. In addition to being an extremely efficient light (photon) absorbing molecule, exhibiting extraordinary photon-phonon conversion processes, melanin transduces both *acoustic* and *electric* energy fields and it can generate enough heat to effect metabolic processes. In addition to responding functionally to both light and sound (and being abundant in both the eyes and inner ears), melanin and neuro-melanin (the form of melanin found in the central nervous system) are located in highly strategic functional regions of the central and peripheral nervous systems....*In vitro* studies have shown that melanin functions as an amorphous semiconductor within physiological ranges of neuronal electrical potentials. *Electrotonic* (graded potential) *processing* in neuronal systems may be effectively triggered by as little as *one photon* or by an *auditory (phononic) input near that of mere Brownian motion.* Melanin's unique combination of photon-(electron)-phonon and electromagnetic semiconductive properties may serve *in vivo* to continuously regulate both the axonal action potentials as well as the glial-dendritic local circuit graded potentials, both of which are necessary for nervous system functioning.

... melanin can continuously produce and scavenge highly reactive free radicals, simultaneously oxidizing one substance while reducing another....

... melanin is the most primitive and universal pigment in living organisms, present since the inception of life.... In searching for a basic organizational molecule, it would seem to make sense to identify a primitive polymer which appears early in the evolutionary process and which subsequently develops an impressive functional repertoire ... melanin/neuromelanin presents itself as a singular candidate for such a role.

Second, melanin seems the principle organizing molecule because of an impressive body of circumstantial evidence, especially because of its participation in what are described here as "melanocentric systems."...

... melanin ... appears to have the potential to bind, rearrange, polymerize and release virtually any molecular ring structure. Melanin, using such internal capabilities, seems to function as an organizational "trigger." Sensitive hierarchies of strategically arranged cellular protein enzyme cascades, controlled by reversible covalent modifications (and in turn presumably by melanin), appear to provide the means for instantly activating and amplifying both the signal response to and catalytic potential necessary for diverse cellular organizational tasks.

Third, during embryological development, melanin is present in every stage from the oocyte to the mature adult organism.... The fact that brain melanin ... increases with ascent up the phylogenetic ladder, reaching a culmination in man, gives additional support to the hypothesis that melanin is performing some as yet unrecognized major function within living systems... ("Melanin," pp. 2–4).

20. Ray, *Book Three,* p. 900.

21. Barr et al. ("Melanin," p. 4) state that "melanin exhibits an extreme stability, both *in vivo* and *in vitro.* Melanin is an *extremely stable* molecule, highly resistant to digestion by most acids and bases, and even quite resistant to advanced techniques of analysis such as electron spin resonance, x-ray diffraction, and synchroton radiation studies. This stability, which is remarkable for molecular structures, gives it a durability and permanence that ideally suits it for its organizational role but which simultaneously renders it relatively inaccessible to analysis—making it a kind of molecular 'black box.' As a result, the synthesis and exact structure of melanin remain unknown."

22. Ray, *Book Three,* p. 904.

23. Talbot, *The Holographic Universe,* p 27.

24. From personal correspondence with Dr. Ray.

Bibliography

Airola, Paavo O. *There Is A Cure For Arthritis*. West Nyack, NY: Parker Publishing Company, Inc., 1968.

Alexander, Caroline. *The Endurance: Shackleton's Legendary Antarctic Expedition*. New York, NY: Alfred A. Knopf, 1999.

Alexandersson, Olof. *Living Water*. Dublin, Ireland: Gill & Macmillan, 1990.

Archer, John. *On the Water Front: Making Your Drinking Water Safe*. Brunswick Heads, NSW, Australia: Pure Water Press, 1991.

Ashmead, DeWayne. *Chelated Mineral Nutrition*. Huntington Beach, CA: Institute Publishers, 1981.

Barr, F.E. (with Saloma, J.S. and Buchele, M.J.) "Melanin: The Organizing Molecule." *Medical Hypothesis* 11 (1983): 1–140.

Batmanghelidj, F. "A New and Natural Method of Treatment of Peptic Ulcer Disease." *Journal of Gastroenterology* 5 (1983): 203–205.

——. *Your Body's Many Cries for Water*. Falls Church, VA: Global Health Solutions, 1997.

Becker, Robert O. *Cross Currents*. New York, NY: St. Martins Press, 1990.

The Boston Globe, 23 December 1999.

Brodeur, Paul. *Currents of Death*. New York, NY: Simon and Schuster, 1989.

Budwig, Johanna. *Flax Oil as a True Aid Against Arthritis, Heart Infarction, Cancer, and Other Diseases*. Vancouver, B.C., Canada: Apple Publishing, 1992.

——. *The Oil-Protein Diet Cookbook*. Vancouver, B.C., Canada: Apple Publishing, 1994.

Camus, Albert. *The Myth of Sisyphus & Other Essays*. New York, NY: Vintage Books, Random House, 1955.

Carter, Albert. *The Miracles of Rebound Exercise.* The National Institute of Reboundology and Health, 1979 (n.p., n.d.).

Chopra, Deepak. *Perfect Health.* New York, NY: Harmony Books, 1991.

Cousens, Gabriel. *Conscious Eating.* Berkeley, CA: North Atlantic Books, 2000.

Covey, Stephen R. *The Seven Habits of Highly Effective People.* New York, NY: Simon & Schuster, 1989.

D'Adamo, Peter J. *Eat Right For Your Type.* New York, NY: G.P. Putnam's Sons, 1996.

Dement, William C. (with Christopher Vaughan). *The Promise of Sleep.* New York, NY: Delacorte Press, 1999.

Dufty, William. *Sugar Blues.* New York, NY: Warner Books, 1993.

Erasmus, Udo. *Fats and Oils: The Complete Guide to Fats and Oils in Health and Nutrition.* Burnaby, B.C., Canada: Alive Books, 1986.

——. *Healing Newsletter* 1988 (from the Gerson Institute P.O. Box 430, Bonita, CA 91908-0430).

——. *Fats that Heal, Fats that Kill.* Burnaby, B.C., Canada: Alive Books, 1993.

Fallon, Sally (with Pat Connolly and Mary G. Enig). *Nourishing Traditions.* San Diego, CA: ProMotion Publishing, 1995.

Finkel, Maurice. *Fresh Hope With New Cancer Treatments.* Englewood Cliffs, NJ: Prentice-Hall, Inc., 1984.

Flanagan, Patrick and Gael Crystal. *Elixir of the Ageless.* Flagstaff, AZ: Vortex Press, 1986.

Frankl, Viktor E. *Man's Search for Meaning.* New York, NY: Pocket Books, Simon & Schuster, 1963.

Gerson, Max. *Healing Newsletter* 1988 (from the Gerson Institute, P.O. Box 430, Bonita, CA 91908-0430).

Gray, Henry. *Gray's Anatomy.* Philadelphia, PA: Running Press, 1974.

Hamaker, John D. and Weaver, Donald A. *The Survival of Civilization.* Michigan and California: Hamaker-Weaver Publishers, 1982.

Heinerman, John. *Heinerman's Encyclopedia of Fruits, Vegetables and Herbs.* West Nyack, NY: Parker Publishing Company, 1988.

Houston, F.M. *The Healing Benefits of Acupressure.* New Canaan, CT: Keats Publishing, 1958.

Howell, Edward. *Food Enzymes for Health and Longevity.* Woodstock Valley, CT: Omangod Press, 1946.

——. *Enzyme Nutrition.* Wayne, NJ: Avery Publishing Group Inc., 1985.

Huggins, Hal A. *It's All In Your Head.* Garden City Park, NY: Avery Publishing Group, 1993.

Jensen, Bernard. *Iridology: The Science and Practice in the Healing Arts.* Escondido, CA: Bernard Jensen, Publisher, 1982.

Jensen, Bernard. *Tissue Cleansing Through Bowel Management.* Escondido, CA: Bernard Jensen, Publisher, 1981.

Kervran, Louis C. *Biological Transmutations.* Brooklyn, NY: Swan House Publishing Company, 1972.

Keyes, Ken Jr. *The Hundredth Monkey.* Coos Bay, Oregon: Vision Books, 1982.

Kupsinel, Roy. *A Patient's Guide to Mercury-Amalgam Toxicity.* PO Box 550, Oviedo, FL 32765, USA: 1992.

Kronberger, Hans and Lattacher, Siegbert. *On the Track of Water's Secret.* Vienna, Austria: Uranus Verlagsgesellschaft m.b.h., 1995.

Levy, Stuart B. "The Challenge of Antibiotic Resistance." *Scientific American,* March 1998.

Lynes, Barry. *The Healing of Cancer.* Queensville, Ontario, Canada: Marcus Books, 1989.

Magoun, Harold Ives. *Osteopathy in the Cranial Field.* Kirksville, MO: The Cranial Academy, 1966.

McBean, Eleanora. *The Poisoned Needle.* Health Research, 1993.

McCabe, Ed. *Oxygen Therapies: A New Way of Approaching Disease.* Morrisville, NY: Energy Publications, 1988.

McDougall, John A. and Mary A. *The McDougall Plan.* Clinton, NJ: New Win Publishing, 1983.

Meinig, George E. *Root Canal Cover-Up.* Ojai, CA: Bion Publishing, 1998.

Morell, Franz. "The Bio-Electronic Method of Prof. Vincent." Paper presented at the O.I.C.S. (Occidental Institute Research Foundation of Bellingham, WA) Alumni Association's German Electro-Acupuncture Week. Millbrae, CA: July 1982.

Mullins, Eustace. *Murder By Injection: The Story of the Medical Conspiracy Against America.* Staunton, VA: National Council for Medical

Research, 1988.

Nelson, Dennis. *Food Combining Simplified*. Santa Cruz, CA: Dennis Nelson, Publisher, 1983.

Oster, Kurt A. and Ross, Donald J. *The XO Factor*. New York, NY: Park City Press, 1983.

Ott, John N. *Light, Radiation, & You*. Greenwich, CT: Devin-Adair Publishers, 1982.

Page, Melvin E. *Degeneration—Regeneration*. La Mesa, CA: Price-Pottenger Nutrition Foundation, 1951.

Pitchford, Paul. *Healing with Whole Foods*. Berkeley, CA: North Atlantic Books, 1993.

Pottenger, Francis M., Jr. *Pottenger's Cats: A Study in Cat Nutrition*. La Mesa, CA: Price-Pottenger Nutrition Foundation, 1995.

Price, Weston A. *Nutrition and Physical Degeneration*. New Canaan, CT: Keats Publishing, 1989.

——. (Compiled by Hal Huggins.) *The Price of Root Canals*. Colorado Springs, CO: Huggins Diagnostic Center, 1995.

Ray, John Whitman. *Logic In Sequence: Book One: The Laws of Perfection*. Keri Keri, New Zealand: John Whitman Ray Publications, 1990.

——. *Logic In Sequence: Book Two: The Healing Crisis*. Keri Keri, New Zealand: John Whitman Ray Publications, 1994.

——. *Logic In Sequence: Book Three: The Electrification of Matter*. Keri Keri, New Zealand: John Whitman Ray Publications, 1995.

Rodale, J.I., et al. *The Complete Book of Minerals for Health*. Emmaus, PA: Rodale Books, Inc., 1976.

de Sainte Exupery, Antoine. *The Little Prince*. San Diego, CA: Harcourt Brace Jovanovich, 1971.

Sheldrake, Rupert. *A New Science of Life: The Hypothesis of Formative Causation*. London: Blond & Briggs, 1981.

——. *The Presence of the Past: Morphic Resonance and the Habits of Nature*. London: Collins, 1988.

Shelton, Herbert M. *Food Combining Made Easy*. San Antonio, TX: Natural Hygiene Press, 1951.

Skarin, Annalee. *Ye Are Gods*. Marina del Rey, CA: DeVorss & Company, 1952.

——. *The Book of Books*. Marina del Rey, CA: DeVorss & Company, 1972.

——. *The Celestial Song of Creation*. Marina del Rey, CA: DeVorss & Company, (n.d.).

Szekely, Edmond Bordeaux, trans. *Medicine Tomorrow*. Ashingdon, Rochford, Essex, England: C.W. Daniel Company, 1951.

——. *The Essene Gospel of Peace, Book One*. Matsqui, B.C., Canada: International Biogenic Society, 1981.

Talbot, Michael. *The Holographic Universe*. New York, NY: Harper-Perennial, 1991.

Tietze, Harald W. *Papaya: The Medicine Tree*. Bermagui South, NSW, Australia: Harald W. Tietze Publishing, 1997.

Tips, Jack. *Insights in the Eyes*. Austin, TX: Life Resources, 1999.

Walker, Norman. *Colon Health: The Key to a Vibrant Life*. Prescott, AZ: Norwalk Press, 1979.

Whiteside, Robert. *Face Language II*. Hollywood, FL: Frederick Fell Publishers, 1988.

Yiamouyiannis, John. *Fluoride the Aging Factor*. Delaware, OH: Health Action Press, 1986.

Ziff, Sam. *Silver Dental Fillings: The Toxic Time Bomb*. Santa Fe, N.M.: Aurora Press, 1984.

Resources and Suppliers

Visit Doug's Web Site on nutrition, health, and healing at *www.d-w-m.com*.

For details on how to receive free e-mail updates on health, nutrition and related topics, please visit *www.d-w-m.com* or send an e-mail entitled UPDATES to *updates@d-w-m.com*. Please include your name, postal address, and country.

For information on how to obtain enzymes, minerals, and most of the other supplements referred to in this book, please visit *www.d-w-m.com* or send an e-mail entitled SUPPLEMENTS to *supplements@d-w-m.com*. Please include your name, postal address, and country.

For information on how to obtain the various Grainfields products developed by Alan Meyer of AGM Foods, please visit *www.d-w-m.com* or send an e-mail entitled AGM to *agm@d-w-m.com*. Please include your name, postal address, and country.

For information on how to obtain the Grander Water Units, please visit *www.d-w-m.com* or send an e-mail entitled GRANDER to *grander@d-w-m.com*. Please include your name, postal address, and country.

For information on private consultations with Doug Morrison, please visit *www.d-w-m.com* or send an e-mail entitled CONSULTATION to *consultation@d-w-m.com* or fax +1-603-584-8592. Please include your name, postal address, and country.

For Doug's seminar schedule, please visit *www.d-w-m.com*.

For information on organizing a seminar with Doug, please send an e-mail entitled SEMINAR to *seminar@d-w-m.com* or fax +1-603-584-8592. Please include your name, postal address, and country.

To obtain the eye charts found in this book or to contact those who devised them:

BERNARD JENSEN'S EYE CHART IS AVAILABLE FROM:

Bernard Jensen International
24360 Old Wagon Road
Escondido CA 92027
Phone: (760)749-2727
Fax: (760)749-1248.

HARRI WOLF'S EYE CHART IS AVAILABLE FROM:

Harri Wolf
c/o Healthbuilders
23232 Paseo De Peralta suite 205
Laguna Hills, California 92653
Wolf1Angel@aol.com

DAVID PESEK'S EYE CHART IS AVAILABLE FROM:

David J. Pesek, Ph.D.
International Institute of Iridology
375 Paradise Lane
Waynesville, North Carolina 28785-8275
Office: (828) 926-6100
Fax: (828) 926-6084
drpesek@holisticiridology.com
www.holisticiridology.com

JACK TIP'S EYE CHART IS AVAILABLE FROM:

International Sclerology Institute
3654 Bee Caves Road Suite D
Austin, Texas 78746
Phone: 512.328.3996
Fax: 512.328.0812
apple-a-day@jacktips.com
www.sclerology-institute.com

INDEX

A

acidophilus, 211

actinidin, 149, 150, 366

adrenal glands, 18, 127, 163, 169, 190, 214, 262, 331, 349, 365

air, xxxvi, 70, 71, 82, 90, 91, 119, 224, 225, 238, 413

Airola, Paavo O., 222, 226, 236, 418, 419, 427

alcohol, 67, 75, 99, 151, 190, 192, 193, 256, 341

aluminum cookware, 193, 205

amalgams—*see* "mercury"

amino acids, 103, 144, 145, 146, 147, 158, 160, 161, 162, 167, 171, 201, 207, 210, 213, 217, 365, 366, 368

amylase, 110, 143, 145, 148, 209, 213

anaerobic, 163, 175

anemia in the extremities, 361

anemia ring, 339, 345, 346, 360

anesthesia, 29, 223, 256, 271

anger, 16, 17, 19, 20, 25, 224, 243, 247, 248, 256, 284, 289, 339, 362, 369, 372

animal protein, 127, 162, 201

anion, 83, 407

anterior layer of iris, 338, 346

antibiotics, 137, 152, 188, 211, 411, 417, 429

antioxidants, 168, 169, 173, 174

ANW, 338, 343, 344, 347, 351

apathy, 16, 18, 19, 20, 24, 25, 243, 247, 256, 284, 289, 339, 369, 372

Archer, John, 407, 427

arcus senilus, 339, 345, 361

arteriosclerosis, 187, 416

arthritis, 116, 120, 122, 156, 166, 222, 226, 232, 236, 275, 414, 418, 419, 427

artificial colorings, 192, 193

artificial sweeteners, 192, 193

ascorbic acid, 152

aspartame, 192

assimilation, xxxvii, 134, 137, 141, 142, 144, 151, 153, 181

attachment, 36, 37, 38, 46, 249, 314

attitude, xxxvii, 24, 35, 36, 39, 42, 49, 58, 59, 60, 63, 91, 94, 104, 106, 108, 109, 130, 221, 224, 225, 226, 238, 286, 289, 313, 317, 318, 342, 351

Auerbach, Arnold "Red," 309

autonomic nerve wreath—*see* "ANW"

awareness, 16, 17, 18, 19, 23, 24, 25, 26, 31, 42, 43, 44, 45, 247, 288, 298, 312, 313, 317, 377, 381, 382, 386, 387

Ayurveda, 110

dependency relationships, 308

desire, 11, 36, 37, 38, 61, 113, 114, 122, 148, 314, 371, 372, 373, 374, 375

desire and will—*see* "will and desire"

detoxification—*see* "cleansing"

diabetes, 76, 116, 120, 156, 166, 178, 213, 275, 350, 420

digestion, xxxiii, 64, 68, 74, 75, 76, 81, 108, 110, 127, 128, 134, 137, 141, 142, 143, 144, 145, 146, 147, 148, 149, 151, 154, 159, 160, 161, 162, 168, 169, 202, 209, 211, 212, 214, 329, 351, 361, 365, 366, 394, 395, 399, 413

digestive enzymes, 145, 146

dipole, 79, 83, 84, 85

disease crisis, 96, 341

dissolved oxygen content, 81, 82

DNA, 5, 6, 27, 32, 106, 374

drugs, 222, 223, 229, 239, 256, 279, 411

duality, 21, 25, 42, 46, 54, 104, 248, 285, 290, 291, 372, 373

Dufty, William, 178, 428

E

Edison, Thomas A., 207

EFAs—*see* "essential fatty acids"

effect (*see* "outer" and "manifestation"), 13, 17, 23, 27, 29, 58, 61, 62, 63, 100, 153, 187, 245, 307, 381, 386

Einstein, Albert, 3

electromagnetic pollution, 87, 228

electrons, 80, 83, 158, 171, 172, 174, 183, 257, 364, 379, 407, 424, 425

elimination, xxxvi, xxxvii, 22, 64, 78, 91, 109, 110, 127, 134, 137, 141, 142, 144, 151, 156, 157, 188, 214, 218, 225, 236, 237, 329, 351, 399

Eliot, T. S., xxix

Emerson, Ralph Waldo, 13

emotional body—*see* "emotional level"

emotional level, xxxviii,14, 16, 18, 19, 24, 25, 26, 30, 104, 245, 248, 249, 288, 289, 290, 313, 389

emotional patterns—*see* "patterns of thought, word, and emotion"

empathy, 316, 317, 318

encompassment, 19, 21, 25, 30, 46, 104, 248, 285, 289, 290, 291, 313, 387, 388

endocrine system, xxxiv, 17, 70, 71, 160, 190, 262, 264, 266, 273, 276, 280, 329, 351, 352, 365

endogenous enzymes, 145, 394, 399, 415

endothermal reactions (*see* "biological transmutation"), 257, 363, 364, 369, 376

enthusiasm, 16, 18, 19, 20, 24, 25, 30, 43, 52, 55, 70, 103, 104, 226, 243, 247, 248, 256, 284, 285, 286, 289, 290, 304, 313, 339, 369, 372, 381

entities—*see* "Entity Level"

Entity Level, xxxvi, 28, 29, 30, 246, 381, 393, 396

enzymes, xxxvii, 76, 103, 110, 137, 138, 143, 144, 145, 146, 147, 148, 149, 150, 151, 153, 158, 160, 162, 164, 169, 183, 186, 187, 188, 190, 198, 202, 203, 205, 206, 207, 209,

holographic, 281, 285, 287, 387, 406, 425, 431
homogenized dairy products, 186, 187, 193, 416
homogenization, 186, 187, 193, 416
hormones, 146, 147, 160, 161, 262, 364, 365, 366, 368, 376, 379, 415
Howell, Edward, 144, 146, 147, 150, 202, 209, 393, 412, 414, 416, 417, 429
Hubbard, L. Ron, 405
Huggins, Hal A., 230, 231, 419, 429, 430
hundredth monkey, 31, 32, 406, 429
hydration, 73, 74, 75, 77, 83, 84, 85, 86
hydration envelope, 84, 86
hydrogenation (*see* "margarine"), 181, 182, 183, 184, 193, 205, 415
hyperactive, 339
hypoactive, 340

I
imbalance, 93, 96, 97, 99
immune system, 65, 67, 164, 168, 201, 204, 212, 223, 227, 230, 277, 279, 344, 359, 418, 423
indicating lines, 356, 357, 358, 360, 362
individual responsibility, 91, 283, 296, 304, 307, 420
inner (*see* "cause" and "essence"), 8, 17, 19, 21, 27, 30, 41, 58, 60, 61, 62, 93, 105, 245, 246, 249, 251, 265, 267, 285, 296, 300, 317, 321, 323, 362, 371, 372, 373, 374, 375, 385, 386, 424

insulin, 76, 214, 396, 420
intercepted heredity, 117, 118, 267, 409, 410
intestines, xxxiii, xxxiv, 75, 76, 148, 149, 170, 185, 214, 262, 265, 329, 344, 351, 366, 393
iridology, xxxvii, 262, 264, 273, 276, 325, 326, 327, 328, 330, 332, 334, 335, 336, 341, 344, 350, 352, 353, 355, 362, 365, 421, 422, 423, 429, 434
iris, 259, 278, 325, 326, 327, 328, 329, 331, 336, 337, 338, 339, 340, 341, 342, 343, 344, 345, 346, 347, 348, 350, 351, 352, 353, 355, 356, 357, 358, 359, 360, 361, 365, 377, 378, 421
iris fibers, 339, 340, 341, 346, 348, 353
Iris-Sclera Integrated Diagnosis, 259, 325, 326, 350
irradiated foods, 191, 193

J
James, William, 93
Jefferson, Thomas, 41, 283
Jensen, Bernard, 325, 326, 327, 328, 329, 330, 331, 333, 339, 345, 413, 421, 422, 423, 429, 434
judgment, xxxii, 16, 21, 22, 23, 25, 26, 42, 44, 46, 47, 54, 248, 249, 290, 315, 387
Jumanji, 291

K
kelp, 199, 200, 214
Kervran, Louis C., 257, 363, 364,

366, 367, 368, 369, 419, 422, 423, 429

Keyes, Ken Jr., 31, 406, 429

kidneys, 74, 140, 164, 169, 178, 215, 232, 262, 331, 352

kinesiology, 97

Kleitman, Nathaniel 66

Koesel, Kurt, 149, 212, 417

Krishnamurti, J., 371

kundalini, 25, 248, 256, 405

Kupsinel, Roy, 230, 408, 429

L

lactation, 114, 118, 126, 128, 169

lacunae, 339, 342, 343, 347

Law of Attraction, 21, 45, 59, 381

Law of Light, 313

Law of Love, 25, 313

Lee, John, 227

light, xxxi, xxxv, xxxvi, 4, 5, 8, 9, 10, 11, 22, 26, 69, 70, 71, 91, 158, 165, 171, 243, 306, 313, 339, 378, 385, 388, 390, 406, 414, 415, 424, 430

limbus, 338, 344, 355

Lincoln, Abraham, 283

lipase, 145, 209, 213, 399, 417

liver, 140, 168, 169, 170, 171, 180, 183, 215, 262, 331, 348, 349, 352, 361, 399, 414

love, xxxvi, 18, 19, 21, 25, 26, 35, 36, 38, 42, 47, 52, 57, 58, 59, 61, 64, 91, 95, 103, 104, 108, 109, 174, 243, 247, 248, 285, 286, 291, 304, 306, 312, 313, 315, 323, 373, 381, 387, 388, 391, 411

lovingly and willingly endure all things, 58, 59, 285, 351

lungs, 74, 76, 77185, 215, 262, 348, 349, 352

lymphatic rosary, 339, 345, 346

lymphatic system, 22, 64, 78, 109, 185, 213, 218, 237, 329, 333, 339, 345, 346, 351, 365

lysine and tryptophan denatured, 365

M

manifestation (see "outer" and "effect"), 17, 21, 27, 30, 36, 41, 43, 58, 100, 105, 245, 251, 285, 296, 317, 321, 323, 371, 372, 373, 382, 385, 386, 423

Marcus Aurelius, 41

margarine (see "hydrogenation"), 181, 182, 184, 185, 187, 191, 193, 415

mastication, 110, 233, 271, 394

mature green papaya—see "papaya"

maxilla, 271

McBean, Eleanora, 234, 429

McCabe, Ed, 173, 417, 429

Meinig, George E., 179, 231, 408, 415, 418, 419, 429

melanin, 247, 347, 368, 371, 375, 376, 377, 378, 379, 380, 381, 382, 385, 386, 423, 424, 425, 427

melanin-protein complex, xxxvi, 22, 24, 49, 245, 246, 247, 248, 249, 251, 284, 285, 291, 305, 368, 371, 375, 376, 377, 378, 380, 381, 382, 385, 386, 387, 423

memory, 25, 27, 28, 30, 47, 48, 63, 82, 83, 85, 86, 88, 89, 95, 169, 243, 247, 248, 254, 256, 284, 286, 287, 288, 291, 304, 310, 311, 312, 350, 376, 405, 420 mental body—*see* "mental level"

mental level, 14, 19, 21, 25, 104, 248, 249, 289, 290, 313, 372, 373, 374, 380

mercury, 230, 429

metabolic enzymes, 145, 146

Metchnikoff, 398

Meyer, Alan G., 152, 170, 191, 210, 211, 433

Michelangelo, 155

microbes—*see* "friendly microbes"

microendocrinology, 415

microwaved foods, 132, 191, 193

mineral ring, 345, 346

minerals, 87, 103, 122, 123, 124, 134, 135, 136, 137, 139, 140, 146, 147, 158, 159, 160, 162, 171, 202, 203, 207, 209, 216, 218, 247, 346, 367, 376, 411, 413, 419, 430, 433

moderate quantities of high quality food, 141

monopoles, 368, 371, 374, 375, 376, 380, 381, 382, 383, 385, 386, 423

monounsaturated fatty acids, 182

morphic resonance, 31, 32, 430

morphogenetic fields, 32, 374, 383

motilin, 76

Mullins, Eustace 223, 418, 429

muscle testing, 97, 98, 99

muscles, 64, 65, 189, 218, 260, 265, 267, 269, 270, 271, 272, 273, 279, 420

N

Nelson, Dennis, 412, 430

nerve rings, 339, 345, 347, 351

nerve supply, xxxiv, 22, 237, 253, 259, 260, 262, 264, 266, 268, 276, 280

neuromelanin, 377, 378, 424

nutrasweet, 192

nutrient saturation, xxxvii, 103, 104, 158, 207, 208, 240, 243, 246, 247, 276, 277, 280, 284, 353, 376, 405, 419, 420

nutrition, xxxvi, xxxvii, 13, 22, 24, 30, 64, 70, 91, 94, 95, 101, 103, 104, 105, 106, 113, 115, 117, 118, 120, 121, 124, 125, 129, 131, 132, 135, 137, 138, 144, 153, 154, 155, 156, 157, 163, 178, 179, 180, 186, 191, 197, 198, 204, 235, 236, 249, 266, 267, 268, 274, 284, 323, 326, 327, 328, 341, 363, 389, 390, 391, 408, 409, 410, 411, 413, 415, 416, 418, 420, 427, 428, 429, 430, 433

O

observe, receive, recreate, and release, 251, 285, 313

omega-3, 163, 164, 165, 210

omega-6, 163, 164, 165, 210, 213

organic foods, 188

osteoporosis, 116, 140, 156, 205, 253, 277

Oster, Kurt A., 187, 415, 416, 430

Ott, John N., 70, 414, 430

outer (*see* "effect" and "manifestation"), xxxiv, 8, 14, 17, 19, 21, 23, 24, 26, 27, 30, 31, 36, 41, 43, 50, 58, 60, 61, 62, 63, 93, 100, 105, 245, 246, 249, 251, 265, 285, 296, 300, 315, 317, 321, 323, 338, 361, 362, 363, 371, 372, 373,

374, 375, 381, 382, 385, 386, 423
ovary, 349
overhead projector, 7, 9, 23, 26, 383
overlays, 27, 28, 30, 267, 383
oxygenation, 81, 89, 173, 174, 186,
   216, 360, 369

P
Page, Melvin E., 119, 179, 180, 196,
   233, 236, 409, 415, 416, 419, 420,
   430
pain, xxx, xxxii, xxxiii, xxxiv, 16, 17,
   19, 20, 25, 32, 41, 72, 76, 77, 226,
   243, 247, 248, 251, 252, 253, 254,
   256, 262, 264, 266, 273, 275, 276,
   284, 289, 309, 339, 362, 369, 372,
   405, 407
Paine, Thomas, 35, 295
palatine bones, 271
pancreas, 18, 75, 127, 180, 214, 262,
   331, 349, 362, 394, 395, 396, 420
papain, 149, 150, 215, 366
papaya, 149, 150, 212, 215, 351, 366,
   412, 417, 431
parasites, 22, 87, 163, 189, 215, 237,
   344, 351
parathyroid, 17, 262
parietal bones, 269, 271
past lives—see "Soul Level"
pasteurization, 171, 188, 190, 193,
   398
patience, xxxvii, 24, 50, 107, 238,
   269, 288, 306
patterns of thought, word, and
   emotion, xxxii, 17, 18, 21, 22, 23,
   24, 25, 26, 27, 28, 29, 30, 32, 41,
   42, 44, 62, 88, 100, 105, 141, 142,

208, 226, 236, 238, 243, 245, 246,
   247, 248, 249, 251, 254, 256, 275,
   280, 284, 285, 287, 288, 291, 304,
   310, 311, 314, 336, 351, 362, 371,
   372, 373, 375, 378, 381, 382, 383,
   384, 385, 387, 406, 418
perception, 16, 25, 46, 47, 50, 286,
   292, 381
personal mission statement, 300
Pesek, David J., 325, 328, 329, 331,
   333, 334, 335, 421, 434
pH, 75, 80, 82, 142, 143, 148, 149,
   213, 376
photons, 172, 379, 424
physical body—see "physical level"
physical level, xxxviii, 4, 5, 6, 7, 8,
   11, 14, 21, 22, 24, 26, 30, 91, 96,
   100, 103, 114, 126, 222, 245, 246,
   248, 249, 284, 288, 326, 364, 366,
   376, 381, 383, 384, 386, 389, 391,
   405, 410
phytic acid, 202, 203, 206, 416
pigment spots, 339, 343, 344, 347,
   353
pineal gland, 17, 70, 71, 262, 271,
   273, 333, 349, 381
pituitary gland, 17, 230, 262, 265,
   271, 333, 349, 362
Planck, Max, 195
plasmalogen, 187
pointholdee, 254, 255, 256, 258, 260,
   277, 283, 284, 285, 287, 304, 305,
   306, 309, 311, 312, 314, 420
pointholders, 246, 252, 254, 255,
   257, 258, 260, 262, 271, 275, 279,
   284, 292, 303, 304, 306, 307, 309,
   316

Vincent, Professor—*see* "BEV"

violet flame, 313

vitamins, 71, 103, 117, 122, 123, 139, 146, 147, 151, 152, 158, 167, 168, 169, 170, 171, 207, 210, 216, 217, 219, 393, 394, 398, 409, 411, 424

vitamin A, 122, 123, 168, 409

vitamin B complex 168, 170, 217

vitamin B12, 169, 411

vitamin B6, 169, 210

Vitamin B6, 169

vitamin C, 152, 168, 169, 170

vitamin D, 123, 168, 169, 171, 219

vitamin D3, 71, 123, 169, 219

vitamin E, 168, 169

vitamin K, 168, 170

vitamin P, 168, 170

vomer, 271

W

water, xxxvi, 64, 70, 72, 73, 74, 75, 76, 77, 78, 79, 80, 81, 82, 83, 84, 85, 86, 87, 88, 89, 90, 91, 123, 138, 139, 140, 141, 166, 168, 171, 180, 183, 185, 190, 191, 201, 202, 205, 213, 216, 217, 218, 224, 225, 227, 228, 238, 306, 406, 407, 408, 413, 418, 427, 429

water quality, 72, 77, 78, 79, 80, 81, 82, 88, 91

water quantity, 72, 91

Weaver, Donald A., 135, 410, 411, 428

white flour, 115, 131, 178, 180, 181, 184, 188, 191, 193, 416

white sugar—*see* "sugar"

Whiteside, Robert, 268, 431

will and desire, 371, 372, 373, 374, 375, 382

willingness, 36, 91, 243, 280, 307, 318, 352

Wolf, Harri, 328, 329, 331, 332, 333, 421, 434

word patterns—*see* "patterns of thought, word, and emotion"

X

xanthine oxidase ("XO"), 187, 415, 416, 430

Y

Yiamouyiannis, John, 226, 418, 431

Z

Ziff, Sam, 230, 431

zone 1, 329, 350

zone 2, 329

zone 3, 329

zone 6, 329

zone 7, 329, 345, 350

zones 4 and 5, 329

About the Author

Doug is a native of Massachusetts in the USA, where he was a high school valedictorian and National Merit Scholar. Shortly after graduation from Harvard University with a BA in Applied Mathematics, chronic health problems turned him to the study of natural health alternatives. This led him in 1985 to Body Electronics. Doug spent much of the next four years studying Body Electronics with its founder, Dr. John Whitman Ray, living most of this time in Maui, Hawaii. Finding that the process of resolving his own health challenges was deeply intertwined with the release of his own resistance patterns, Doug continued his involvement with Body Electronics long after his original health goals had been fulfilled. In addition to the immense personal satisfaction he has found in working through many of his own resistances, he has also found great enjoyment in helping others to do the same. To provide others with the tools and the guidance to release their own resistances and regain their health on all levels, Doug began teaching seminars in Body Electronics in 1988. For the next twelve years, he taught Body Electronics extensively throughout the United States, Australia, New Zealand, Europe, and Africa. In addition, he has assisted thousands of individuals through private consultations in person as well as by letter, phone, and e-mail.

Doug has also continued to pursue studies in various fields, eventually receiving doctorate degrees in naturopathy, nutritional counseling, and alternative medicine. Doug's articles on Body Electronics, health, and nutrition have appeared in various magazines, journals, and newsletters around the world. Doug is also the author of a previous book *Body Electronics Fundamentals,* which first appeared in 1993. Since 1997, Doug has also sent out free e-mail updates on nutrition, health, and Body Electronics to interested people worldwide. Doug maintains a web site at *www.d-w-m.com* which covers these same topics.

In addition to his passions for natural health, nutrition, and spiritual growth, Doug greatly enjoys travel, reading, music, and time in the great outdoors. He is the very proud father of Meghan Rose Morrison and Andrew John Morrison.

Seminars, Conferences, and Private Consultations

Seminars

Interested in learning more about how to put the ideas in this book into practice? There is no substitute for experience, and Doug is happy to offer seminars where all present can benefit from his wealth of experience. Participants have the opportunity to apply these ideas under Doug's expert supervision, thus rapidly learning from their own experience. Skillfully integrating theory and practice, Doug combines lecture and practical application with ample time for questions and answers to provide a wonderful learning opportunity for all concerned.

If you are interested in having him come to your area to conduct a seminar, please send an e-mail entitled SEMINAR to *seminar@d-w-m.com* or fax +1-603-584-8592 for details. If you would like to receive notification by e-mail of Doug's upcoming seminars, please send an e-mail entitled UPDATES to *updates@d-w-m.com* and you will be added to the e-mailing list. Please include your name, postal address, and country. Upcoming seminars will also be posted at *www.d-w-m.com.*

Conferences

Would you like to see the ideas in this book presented to a wider audience? Doug is available as a guest speaker for conferences and is most happy to speak on these or related topics.

Private Consultations

A private telephone consultation allows you to take advantage of Doug's many years of experience while avoiding the high cost of travel. Doug is available for both individual and group consultations, and with his insight and experience he is able to shed light on your situation, answer your questions, and help steer you in the right direction for better health on all levels. These telephone consultations can also include iris-sclera analysis using iris and sclera photos that can be posted or e-mailed to Doug. For details on scheduling an appointment, please send an e-mail entitled CONSULTATION to *consultation@d-w-m.com* or fax at +1-603-584-8592.